Air Fryer Cookbook

700+ Effortless Air Fryer Recipes for Beginners and Advanced Users

Maria Borkowski

Table of Contents

INTRODUCTION		9
BREAKFAST RECIPES		10
1.	Protein Egg Cups	10
2.	Pumpkin Pancakes	10
3.	Shrimp Frittata	10
4.	Tuna Sandwiches	10
5.	Shrimp Sandwiches	10
6.	Chicken & Zucchini Omelet	10
7.	Zucchini Fritters	11
8.	Onion Omelet	11
9.	Breakfast Pea Tortilla	11
10.	Almond Crust Chicken	11
11.	Breakfast Fish Tacos	11
12.	Garlic Potatoes with Bacon	12
13.	Zucchini Squash Mix	12
14.	Spiced Chicken Omelet	12
15.	Mushroom Cheese Salad	12
16.	Fennel Frittata	12
17.	Strawberries Oatmeal	12
18.	Asparagus Salad	13
19.	Lemony Raspberries Bowls	13
20.	Spaghetti Squash Fritters	13
21.	Mushrooms And Cheese Spread	13
22.	Tuna and Spring Onions Salad	13
23.	Cinnamon Pudding	13
24.	Tomatoes and Swiss chard Bake	13
25.	Egg, Bacon and Cheese Roll Ups	14
26.	Crispy Ham Egg Cups	14
27.	Olives and Kale	14
28.	Stuffed Poblanos	14
29.	Raspberries Oatmeal	14
30.	Easy Scotch Eggs	15
31.	Strawberry Toast	15
32.	Cinnamon Sweet-Potato Chips	15
33.	Quiche Muffin Cups	15
34.	Vegetable and Ham Omelet	15
35.	Cheesy Canadian bacon English muffin	16
36.	Asparagus, Cheese and Egg Strata	16
37.	Shrimp, Spinach And Rice Frittata	16
38.	Tender Monkey Bread With Cinnamon	16
39.	Pesto Cheese Gnocchi	17
40.	Ham in a Cup	17
41.	Cheese Sticks	17
42.	Broccoli Cheese Quiche	17
43.	Onion and Cheese Omelet	17
44.	Air Fried Shirred Eggs	18
45.	Cheesy Hash Brown	18
46.	Cream Bread	18
47.	Sunflower Seeds Bread	18
48.	Date Bread	19
49.	Banana Bread	19
50.	Nutty Banana Bread	19
51.	Yogurt Banana Bread	19
52.	Peanut Butter Banana Bread	20
53.	Chocolate Banana Bread	20
54.	Nutty Zucchini Bread	20
55.	Zucchini & Apple Bread	21
56.	Pumpkin & Yogurt Bread	21
57.	Spiced Pumpkin Bread	21
58.	Chocolate Peanut Butter Bread	21
59.	Simple Cornbread	22
60.	Pineapple Cornbread	22
61.	Banana Oats	22
62.	Cheesy Bread And Eggs Bowls	22
63.	Creamy Carrots Hash Mix	22
64.	Tomato Frittata	23
65.	Strawberry Oatmeal	23
66.	Peppers and Tomato Eggs	23
67.	Mushroom Oatmeal	23
68.	Cauliflower Hash	23
69.	Pesto Scramble	23
70.	Eggplant And Sausage Hash	24
71.	Salmon Eggs	24
72.	Vanilla and Mango Bowls	24
73.	Chili Bowls	24
74.	Mushroom, Potato and Beef Bowls	24
75.	Carrot Muffins	24
76.	Breakfast Peppers Frittata	25
77.	Scrambled Eggs	25
78.	Sausage Egg Cups	25
79.	Cheese Stuff Peppers	25
80.	Roasted Pepper Salad	25
81.	Crust-Less Quiche	25
82.	Milky Scrambled Eggs	26
83.	Toasties and Sausage In Egg Pond	26
84.	Flavorful Bacon Cups	26
85.	Crispy Potato Rosti	26
86.	Stylish Ham Omelet	26
87.	Healthy Tofu Omelet	27
88.	Yummy Savory French Toasts	27
89.	Flaky Maple Donuts	27
90.	Coffee cake Muffins	27
91.	Baked Oatmeal Apple Cups	28
92.	Bacon-Roasted Fruit with Yogurt	28
93.	Scrambled Eggs with Cheese	28
94.	Soda Bread Currant Muffins	28
95.	Raspberry-Stuffed French toast	29
96.	Apple Roll-Ups	29
97.	Pepper Egg Bites	29
98.	Crunchy Nut Granola	29
99.	Breakfast Pizza	30
100.	Veggie Frittata	30
101.	Spicy Hash Brown Potatoes	30
102.	Sage and Pear Sausage Patties	30
103.	Bacon Bombs	31
104.	Morning Potatoes	31
105.	Breakfast Pockets	31
106.	Avocado Flautas	31
107.	Cheese Sandwiches	31
108.	Sausage Cheese Wraps	32
109.	Chicken Omelet	32
110.	Sausage Burritos	32
111.	Sausage Patties	32
112.	Spicy Sweet Potato Hash	32
113.	Cinnamon Cream Doughnuts	33

#	Recipe	Page
114.	Sausage Frittata	33
115.	Potato Jalapeno Hash	33
116.	Bread Rolls	33

LUNCH RECIPES — 34

#	Recipe	Page
117.	Vegetable Egg Rolls	34
118.	Veggies on Toast	34
119.	Jumbo Stuffed Mushrooms	34
120.	Mushroom Pita Pizzas	34
121.	Spinach Quiche	34
122.	Yellow Squash Fritters	35
123.	Pesto Gnocchi	35
124.	English Muffin Tuna Sandwiches	35
125.	Tuna Zucchini Melts	35
126.	Shrimp and Grilled Cheese Sandwiches	35
127.	Shrimp Croquettes	36
128.	Dutch Pancake With Shrimp Salsa	36
129.	Steamed Scallops With Dill	36
130.	Chicken Pita Sandwiches	36
131.	Chicken À La King	37
132.	Sweet Sour Pork	37
133.	Chicken Carnitas	37
134.	Beef Stroganoff	38
135.	Chicken Cacciatore	38
136.	Salsa Chicken	38
137.	Corned Beef	38
138.	Chicken Curry	38
139.	Pork Chops with Gravy	39
140.	Beef Stew	39
141.	Salisbury Steak	39
142.	Pot Roast with Veggies	40
143.	Mexican Rice	40
144.	Hamburger Soup	40
145.	Roasted Brussels sprouts	40

DINNER RECIPES — 42

#	Recipe	Page
146.	Crispy Salt and Pepper Tofu	42
147.	Crispy Indian Wrap	42
148.	Easy Peasy Pizza	42
149.	Eggplant Parmigiana	42
150.	Luscious Lazy Lasagna	43
151.	Pasta With Creamy Cauliflower Sauce	43
152.	Lemony Lentils With "Fried" Onions	44
153.	Our Daily Bean	44
154.	Taco Salad with Creamy Lime Sauce	44
155.	Bbq Jackfruit Nachos	44
156.	10-Minute Chimichanga	45
157.	Mexican Stuffed Potatoes	45
158.	Kids' Taquitos	45
159.	Immune-Boosting Grilled Cheese Sandwich	45
160.	Tamale Pie With Cilantro Lime Cornmeal Crust	46
161.	Air Fryer Chicken Wings	46
162.	Parmesan Chicken Wings	46
163.	Buffalo Cauliflower Bites	47
164.	Spicy Dry-Rubbed Chicken Wings	47
165.	Air Fryer Steak Bites and Mushrooms	47
166.	Pecan Crusted Chicken	47
167.	Chicken Tikka Kebab	48
168.	Air Fryer Brussels sprouts	48
169.	Crispy Air Fried Tofu	48
170.	Buttermilk Fried Mushrooms	48
171.	Crispy Baked Avocado Tacos	49
172.	Buttery Cod	49
173.	Creamy Chicken	49
174.	Mushroom and Turkey Stew	49
175.	Basil Chicken	49
176.	Eggplant Bake	49
177.	Meatball Casserole	50
178.	Herbed Lamb Rack	50
179.	Baked Beef	50
180.	Crispy Pork Chops	50
181.	Turkey Pillows	50
182.	Chicken Wings	51
183.	Chicken Cordon Bleu	51
184.	Fried Chicken	51
185.	Sesame Chicken	51
186.	Chicken and Potatoes	51
187.	Coconut-Crusted Chicken Tenders	51
188.	Crispy Chicken Sliders	52
189.	Garlic Herb Turkey Breast	52
190.	Honey-Lime Chicken Wings	52
191.	Rotisserie-Style, Whole Chicken	52
192.	Tarragon Chicken	52
193.	Beef and Potato	52
194.	Beef Roll-Ups	53
195.	Breaded Beef Schnitzel	53
196.	Cheeseburger 'Mini' Sliders	53
197.	Quick and Easy Rib Eye Steak	53
198.	Roast Beef	53
199.	Sweet and Spicy Montreal Steak	53
200.	Bacon-Wrapped Pork Tenderloin	54
201.	Bratwurst and Veggies	54
202.	Crispy Dumplings	54
203.	Spicy Green Crusted Chicken	54
204.	Cheesy Chicken Drumsticks	54
205.	Jamaican Pork Roast	54
206.	Lime Chicken	55
207.	Swiss Bacon Pork Chops	55
208.	Mustard Pork Chops	55
209.	Buttery Scallops	55
210.	Herbed Buttery Chicken	55
211.	Coconut Crusted Prawns	55
212.	Turmeric Beef	56
213.	Beef Tongue	56
214.	Crispy Parmesan Crusted Pork Chops	56
215.	Easy Air Fried Catfish	56
216.	Lemon Fish Fillet	56
217.	Pork Carnitas	57
218.	Garlic Pork Roast	57
219.	Grilled Skirt Steak with Sauce	57
220.	Cheesy Beef and Mushroom Calzones with Sauce	57
221.	Mexican Stuffed Beef Fajitas	57
222.	Pork Chops With Ranch Dressing	58
223.	Beef Sirloin Steak with Mushrooms	58

SEAFOOD RECIPES — 59

#	Recipe	Page
224.	Air Fried Cod with Basil Vinaigrette	59
225.	Almond Flour Coated Crispy Shrimps	59
226.	Another Crispy Coconut Shrimp Recipe	59
227.	Apple Slaw Topped Alaskan Cod Filet	59
228.	Baked Cod Fillet Recipe From Thailand	59

#	Recipe	Page
229.	Baked Scallops With Garlic Aioli	59
230.	Basil 'N Lime-Chili Clams	60
231.	Bass Filet In Coconut Sauce	60
232.	Beer Battered Cod Filet	60
233.	Buttered Baked Cod with Wine	60
234.	Buttered Garlic-Oregano On Clams	60
235.	Butterflied Prawns with Garlic-Sriracha	61
236.	Cajun Seasoned Salmon Filet	61
237.	Cajun Spiced Lemon-Shrimp Kebabs	61
238.	Cajun Spiced Veggie-Shrimp Bake	61
239.	Tempura Shrimp	61
240.	Tuna Patties	61
241.	Crusted Tilapia Coconut Flavour	62
242.	Fried French Mussels	62
243.	Crab Cakes	62
244.	Lobster Tails	62
245.	Breaded Shrimp	62
246.	Salmon with Mustard Sauce	63
247.	Sweet And Sour Shrimp	63
248.	Fish Cakes	63
249.	Cod	63
250.	Broiled Tilapia	63
251.	Cod Nuggets	63
252.	Air Fryer Cajun Shrimp	64
253.	Grilled Salmon	64
254.	Crispy Paprika Fish Fillets	64
255.	Bacon Wrapped Shrimp	64
256.	Bacon-Wrapped Scallops	64
257.	Air Fryer Salmon	65
258.	Lemon Pepper, Butter and Cajun Cod	65
259.	Steamed Salmon & Sauce	65
260.	Salmon Patties	65
261.	Sweet and Savory Breaded Shrimp	65
262.	Healthy Fish And Chips	66
263.	Indian Fish Fingers	66
264.	Spicy Shrimp Kebab	66
265.	Crumbed Fish Fillets with Tarragon	66
266.	Smoked And Creamed White Fish	67
267.	Parmesan and Paprika Baked Tilapia	67
268.	Tangy Cod Fillets	67
269.	Fish and Cauliflower Cakes	67
270.	Marinated Scallops with Butter And Beer	67
271.	Cheesy Fish Gratin	68
272.	Fijian Coconut Fish	68
273.	Sole Fish and Cauliflower Fritters	68
274.	French-Style Sea Bass	68
275.	Asian-Style Salmon Burgers	68
276.	Crusted Flounder Fillets	69
277.	Pecan Crusted Tilapia	69
278.	Grilled Salmon with Butter And Wine	69
279.	Ranch Flavored Tilapia	69
280.	Butter Up Salmon	69
281.	Coconut Lime Shrimp	70
282.	Prosciutto Wrapped Shrimp	70
283.	Shrimp Spring Rolls	70
284.	Flakey Fried Whitefish	70
285.	Cod with Simple Olive Caper Sauce	71
286.	Sesame Soy Striped Bass	71
287.	Crab And Herb Croquettes	71
288.	Garlic Tarragon Buttered Salmon	72
289.	Crab-Stuffed Mushrooms	72
290.	Oysters Rockefeller	72
291.	Steamer Clams	72
292.	Bay Scallops	72
293.	Smoky Fried Calamari	73
294.	Breaded Fish Sticks with Tartar Sauce	73
295.	Crab Cakes With Arugula And Blackberry Salad	73
296.	Bacon-Wrapped Stuffed Shrimp	73
297.	Simply Shrimp	74
298.	Chili Lime–Crusted Halibut	74
299.	Tuna Croquettes	74
300.	Tuna Melts On Tomatoes	74
301.	Classic Lobster Salad	74
302.	Baked Avocados with Smoked Salmon	75
303.	Breaded Cod Sticks	75
304.	Cod Fish Nuggets	75
305.	Easy Crab Sticks	75
306.	Caspian Cod	75
307.	Sesame Seeds Fish Fillet	76
308.	Chili Tuna Puff	76
309.	Shrimp Spring Rolls with Sweet Chili Sauce	76
310.	Gambas with Sweet Potato	76
311.	Wasabi Crab Cakes	77
312.	Crab Legs	77
313.	Avocado Shrimp	77
314.	Cheesy Lemon Halibut	77
315.	Spicy Mackerel	78
316.	Thyme Scallops	78
317.	Whitefish Cakes	78
318.	Marinated Sardines	78
319.	Halibut Steaks	78
320.	Fish Taco	79
321.	Seafood Fritters	79

POULTRY RECIPES 80

#	Recipe	Page
322.	Pretzel Crusted Chicken with Spicy Mustard Sauce	80
323.	Chinese-Style Sticky Turkey Thighs	80
324.	Easy Hot Chicken Drumsticks	80
325.	Crunchy Munchy Chicken Tenders With Peanuts	80
326.	Tarragon Turkey Tenderloins with Baby Potatoes	81
327.	Mediterranean Chicken Breasts with Roasted Tomatoes	81
328.	Thai Red Duck with Candy Onion	81
329.	Rustic Chicken Legs With Turnip Chips	81
330.	Old-Fashioned Chicken Drumettes	81
331.	Easy Ritzy Chicken Nuggets	82
332.	Asian Chicken Filets With Cheese	82
333.	Paprika Chicken Legs With Brussels Sprouts	82
334.	Chinese Duck	82
335.	Turkey Bacon with Scrambled Eggs	83
336.	Italian Chicken And Cheese Frittata	83
337.	Parmigiana Chicken	83
338.	Easy Paprika Chicken	83
339.	Spinach and Cheese Stuffed Chicken Breasts	84
340.	Texas Thighs	84
341.	Chicken Wings with Sweet Chili Sauce	84
342.	Crunchy Golden Nuggets	84

#	Recipe	Page
343.	Roasted Whole Chicken	84
344.	Cheesy Chicken Thighs With Marinara Sauce	85
345.	Chicken In Bacon Wrap	85
346.	Chicken Thighs With Honey-Dijon Sauce	85
347.	Lemon and Honey Glazed Game Hen	85
348.	Cheesy Spinach Stuffed Chicken Breasts	86
349.	Turkey And Pepper Sandwich	86
350.	Spicy Turkey Breast	86
351.	Chicken, Mushroom, And Pepper Kabobs	86
352.	Chicken & Zucchini	87
353.	Chicken Quesadilla	87
354.	Buffalo Chicken Wings	87
355.	Mustard Chicken	87
356.	Honey & Rosemary Chicken	87
357.	Grilled Chicken with Veggies	88
358.	Grilled Garlic Chicken	88
359.	Grilled Balsamic Chicken Breast	88
360.	Barbecue Chicken Breast	88
361.	Chicken, Potatoes & Cabbage	88
362.	Roasted Chicken	88
363.	Sugar Glazed Chicken	89
364.	Lemon Garlic Chicken	89
365.	Grilled Ranch Chicken	89
366.	Chicken Breast Pita Sandwiches	89
367.	Asian Style Turkey Meatballs	90
368.	Sweet and Spicy Chicken Stir-Fry	90
369.	Crispy Chicken Parmigiana	90
370.	Chicken Fajitas With Avocados	90
371.	Fried Chicken with Buttermilk	91
372.	Panko-Crusted Chicken Nuggets	91
373.	Crusted Chicken Tenders	91
374.	Chicken With Greek Yogurt Buffalo Sauce	91
375.	Baked Chicken Fajita Roll-Ups	92
376.	Garlicky Chicken and Potatoes	92
377.	Chicken Thighs with Lemon Garlic	92
378.	Lemony Chicken with Barbecue Sauce	92
379.	Chicken Popcorn	93
380.	Quick & Easy Meatballs	93
381.	Lemon Pepper Chicken Wings	93
382.	Bbq Chicken Wings	93
383.	Yummy Chicken Nuggets	93
384.	Italian Seasoned Chicken Tenders	94
385.	Classic Chicken Wings	94
386.	Simple Spice Chicken Wings	94
387.	Herb Seasoned Turkey Breast	94
388.	Tasty Rotisserie Chicken	94
389.	Spicy Asian Chicken Thighs	95
390.	Tomato, Eggplant 'n Chicken Skewers	95
391.	Teriyaki Glazed Chicken Bake	95
392.	Sriracha-Ginger Chicken	95
393.	Naked Cheese, Chicken Stuffing 'n Green Beans	95
394.	Grilled Chicken Pesto	96
395.	Healthy Turkey Shepherd's Pie	96
396.	Chicken Fillet Strips	96
397.	Chicken Chili Verde	96
398.	Lemon Curry Chicken	96
399.	Turkey Joint	97
400.	Cilantro Drumsticks	97
401.	Mozzarella Turkey Rolls	97
402.	Sage & Onion Turkey Balls	97
403.	Turkey Loaf	97
404.	Moroccan Chicken	98

MEAT RECIPES 99

#	Recipe	Page
405.	Pork And Mixed Greens Salad	99
406.	Pork Satay	99
407.	Pork Burgers With Red Cabbage Salad	99
408.	Crispy Mustard Pork Tenderloin	99
409.	Apple Pork Tenderloin	99
410.	Espresso-Grilled Pork Tenderloin	100
411.	Pork And Potatoes	100
412.	Pork And Fruit Kebabs	100
413.	Steak And Vegetable Kebabs	100
414.	Spicy Grilled Steak	100
415.	Greek Vegetable Skillet	101
416.	Light Herbed Meatballs	101
417.	Brown Rice And Beef-Stuffed Bell Peppers	101
418.	Beef And Broccoli	101
419.	Beef And Fruit Stir-Fry	102
420.	Simple Beef Sirloin Roast	102
421.	Seasoned Beef Roast	102
422.	Bacon Wrapped Filet Mignon	102
423.	Beef Burgers	103
424.	Beef Jerky	103
425.	Sweet & Spicy Meatballs	103
426.	Spiced Pork Shoulder	104
427.	Seasoned Pork Tenderloin	104
428.	Garlicky Pork Tenderloin	104
429.	Glazed Pork Tenderloin	104
430.	Honey Mustard Pork Tenderloin	105
431.	Seasoned Pork Chops	105
432.	Breaded Pork Chops	105
433.	Crusted Rack Of Lamb	105
434.	Lamb Burgers	106
435.	Pork Taquitos	106
436.	Cajun Bacon Pork Loin Fillet	106
437.	Panko-Breaded Pork Chops	106
438.	Porchetta-Style Pork Chops	107
439.	Apricot Glazed Pork Tenderloins	107
440.	Sweet & Spicy Country-Style Ribs	107
441.	Pork Tenders With Bell Peppers	107
442.	Wonton Meatballs	108
443.	Barbecue Flavored Pork Ribs	108
444.	Easy Air Fryer Marinated Pork Tenderloin	108
445.	Balsamic Glazed Pork Chops	108
446.	Perfect Air Fried Pork Chops	108
447.	Rustic Pork Ribs	109
448.	Air Fryer Baby Back Ribs	109
449.	Parmesan Crusted Pork Chops	109
450.	Pork Joint	109

VEGETABLES RECIPES 110

#	Recipe	Page
451.	Air Fryer Asparagus	110
452.	Spicy Sweet Potato Fries	110
453.	Air Fryer Cauliflower Rice	110
454.	Air Fried Carrots, Yellow Squash & Zucchini	110
455.	Air Fried Kale Chips	110
456.	Cheesy Cauliflower Fritters	111
457.	Avocado Fries	111
458.	Zucchini Parmesan Chips	111
459.	Crispy Roasted Broccoli	111

#	Recipe	Page	#	Recipe	Page
460.	Crispy Jalapeno Coins	111	517.	Pizza Rolls	124
461.	Buffalo Cauliflower	111	518.	Bacon Cheeseburger Dip	124
462.	Jicama Fries	112	519.	Pork Rind Tortillas	124
463.	Air Fryer Brussels Sprouts	112	520.	Mozzarella Sticks	124
464.	Spaghetti Squash Tots	112	521.	Bacon-Wrapped Onion Rings	125
465.	Cinnamon Butternut Squash Fries	112	522.	Mini Sweet Pepper Poppers	125
466.	Sweet Potato Chips	112	523.	Spicy Spinach Artichoke Dip	125
467.	Fried Zucchini	112	524.	Personal Mozzarella Pizza Crust	125
468.	Fried Avocado	113	525.	Garlic Cheese Bread	125
469.	Vegetables In Air Fryer	113	526.	Crustless Three-Meat Pizza	126
470.	Crispy Rye Bread Snacks With Guacamole And Anchovies	113	527.	Bacon Snack	126
471.	Mushrooms Stuffed With Tomato	113	528.	Shrimp Snack	126
472.	Spiced Potato Wedges	113	529.	Avocado Wraps	126
473.	Egg Stuffed Zucchini Balls	114	530.	Cheesy Meatballs	126
474.	Vegetables With Provolone	114	531.	Tuna Appetizer	126
475.	Spicy Potatoes	114	532.	Cheese And Leeks Dip	127
476.	Scrambled Eggs With Beans, Zucchini, Potatoes And Onions	114	533.	Cucumber Salsa	127
477.	French Toast	115	534.	Chicken Cubes	127
478.	Sweet Potato Salt And Pepper	115	535.	Salmon Spread	127
479.	Basil Tomatoes	115	536.	Crustless Pizza	127
480.	Pesto Tomatoes	115	537.	Olives And Zucchini Cakes	127
481.	Stuffed Tomatoes	116	538.	Fluffy Strawberry Muffins	127
482.	Parmesan Asparagus	116	539.	Paleo Blueberry Muffins	128
483.	Almond Asparagus	116	540.	Orange Cardamom Muffins With Coconut Butter Glaze	128
484.	Spicy Butternut Squash	116	541.	Bacon And Egg Cups	128
485.	Sweet & Spicy Parsnips	116	542.	Breadsticks	128
486.	Caramelized Baby Carrots	117	543.	Butter Crackers	129
487.	Carrot With Spinach	117	544.	Homemade Almond Crackers	129
488.	Broccoli With Sweet Potatoes	117	545.	Pepperoni Chips	129
489.	Broccoli With Olives	117	546.	3-Ingredient Flourless Cheesy Breadsticks	129
490.	Broccoli With Cauliflower	118	547.	Cauliflower Breadsticks	130
491.	Cauliflower In Buffalo Sauce	118	548.	Breadsticks With Mozzarella Dough	130
492.	Curried Cauliflower	118	549.	Bacon Onion Cookies	130
493.	Lemony Green Beans	118	550.	Cinnamon Swirl Cookies	130
494.	Roasted Okra	119	551.	Peanut Butter Cookies	131
495.	Artichoke Hearts	119	552.	Cranberry Pistachio Vegan Shortbread Cookies	131
496.	Jalapeno Poppers	119	553.	Garlic Edamame	131
497.	Asparagus Fries	119	554.	Spicy Chickpeas	131
498.	Vegan Veggie Balls	119	555.	Black Bean Corn Dip	132
499.	Spinach Sauté	120	556.	Crunchy Tex-Mex Tortilla Chips	132
500.	Paprika Tomatoes	120	557.	Egg Roll Pizza Sticks	132
501.	Cilantro Beets	120	558.	Cajun Zucchini Chips	132
502.	Kale Sauté	120	559.	Mexican Potato Skins	133
503.	Mustard Beets	120	560.	Crispy Old Bay Chicken Wings	133
504.	Cabbage Sauté	120	561.	Cinnamon Apple Chips	133
505.	Turmeric Carrots	121	562.	Cinnamon and Sugar Peaches	133
506.	Coriander Endives	121	563.	Spicy Dill Pickle Fries	133
507.	Lemon Fennel	121	564.	Carrot Chips	134
508.	Turmeric Kale	121	565.	Spicy Corn On The Cob	134
509.	Garlic Corn	121	566.	Pickle Chips	134
510.	Lemon Tomatoes	121	567.	Potato Chips	134
511.	Garlic Carrots	121	568.	Dehydrated Coconut Wrap	134

SNACK RECIPES — 123

#	Recipe	Page
512.	Prosciutto-Wrapped Parmesan Asparagus	123
513.	Bacon-Wrapped Jalapeño Poppers	123
514.	Garlic Parmesan Chicken Wings	123
515.	Spicy Buffalo Chicken Dip	123
516.	Bacon Jalapeño Cheese Bread	123
569.	Dehydrated Banana Chips	134
570.	Dehydrated Banana Candy	135
571.	Garlic Jerky	135
572.	Sweet & Tangy Mango Slices	135
573.	Dehydrated Bananas	135
574.	Canned Peaches	135

#	Recipe	Page
575.	Peach Wedges	135
576.	Cinnamon & Vinegar Apple Chips	135
577.	Green Apple Chips	135
578.	Sliced Strawberries	136
579.	Dried Raspberries	136
580.	Bite-Sized Blooming Onions	136
581.	Mini Scotch Eggs	136
582.	Pimiento Cheese-Stuffed Jalapeños	136
583.	Jalapeño Popper Bombs	137
584.	Cheddar Biscuit-Breaded Green Olives	137
585.	Fried Feta-Dill-Breaded Kalamata Olives	137
586.	Buffalo-Honey Chicken Wings	137
587.	Peanut Butter And Strawberry Jelly Wings	137
588.	Thai Sweet Chili Wings	138
589.	Salmon Croquettes	138
590.	Pepperoni Pizza Bites	138
591.	Broccoli Snackers	138
592.	Bite-Sized Pork Egg Rolls	138
593.	Green Chili Crispy Wonton Squares	139
594.	Brie And Red Pepper Jelly Triangles	139
595.	Reuben Pizza For One	139
596.	Parsnip Sticks	139
597.	Turmeric Sweet Potato Bites	139
598.	Avocado Balls	140
599.	Hard-Boiled Egg Halves with Bacon	140
600.	Stuffed Figs with Almonds	140
601.	Pear Chips	140
602.	Peach Chips	140
603.	Garlic Tomato Circles	140
604.	Beef Muffins	141
605.	Trout Balls	141
606.	Papaya Sticks	141
607.	Beet Chips	141
608.	Broccoli Steaks	141
609.	Devil Eggs with Pesto	141
610.	Crab Balls	142

DESSERTS RECIPES — 143

#	Recipe	Page
611.	Tasty Banana Cake	143
612.	Simple Cheesecake	143
613.	Bread Pudding	143
614.	Bread Dough And Amaretto Dessert	143
615.	Wrapped Pears	143
616.	Air Fried Bananas	143
617.	Cocoa Cake	144
618.	Apple Bread	144
619.	Mini Lava Cakes	144
620.	Crispy Apples	144
621.	Ginger Cheesecake	144
622.	Cocoa Cookies	145
623.	Special Brownies	145
624.	Blueberry Scones	145
625.	Half Dipped Chocolate Biscuits	145
626.	Chocolate Cake	145
627.	Chocolate Cupcakes With Cream Cheese Frosting	146
628.	Almost Guilt-Free Cinnamon Doughnut	146
629.	Donuts Recipe	146
630.	Peach Hand Pies	146
631.	Honey Glazed Pineapple Fries	147
632.	Baked Apple	147
633.	Mini Apple Pie	147
634.	Flourless Chocolate Cake	147
635.	Butter Cake	147
636.	Lime Mousse	148
637.	Mini Cheesecakes	148
638.	Cherry Crumble	148
639.	Blackberries Cobbler	148
640.	Glazed Bananas	149
641.	Banana Muffins	149
642.	Chocolate Muffins	149
643.	Banana-Choco Brownies	150
644.	Blueberry & Lemon Cake	150
645.	Bread Pudding with Cranberry	150
646.	Cherries 'n Almond Flour Bars	150
647.	Cherry-Choco Bars	150
648.	Coffee 'n Blueberry Cake	151
649.	Crisped 'n Chewy Chonut Holes	151
650.	Leche Flan Filipino Style	151
651.	Maple Cinnamon Buns	151
652.	Poppy Seed Pound Cake	152
653.	Banana Smores	152
654.	Fluffy Peanut Butter Marshmallow Turnovers	152
655.	Yogurt Pineapple Sticks	152
656.	Low Carb Snickerdoodle Cookies	152
657.	White Chocolate Raspberry Fat Bombs	153
658.	Sponge Ricotta Cake	153
659.	Plum Cake	153
660.	Baked Plums	153
661.	Walnut and Vanilla Bars	153
662.	Plum Cream	153
663.	Currant Pudding	154
664.	Currant Cookies	154
665.	Fruity Oreo Muffins	154
666.	Doughnuts Pudding	154
667.	Marshmallow Pastries	154
668.	Cinnamon Doughnuts	155
669.	Tea Cookies	155
670.	Zucchini Brownies	155
671.	Lemon Mousse	155
672.	Pear Delight	155
673.	Pumpkin Muffins	155
674.	Cranberry Muffins	156
675.	Apple Cinnamon Dessert Empanadas	156
676.	Apple Dumplings	156
677.	Pineapple with Honey and Coconut	156
678.	Tasty Cheese Bites	157
679.	Coconut Pie	157
680.	Pecan Muffins	157
681.	Cappuccino Muffins	157
682.	Almond Bars	157
683.	Coffee Cookies	158
684.	Berry Cobbler	158
685.	Cashew Pie	158
686.	Almond Pumpkin Cookies	158
687.	Vanilla Butter Pie	158
688.	Poppy seed Muffins	159
689.	Chia Chocolate Cookies	159
690.	Cinnamon Ginger Cookies	159
691.	Crustless Pie	159
692.	Tasty Peanut Butter Bars	159

693.	Apple Fritters	160	700.	Grilled Pineapple	161
694.	Churros	160	701.	Chocolate Covered Strawberry S'more	161
695.	Beignets	160	**CONCLUSION**		**162**
696.	Cinnamon Rolls	160			
697.	S'more	161			
698.	Fried Oreos	161			
699.	Fig Egg Rolls	161			

INTRODUCTION

In 2008, a company in England invented the air fryer as an alternative to deep fat fryers. An air fryer is a stand-alone appliance that uses a fan to blow hot air on and around your food, cooking it rapidly, while a vent removes moisture and keeps the temperature inside the appliance constant.

To compare:

Hot oil conducts heat very well and cooks food quickly. When you put food into a deep-fat fryer, the water on the food's surface instantly evaporates. Water from inside the food is released, which rapidly moves the oil around, causing the bubbling action of the oil. The food's interior is cooked as the heat moves through the food. The crust starts to brown due to a chemical reaction called the Maillard reaction, in which sugars and proteins on the crust break down and recombine to form compounds that look brown and taste great.

Hot air cooks food more slowly because it does not conduct heat as well as oil or water. To understand the difference, think of how you can put your hand into a 350°F oven for a few seconds, but you cannot put it into boiling water (212°F). To mimic deep-frying, but without all the unhealthy oil, an air fryer uses a fan to push the air around the food to dramatically speed the cooking process. So, just as in a deep-fat fryer, in an air fryer, the surface of the food dehydrates, water is released, and the interior cooks in a few minutes. Foods cooked in an air fryer cook 25 percent faster than foods cooked in a conventional oven.

And because little or no oil is used, cooking with an air fryer is a much more versatile way to cook food than cooking with a deep fryer. You can bake, roast, grill, stir-fry, and even steam foods in an air fryer. So instead of just cooking alternatives to fried foods, use this appliance to make foods without those hundreds of added fat calories; it actually will help improve your health and well-being.

While other air fryer cookbooks offer recipes that are certainly healthier than their deep-fried counterparts, this book is the only one that offers truly healthy recipes. If you look at all other air fryer cookbooks' nutrition content, you will see that the recipes are still very high in fat, sodium, and sugars. I developed the recipes in this book to be as low in fat, sodium, and sugars as possible, and high in vitamins and fiber.

Air Fryer: Step by Step:

You can think of an air fryer as a miniature convection oven. Inside the air fryer, a heater underneath the food heats the air. A slotted pan over the heater lets the superheated air move quickly around the food. A fan keeps the air circulating, and a vent pulls moisture and cooler air out of the appliance, so the temperature inside stays high and constant.

Just as in deep-frying, a crust immediately forms on the food in the air fryer. This helps seal in moisture so the interior of the food can cook. The starches inside the food gelatinize, the proteins denature, and the fiber softens as the outside browns—all fancy terms meaning the food cooks as it heats.

Most recipes for air fryers are very similar to recipes cooked in ovens or deep-fried in oil. But there are some essential differences.

Batter: Hot oil instantly solidifies a batter. But in an air fryer, the liquid runs off in the few seconds intakes for the air to heat it. Wet foods will not work in an air fryer.

Shape: Cut foods into similarly sized pieces, so everything cooks evenly in your air fryer.

Coatings: Foods coated with bread crumbs, ground nuts, or grated cheeses should be moist enough to ensure those small particles stay on the food and do not drop off into the air fryer and burn.

Once the food is prepared according to the recipe, the air fryer is usually preheated following the Directions: that came with your appliance. The food is placed in a basket and inserted into the air fryer before you start timing. In just a few minutes, outcomes perfectly cooked, hot, crisp food that is ready to eat.

BREAKFAST RECIPES

1. Protein Egg Cups

Preparation Time: 10 minutes
Cooking Time: 9 minutes
Servings: 2

Ingredients:
- 3 eggs, lightly beaten
- 4 tomato slices
- 4 tsp cheddar cheese, shredded
- 2 bacon slices, cooked and crumbled
- Pepper
- Salt

Directions:
1. Spray silicone muffin molds with cooking spray. In a small bowl, whisk the egg with pepper and salt. Preheat the air fryer to 350 F. Pour eggs into the silicone muffin molds. Divide cheese and bacon into molds. Top each with tomato slice and place in the air fryer basket. Cook for 9 minutes. Serve and enjoy.

Nutrition: Calories 67 Fat 4 g Carbohydrates 1 g Sugar 0.7 g Protein 5.1 g Cholesterol 125 mg

2. Pumpkin Pancakes

Preparation Time: 15 minutes
Cooking Time: 12 minutes
Servings: 2

Ingredients:
- 1 square puff pastry
- 3 tablespoons pumpkin filling
- 1 small egg, beaten

Directions:
1. Roll out a square of puff pastry and layer it with pumpkin pie filling, leaving about ¼-inch space around the edges. Cut it up into 8 equal sized square pieces and coat the edges with beaten egg.
2. Press "Power Button" of Air Fry Oven and turn the dial to select the "Air Fry" mode. Press the Time button and again turn the dial to set the cooking time to 12 minutes. Now push the Temp button and rotate the dial to set the temperature at 355 degrees F. Press "Start/Pause" button to start. When the unit beeps to show that it is preheated, open the lid. Arrange the squares into a greased "Sheet Pan" and insert in the oven. Serve warm.

Nutrition: Calories 109 Total Fat 6.7 g Saturated Fat 1.8 g Cholesterol 34 mg Sodium 87 mg Total Carbs 9.8 g Fiber 0.5 g Sugar 2.6 g Protein 2.4 g

3. Shrimp Frittata

Preparation time: 10 minutes
Cooking time: 15 minutes
Servings: 2

Ingredients:
- 4 eggs
- ½ teaspoon basil, dried
- Cooking spray
- Salt and black pepper to the taste
- ½ cup rice, cooked
- ½ cup shrimp, cooked, peeled, deveined and chopped
- ½ cup baby spinach, chopped
- ½ cup Monterey jack cheese, grated

Directions:
1. In a bowl, mix eggs with salt, pepper and basil and whisk. Grease your air fryer's pan with cooking spray and add rice, shrimp and spinach. Add eggs mix, sprinkle cheese all over and cook in your air fryer at 350 degrees F for 10 minutes. Divide among plates and serve for breakfast. Enjoy!

Nutrition: Calories 162 Fat 6 Fiber 5 Carbs 8 Protein 4

4. Tuna Sandwiches

Preparation time: 10 minutes
Cooking time: 5 minutes
Servings: 2

Ingredients:
- 16 ounces canned tuna, drained
- ¼ cup mayonnaise
- 2 tablespoons mustard
- 1 tablespoons lemon juice
- 2 green onions, chopped
- 3 English muffins, halved
- 3 tablespoons butter
- 6 provolone cheese

Directions:
1. In a bowl, mix tuna with mayo, lemon juice, mustard and green onions and stir. Grease muffin halves with the butter, place them in preheated air fryer and bake them at 350 degrees F for 4 minutes. Spread tuna mix on muffin halves, top each with provolone cheese, return sandwiches to air fryer and cook them for 4 minutes, divide among plates and serve for breakfast right away. Enjoy!

Nutrition: Calories: 182 Fat: 4 Fiber: 7 Carbs: 8 Protein: 6

5. Shrimp Sandwiches

Preparation time: 10 minutes
Cooking time: 5 minutes
Servings: 2

Ingredients:
- 1 and ¼ cups cheddar, shredded
- 6 ounces canned tiny shrimp, drained
- 3 tablespoons mayonnaise
- 2 tablespoons green onions, chopped
- 4 whole wheat bread slices
- 2 tablespoons butter, soft

Directions:
1. In a bowl, mix shrimp with cheese, green onion and mayo and stir well. Spread this on half of the bread slices, top with the other bread slices, cut into halves diagonally and spread butter on top. Place sandwiches in your air fryer and cook at 350 degrees F for 5 minutes. Divide shrimp sandwiches on plates and serve them for breakfast. Enjoy!

Nutrition: Calories: 162 Fat: 3 Fiber: 7 Carbs: 12 Protein: 4

6. Chicken & Zucchini Omelet

Preparation Time: 15 minutes
Cooking Time: 35 minutes
Servings: 2

Ingredients:
- 8 eggs
- ½ cup milk
- Salt and ground black pepper, as required
- 1 cup cooked chicken, chopped
- 1 cup Cheddar cheese, shredded
- ½ cup fresh chives, chopped
- ¾ cup zucchini, chopped

Directions:

1. In a bowl, add the eggs, milk, salt and black pepper and beat well. Add the remaining ingredients and stir to combine. Place the mixture into a greased baking pan. Press "Power Button" of Air Fry Oven and turn the dial to select the "Air Bake" mode. Press the Time button and again turn the dial to set the cooking time to 35 minutes. Now push the Temp button and rotate the dial to set the temperature at 315 degrees F. Press "Start/Pause" button to start. When the unit beeps to show that it is preheated, open the lid. Arrange pan over the "Wire Rack" and insert in the oven. Cut into equal-sized wedges and serve hot.

Nutrition: Calories: 209 Total Fat: 13.3 g Saturated Fat: 6.3 g Cholesterol: 258 mg Sodium: 252 mg Total Carbs: 2.3 g Fiber: 0.3 g Sugar: 1.8 g Protein: 9.8 g

7. Zucchini Fritters

Preparation Time: 15 minutes
Cooking Time: 7 minutes
Servings: 2

Ingredients:
- 10½ oz. zucchini, grated and squeezed
- 7 oz. Halloumi cheese
- ¼ cup all-purpose flour
- 2 eggs
- 1 teaspoon fresh dill, minced
- Salt and ground black pepper, as required

Directions:
1. In a large bowl and mix together all the ingredients. Make a small-sized fritter from the mixture. Press "Power Button" of Air Fry Oven and turn the dial to select the "Air Fry" mode. Press the Time button and again turn the dial to set the cooking time to 7 minutes. Now push the Temp button and rotate the dial to set the temperature at 355 degrees F. Press "Start/Pause" button to start. When the unit beeps to show that it is preheated, open the lid. Arrange fritters into grease "Sheet Pan" and insert in the oven. Serve warm.

Nutrition: Calories: 253 Total Fat: 17.2 g Saturated Fat: 11 g Cholesterol: 121 mg Sodium: 333 mg Total Carbs: 10 g Fiber: 1.1 g Sugar: 2.7 g Protein: 15.2 g

8. Onion Omelet

Preparation Time: 10 minutes
Cooking Time: 15 minutes
Servings: 2

Ingredients:
- 4 eggs
- ¼ teaspoon low-sodium soy sauce
- Ground black pepper, as required
- 1 teaspoon butter
- 1 medium yellow onion, sliced
- ¼ cup Cheddar cheese, grated

Directions:
1. In a skillet, melt the butter over medium heat and cook the onion and cook for about 8-10 minutes. Remove from the heat and set aside to cool slightly. Meanwhile, in a bowl, add the eggs, soy sauce and black pepper and beat well. Add the cooked onion and gently, stir to combine. Place the zucchini mixture into a small baking pan. Press "Power Button" of Air Fry Oven and turn the dial to select the "Air Fry" mode. Press the Time button and again turn the dial to set the cooking time to 5 minutes. Now push the Temp button and rotate the dial to set the temperature at 355 degrees F. Press "Start/Pause" button to start. When the unit beeps to show that it is preheated, open the lid. Arrange pan over the "Wire Rack" and insert in the oven. Cut the omelet into 2 portions and serve hot.

Nutrition: Calories: 222 Total Fat: 15.4 g Saturated Fat: 6.9 g Cholesterol: 347 mg Sodium: 264 mg Total Carbs: 6.1 g Fiber: 1.2 g Sugar: 3.1 g Protein: 15.3 g

9. Breakfast Pea Tortilla

Preparation time: 10 minutes
Cooking time: 7 minutes
Servings: 2

Ingredients:
- ½ pound baby peas
- 4 tablespoons butter
- 1 and ½ cup yogurt
- 8 eggs
- ½ cup mint, chopped
- Salt and black pepper to the taste

Directions:
1. Heat up a pan that fits your air fryer with the butter over medium heat, add peas, stir and cook for a couple of minutes. Meanwhile, in a bowl, mix half of the yogurt with salt, pepper, eggs and mint and whisk well. Pour this over the peas, toss, introduce in your air fryer and cook at 350 degrees F for 7 minutes. Spread the rest of the yogurt over your tortilla, slice and serve. Enjoy!

Nutrition: Calories: 192 Fat: 5 Fiber: 4 Carbs: 8 Protein: 7

10. Almond Crust Chicken

Preparation Time: 10 minutes
Cooking Time: 25 minutes
Servings: 2

Ingredients:
- 2 chicken breasts, skinless and boneless
- 1 tbsp Dijon mustard
- 2 tbsp mayonnaise
- ¼ cup almonds
- Pepper
- Salt

Directions:
1. Add almond into the food processor and process until finely ground. Transfer almonds on a plate and set aside. Mix together mustard and mayonnaise and spread over chicken. Coat chicken with almond and place into the air fryer basket and cook at 350 F for 25 minutes. Serve and enjoy.

Nutrition: Calories 409 Fat 22 g Carbohydrates 6 g Sugar 1.5 g Protein 45 g Cholesterol 134 mg

11. Breakfast Fish Tacos

Preparation time: 10 minutes
Cooking time: 13 minutes
Servings: 2

Ingredients:
- 4 big tortillas
- 1 red bell pepper, chopped
- 1 yellow onion, chopped
- 1 cup corn
- 4 white fish fillets, skinless and boneless
- ½ cup salsa
- A handful mixed romaine lettuce, spinach and radicchio
- 4 tablespoon parmesan, grated

Directions:
1. Put fish fillets in your air fryer and cook at 350 degrees F for 6 minutes. Meanwhile, heat up a pan over medium high heat, add bell pepper, onion and corn, stir and cook for 1-2 minutes. Arrange tortillas on a working surface,

divide fish fillets, spread salsa over them, divide mixed veggies and mixed greens and spread parmesan on each at the end. Roll your tacos, place them in preheated air fryer and cook at 350 degrees F for 6 minutes more. Divide fish tacos on plates and serve for breakfast. Enjoy!

Nutrition: Calories: 200 Fat: 3 Fiber: 7 Carbs: 9 Protein: 5

12. Garlic Potatoes with Bacon

Preparation time: 10 minutes
Cooking time: 20 minutes
Servings: 2

Ingredients:
- 4 potatoes, peeled and cut into medium cubes
- 6 garlic cloves, minced
- 4 bacon slices, chopped
- 2 rosemary springs, chopped
- 1 tablespoon olive oil
- Salt and black pepper to the taste
- 2 eggs, whisked

Directions:
1. In your air fryer's pan, mix oil with potatoes, garlic, bacon, rosemary, salt, pepper and eggs and whisk. Cook potatoes at 400 degrees F for 20 minutes, divide everything on plates and serve for breakfast. Enjoy!

Nutrition: Calories: 211 Fat: 3 Fiber: 5 Carbs: 8 Protein: 5

13. Zucchini Squash Mix

Preparation Time: 10 minutes
Cooking Time: 35 minutes
Servings: 2

Ingredients:
- 1 lb zucchini, sliced
- 1 tbsp parsley, chopped
- 1 yellow squash, halved, deseeded, and chopped
- 1 tbsp olive oil
- Pepper
- Salt

Directions:
1. Add all ingredients into the large bowl and mix well.
2. Transfer bowl mixture into the air fryer basket and cook at 400 F for 35 minutes.
3. Serve and enjoy.

Nutrition: Calories: 49 Fat: 3 g Carbohydrates: 4 g Sugar: 2 g Protein: 1.5 g Cholesterol: 0 mg

14. Spiced Chicken Omelet

Preparation Time: 10 minutes
Cooking Time: 16 minutes
Servings: 2

Ingredients:
- 1 teaspoon butter
- 1 small yellow onion, chopped
- ½ jalapeño pepper, seeded and chopped
- 3 eggs
- Salt and ground black pepper, as required
- ¼ cup cooked chicken, shredded

Directions:
1. In a frying pan, melt the butter over medium heat and cook the onion for about 4-5 minutes. Add the jalapeño pepper and cook for about 1 minute. Remove from the heat and set aside to cool slightly. Meanwhile, in a bowl, add the eggs, salt, and black pepper and beat well. Add the onion mixture and chicken and stir to combine. Place the chicken mixture into a small baking pan. Press "Power Button" of Air Fry Oven and turn the dial to select the "Air Fry" mode. Press the Time button and again turn the dial to set the cooking time to 6 minutes. Now push the Temp button and rotate the dial to set the temperature at 355 degrees F. Press "Start/Pause" button to start. When the unit beeps to show that it is preheated, open the lid. Arrange pan over the "Wire Rack" and insert in the oven. Cut the omelet into 2 portions and serve hot.

Nutrition: Calories: 153 Total Fat: 9.1 g Saturated Fat: 3.4 g Cholesterol: 264 mg Sodium: 196 mg Total Carbs: 4 g Fiber: 0.9 g Sugar: 2.1 g Protein: 13.8 g

15. Mushroom Cheese Salad

Preparation Time: 10 minutes
Cooking Time: 15 minutes
Servings: 2

Ingredients:
- 10 mushrooms, halved
- 1 tbsp. fresh parsley, chopped
- 1 tbsp. olive oil
- 1 tbsp. mozzarella cheese, grated
- 1 tbsp. cheddar cheese, grated
- 1 tbsp. dried mix herbs
- Pepper
- Salt

Directions:
1. Add all Ingredients into the bowl and toss well. Transfer bowl mixture into the air fryer baking dish. Place in the air fryer and cook at 380 F for 15 minutes. Serve and enjoy.

Nutrition: Calories: 90 Fat: 7 g Carbohydrates: 2 g Sugar: 1 g Protein: 5 g Cholesterol: 7 mg

16. Fennel Frittata

Preparation Time: 5 minutes
Cooking Time: 15 minutes
Servings: 6

Ingredients:
- 1 fennel bulb; shredded
- 6 eggs; whisked
- 2 tsp. cilantro; chopped.
- 1 tsp. sweet paprika
- Cooking spray
- A pinch of salt and black pepper

Directions:
1. Take a bowl and mix all the Ingredients except the cooking spray and stir well.
2. Grease a baking pan with the cooking spray, pour the frittata mix and spread well
3. Put the pan in the Air Fryer and cook at 370°F for 15 minutes. Divide between plates and serve them for breakfast.

Nutrition: Calories: 200 Fat: 12g Fiber: 1g Carbs: 5g Protein: 8g

17. Strawberries Oatmeal

Preparation Time: 5 minutes
Cooking Time: 15 minutes
Servings: 4

Ingredients:
- ½ cup coconut; shredded
- ¼ cup strawberries
- 2 cups coconut milk
- ¼ tsp. vanilla extract
- 2 tsp. stevia
- Cooking spray

Directions:

BREAKFAST RECIPES

1. Grease the Air Fryer's pan with the cooking spray, add all the Ingredients inside and toss
2. Cook at 365°F for 15 minutes, divide into bowls and serve for breakfast

Nutrition: Calories: 142 Fat: 7g Fiber: 2g Carbs: 3g Protein: 5g

18. Asparagus Salad

Preparation Time: 5 minutes
Cooking Time: 10 minutes
Servings: 4

Ingredients:
- 1 cup baby arugula
- 1 bunch asparagus; trimmed
- 1 tbsp. balsamic vinegar
- 1 tbsp. cheddar cheese; grated
- A pinch of salt and black pepper
- Cooking spray

Directions:
1. Put the asparagus in your air fryer's basket, grease with cooking spray, season with salt and pepper and cook at 360°F for 10 minutes.
2. Take a bowl and mix the asparagus with the arugula and the vinegar, toss, divide between plates and serve hot with cheese sprinkled on top

Nutrition: Calories: 200 Fat: 5g Fiber: 1g Carbs: 4g Protein: 5g

19. Lemony Raspberries Bowls

Preparation Time: 5 minutes
Cooking Time: 12 minutes
Servings: 2

Ingredients:
- 1 cup raspberries
- 2 tbsp. butter
- 2 tbsp. lemon juice
- 1 tsp. cinnamon powder

Directions:
1. In your air fryer, mix all the Ingredients, toss, cover, cook at 350°F for 12 minutes, divide into bowls and serve for breakfast

Nutrition: Calories: 208 Fat: 6g Fiber: 9g Carbs: 14g Protein: 3g

20. Spaghetti Squash Fritters

Preparation Time: 15 minutes
Cooking Time: 8 minutes
Servings: 4

Ingredients:
- 2 cups cooked spaghetti squash
- 2 stalks green onion, sliced
- 1 large egg.
- ¼ cup blanched finely ground almond flour.
- 2 tbsp. unsalted butter; softened.
- ½ tsp. garlic powder.
- 1 tsp. dried parsley.

Directions:
1. Remove excess moisture from the squash using a cheesecloth or kitchen towel.
2. Mix all Ingredients in a large bowl. Form into four patties
3. Cut a piece of parchment to fit your air fryer basket. Place each patty on the parchment and place into the air fryer basket
4. Adjust the temperature to 400 Degrees F and set the timer for 8 minutes. Flip the patties halfway through the cooking time. Serve warm.

Nutrition: Calories: 131 Protein: 3.8g Fiber: 2.0g Fat: 10.1g Carbs: 7.1g

21. Mushrooms And Cheese Spread

Preparation Time: 5 minutes
Cooking Time: 20 minutes
Servings: 4

Ingredients:
- ¼ cup mozzarella; shredded
- ½ cup coconut cream
- 1 cup white mushrooms
- A pinch of salt and black pepper
- Cooking spray

Directions:
1. Put the mushrooms in your air fryer's basket, grease with cooking spray and cook at 370°F for 20 minutes.
2. Transfer to a blender, add the remaining Ingredients, pulse well, divide into bowls and serve as a spread

Nutrition: Calories: 202 Fat: 12g Fiber: 2g Carbs: 5g Protein: 7g

22. Tuna and Spring Onions Salad

Preparation Time: 5 minutes
Cooking Time: 15 minutes
Servings: 4

Ingredients:
- 14 oz. canned tuna, drained and flaked
- 2 spring onions; chopped.
- 1 cup arugula
- 1 tbsp. olive oil
- A pinch of salt and black pepper

Directions:
1. In a bowl, all the Ingredients except the oil and the arugula and whisk.
2. Preheat the Air Fryer over 360°F, add the oil and grease it. Pour the tuna mix, stir well and cook for 15 minutes
3. In a salad bowl, combine the arugula with the tuna mix, toss and serve.

Nutrition: Calories: 212 Fat: 8g Fiber: 3g Carbs: 5g Protein: 8g

23. Cinnamon Pudding

Preparation Time: 5 minutes
Cooking Time: 12 minutes
Servings: 2

Ingredients:
- 4 eggs; whisked
- 4 tbsp. erythritol
- 2 tbsp. heavy cream
- ½ tsp. cinnamon powder
- ¼ tsp. allspice, ground
- Cooking spray

Directions:
1. Take a bowl and mix all the Ingredients except the cooking spray, whisk well and pour into a ramekin greased with cooking spray
2. Add the basket to your Air Fryer, put the ramekin inside and cook at 400°F for 12 minutes. Divide into bowls and serve for breakfast.

Nutrition: Calories: 201 Fat: 11g Fiber: 2g Carbs: 4g Protein: 6g

24. Tomatoes and Swiss chard Bake

Preparation Time: 5 minutes
Cooking Time: 15 minutes
Servings: 4

Ingredients:
- 4 eggs; whisked
- 3 oz. Swiss chard; chopped.

- 1 cup tomatoes; cubed
- 1 tsp. olive oil
- Salt and black pepper to taste.

Directions:
1. Take a bowl and mix the eggs with the rest of the Ingredients except the oil and whisk well.
2. Grease a pan that fits the fryer with the oil, pour the swish chard mix and cook at 359°F for 15 minutes.
3. Divide between plates and serve.

Nutrition: Calories: 202 Fat: 14g Fiber: 3g Carbs: 5g Protein: 12g

25. Egg, Bacon and Cheese Roll Ups

Preparation Time: 10 minutes
Cooking Time: 25 minutes
Servings: 4

Ingredients:
- 12 slices sugar-free bacon.
- ½ medium green bell pepper; seeded and chopped
- 6 large eggs.
- ¼ cup chopped onion
- 1 cup shredded sharp Cheddar cheese.
- ½ cup mild salsa, for dipping
- 2 tbsp. unsalted butter.

Directions:
1. In a medium skillet over medium heat, melt butter. Add onion and pepper to the skillet and sauté until fragrant and onions are translucent, about 3 minutes
2. Whisk eggs in a small bowl and pour into skillet. Scramble eggs with onions and peppers until fluffy and fully cooked, about 5 minutes. Remove from heat and set aside
3. On work surface, place three slices of bacon side by side, overlapping about ¼-inch. Place ¼ cup scrambled eggs in a heap on the side closest to you and sprinkle ¼ cup cheese on top of the eggs.
4. Tightly roll the bacon around the eggs and secure the seam with a toothpick if necessary. Place each roll into the air fryer basket.
5. Adjust the temperature to 350 Degrees F and set the timer for 15 minutes. Rotate the rolls halfway through the cooking time. Bacon will be brown and crispy when completely cooked. Serve immediately with salsa for dipping.

Nutrition: Calories: 460 Protein: 28.2g Fiber: 0.8g Fat: 31.7g Carbs: 6.1g

26. Crispy Ham Egg Cups

Preparation Time: 5 minutes
Cooking Time: 12 minutes
Servings: 2

Ingredients:
- 4 large eggs.
- 4: 1-oz. slices deli ham
- ½ cup shredded medium Cheddar cheese.
- ¼ cup diced green bell pepper.
- 2 tbsp. diced red bell pepper.
- 2 tbsp. diced white onion.
- 2 tbsp. full-fat sour cream.

Directions:
1. Place one slice of ham on the bottom of four baking cups.
2. Take a large bowl, whisk eggs with sour cream. Stir in green pepper, red pepper and onion
3. Pour the egg mixture into ham-lined baking cups. Top with Cheddar. Place cups into the air fryer basket. Adjust the temperature to 320 Degrees F and set the timer for 12 minutes or until the tops are browned. Serve warm.

Nutrition: Calories: 382 Protein: 29.4g Fiber: 1.4g Fat: 23.6g Carbs: 6.0g

27. Olives and Kale

Preparation Time: 5 minutes
Cooking Time: 20 minutes
Servings: 4

Ingredients:
- 4 eggs; whisked
- 1 cup kale; chopped.
- ½ cup black olives, pitted and sliced
- 2 tbsp. cheddar; grated
- Cooking spray
- A pinch of salt and black pepper

Directions:
1. Take a bowl, mix the eggs with the rest of the Ingredients except the cooking spray, and whisk well.
2. Now, take a pan that fits in your air fryer and grease it with the cooking spray, pour the olives mixture inside, spread
3. Put the pan into the machine and cook at 360°F for 20 minutes. Serve for breakfast hot.

Nutrition: Calories: 220 Fat: 13g Fiber: 4g Carbs: 6g Protein: 12g

28. Stuffed Poblanos

Preparation Time: 10 minutes
Cooking Time: 20 minutes
Servings: 4

Ingredients:
- ½ lb. spicy ground pork breakfast sausage
- 4 large poblano peppers
- 4 large eggs.
- ½ cup full-fat sour cream.
- 4 oz. full-fat cream cheese; softened.
- ¼ cup canned diced tomatoes and green chiles, drained
- 8 tbsp. shredded pepper jack cheese

Directions:
1. In a medium skillet over medium heat, crumble and brown the ground sausage until no pink remains. Remove sausage and drain the fat from the pan. Crack eggs into the pan, scramble and cook until no longer runny
2. Place cooked sausage in a large bowl and fold in cream cheese. Mix in diced tomatoes and chiles. Gently fold in eggs
3. Cut a 4"–5" slit in the top of each poblano, removing the seeds and white membrane with a small knife. Separate the filling into four and spoon carefully into each pepper. Top each with 2 tbsp. pepper jack cheese
4. Place each pepper into the air fryer basket. Adjust the temperature to 350 Degrees F and set the timer for 15 minutes.
5. Peppers will be soft and cheese will be browned when ready. Serve immediately with sour cream on top.

Nutrition: Calories: 489 Protein: 22.8g Fiber: 3.8g Fat: 35.6g Carbs: 12.6g

29. Raspberries Oatmeal

Preparation Time: 5 minutes
Cooking Time: 15 minutes
Servings: 4

Ingredients:
- 1 ½ cups coconut; shredded
- ½ cups raspberries
- 2 cups almond milk
- ¼ tsp. nutmeg, ground

- 2 tsp. stevia
- ½ tsp. cinnamon powder
- Cooking spray

Directions:
1. Grease the air fryer's pan with cooking spray, mix all the Ingredients inside, cover and cook at 360°F for 15 minutes. Divide into bowls and serve

Nutrition: Calories: 172 Fat: 5g Fiber: 2g Carbs: 4g Protein: 6g

30. Easy Scotch Eggs

Preparation Time: 15 minutes
Cooking Time: 15 minutes
Servings: 4

Ingredients:
- 1-pound ground breakfast sausage
- 3 tablespoons flour
- 4 hard-boiled eggs, peeled
- 1 egg
- 1 tablespoon water
- ¾ cup panko bread crumbs

Direction:
1. In a bowl, mix the sausage and one tablespoon flour.
2. Divide the sausage mixture into four equal parts. Lay one hard-boiled egg in the center, then wrap the sausage around the egg, sealing completely. Repeat with remaining sausage parts and hard-boiled eggs.
3. In a small bowl, whisk the egg and water until smooth.
4. Place the remaining flour and bread crumbs into separate bowls large enough to dredge the sausage-wrapped eggs.
5. Dredge the sausage-wrapped eggs in the flour, then in the whisked egg, and finally coat in the bread crumbs.
6. Arrange them in the basket. Put the air fryer lid on and cook in the preheated instant pot at 375°F for 20 minutes. Flip them over when the lid screen indicates 'TURN FOOD' halfway through, or until the sausage is cooked to desired doneness.
7. Remove from the basket and serve on a plate.

Nutrition: Calories: 509 Total Fat: 16g Saturated Fat: 5g Total Carbs: 8g Net Carbs: 2g Fiber: 7g Protein: 24g Sugar: 16g Sodium: 785mg

31. Strawberry Toast

Preparation Time: 8 minutes
Cooking Time: 10 minutes
Servings: 4

Ingredients:
- 4 slices bread, ½-inch thick
- 1 cup sliced strawberries
- 1 teaspoon sugar
- Cooking spray

Direction:
1. On a plate, place the bread slices.
2. Arrange the bread slices (sprayed side down) in the air fryer basket. Evenly spread the strawberries onto them and sprinkle with sugar.
3. Put the air fryer lid on and cook in the preheated instant pot at 375°F for 8 minutes, or until the tops are covered with a beautiful glaze.
4. Remove from the basket and serve on a plate.

Nutrition: Calories: 375 Total Fat: 22g Saturated Fat: 5g Total Carbs: 2g Net Carbs: 2g Fiber: 4g Protein: 14g Sugar: 5g Sodium: 600mg

32. Cinnamon Sweet-Potato Chips

Preparation Time: 7 minutes
Cooking Time: 8 minutes
Servings: 7

Ingredients:
- 1 small sweet potato, cut into 3/8-inch slices
- 2 tablespoons olive oil
- Ground cinnamon

Direction:
1. In a bowl, toss the potato slices in olive oil. Sprinkle with the cinnamon and mix well.
2. Lay the potato slices in the air fryer basket. You may need to work in batches to avoid overcrowding.
3. Put the air fryer lid on and cook in the preheated instant pot at 375°F for 4 minutes. Shake the basket when the lid screen indicates 'TURN FOOD' Cook for an additional 4 minutes or until fork-tender.
4. Remove from the basket and serve on a large dish lined with paper towels.

Nutrition: Calories: 385 Total Fat: 18g Saturated Fat: 2g Total Carbs: 5g Net Carbs: 3g Fiber: 8g Protein: 20g Sugar: 3g Sodium: 518mg

33. Quiche Muffin Cups

Preparation Time: 11 minutes
Cooking Time: 10 minutes
Servings: 10

Ingredients:
- ¼ pound all-natural ground pork sausage
- Three eggs
- ¾ cup milk
- 4 ounces sharp Cheddar cheese, grated
- One muffin pan
- Cooking spray

Direction:
1. On a clean work surface, slice the pork sausage into 2-ounce portions. Shape each portion into a ball and gently flatten it with your palm.
2. Lay the patties in the air fryer basket and cook in the preheated instant pot at 375°F for 6 minutes. Flip the patties over when the lid screen indicates 'TURN FOOD' during cooking time.
3. Remove the patties from the basket to a large dish lined with paper towels. Crumble them into small pieces with a fork. Set aside.
4. Line a muffin pan with ten paper liners. Lightly spray the muffin cups with cooking spray.
5. Divide crumbled sausage equally among the ten muffin cups and sprinkle the tops with the cheese.
6. Arrange the muffin pan in the air fryer basket.
7. Put the air fryer lid on and cook in the preheated instant pot at 375°F for 8 minutes, until the tops are golden and a toothpick inserted in the middle comes out clean.
8. Remove from the basket and let cool for 5 minutes before serving.

Nutrition: Calories: 497 Total Fat: 25g Saturated Fat: 2g Total Carbs: 1g Net Carbs: 1g Fiber: 4g Protein: 28g Sugar: 5g Sodium: 742mg

34. Vegetable and Ham Omelet

Preparation Time: 10 minutes
Cooking Time: 10 minutes
Servings: 6

Ingredients:
- ¼ cup ham, diced
- ¼ cup green or red bell pepper, cored and chopped
- ¼ cup onion, chopped
- 1 teaspoon butter
- 4 large eggs

- 2 tablespoons milk
- 1/8 teaspoon salt
- ¾ cup sharp Cheddar cheese, grated

Direction:
1. Add the ham, bell pepper, onion, and butter into a 6×6×2-inch baking pan. Place the pan inside the air fryer basket.
2. Put the air fryer lid on and cook in the preheated instant pot at 375ºF for 6 minutes. Stir once halfway through the cooking time, or until the vegetables are soft.
3. In a bowl, whisk the eggs, milk, and salt until smooth and creamy. Gently pour over the ham and vegetables in the pan.
4. Put the air fryer lid on and cook at 375ºF for about 13 minutes, or until the top begins to turn brown.
5. Top with the cheese and cook for 1 minute more, or until the cheese is bubbly and melted.
6. Remove from the basket and cool for 5 minutes before serving.

Nutrition: Calories: 367 Total Fat: 14g Saturated Fat: 5g Total Carbs: 13g Net Carbs: 7g Fiber: 6g Protein: 18g Sugar: 2g Sodium: 423mg

35. Cheesy Canadian bacon English muffin

Preparation Time: 5 minutes
Cooking Time: 10 minutes
Servings: 4

Ingredients:
- 4 English muffins
- Eight slices Canadian bacon
- Four slices cheese
- Cooking spray

Direction:
1. On a clean work surface, cut each English muffin in half.
2. To assemble a sandwich, layer two slices of bacon and one cheese slice on the bottom of each muffin and put the other half of the bread on top. Repeat with remaining biscuits, bacon, and cheese slices.
3. Arrange the sandwiches in the air fryer basket and spritz with cooking spray. You may need to work in batches to avoid overcrowding.
4. Put the air fryer lid on and cook in the preheated instant pot at 375ºF for 8 minutes. Flip the sandwiches when it shows 'TURN FOOD' on the air fryer lid screen during cooking time.
5. Let them cool for 3 minutes before serving.

Nutrition: Calories: 322 Total Fat: 15g Saturated Fat: 8g Cholesterol: 58mg Sodium: 119mg Carbohydrates: 27g Fiber: 4g Protein: 24g

36. Asparagus, Cheese and Egg Strata

Preparation Time: 15 minutes
Cooking Time: 10 minutes
Servings: 4

Ingredients:
- 6 asparagus spears, cut into 2-inch pieces
- ½ cup grated Havarti or Swiss cheese
- 4 eggs
- 2 slices whole-wheat bread, cut into ½-inch cubes
- 3 tablespoons whole milk
- 2 tablespoons flat-leaf parsley, chopped
- 1 tablespoon water
- Cooking spray

Direction:
1. Place a 6×6×2-inch baking pan into the air fryer basket. Add one tablespoon water, and asparagus spears into the pan.
2. Put the air fryer lid on and cook in the preheated instant pot at 325ºF for 3 to 5 minutes, or until the asparagus spears are tender.
3. Remove the asparagus spears from the baking pan. Drain and dry them thoroughly. Place the asparagus spears and bread cubes in the pan, then spray with cooking spray. Set aside.
4. Add the cheese, parsley, salt, and pepper.
5. Put the air fryer lid on and bake at 350ºF for 11 to 14 minutes, or until a knife inserted in the center comes out clean.
6. Remove the strata from the pan. Let cool for 5 minutes before serving.

Nutrition: Calories: 1214 Total Fat: 90.11g Saturated Fat: 29.721g Total Carbs: 6.16g Fiber: 0.4g Protein: 32.73g Sugar: 2.68g Sodium: 973.1mg

37. Shrimp, Spinach And Rice Frittata

Preparation Time: 15 minutes
Cooking Time: 15 minutes
Servings: 4

Ingredients:
- ½ cup chopped shrimp, cooked
- ½ cup baby spinach
- ½ cup of rice, cooked
- 4 eggs
- ½ cup grated Monterey Jack cheese
- ½ teaspoon dried basil
- Pinch salt
- Cooking spray

Direction:
1. Spritz a 6×6×2-inch baking pan with cooking spray. Place the cooked shrimp, rice, and spinach into the pan and stir to combine well. Put the pan into the air fryer basket.
2. Put the air fryer lid on and bake in the preheated instant pot at 325ºF for 14 to 18 minutes, or until puffy and golden brown.
3. Remove from the pan and cool for 3 minutes before cutting into wedges to serve.

Nutrition: Calories: 1358 Total Fat: 81.86g Saturated Fat: 29.089g Total Carbs: 8.86g Fiber: 3.1g Protein: 35.54g Sugar: 0.98: g Sodium: 831mg

38. Tender Monkey Bread With Cinnamon

Preparation Time: 5 minutes
Cooking Time: 10 minutes
Servings: 4

Ingredients:
- 1 can (8-ounce) refrigerated biscuits
- 3 tablespoons brown sugar
- ¼ cup white sugar
- ½ teaspoon cinnamon
- ⅛ teaspoon nutmeg
- 3 tablespoons unsalted butter, melted

Direction:
1. On your cutting board, divide each biscuit into quarters.
2. In a mixing bowl, add the brown and white sugar, nutmeg, and cinnamon. Stir well.

BREAKFAST RECIPES

3. Pour the melted butter into a medium bowl. Dip each biscuit in the melted butter, then in the sugar mixture to coat thoroughly.
4. Arrange the coated biscuits in a 6×6×2-inch baking pan and place the container into the air fryer basket.
5. Put the air fryer lid on and bake in batches in the preheated instant pot at 350°F for 6 to 9 minutes until set.
6. Transfer to a serving dish and cool for 5 minutes before serving.

Nutrition: Calories: 1228 Total Fat: 42.64g Saturated Fat: 15.178g Total Carbs: 31.53g Fiber: 1.2g Protein: 49.97g Sugar: 8.74g Sodium: 628mg

39. Pesto Cheese Gnocchi

Preparation Time: 15 minutes
Cooking Time: 10 minutes
Servings: 4
Ingredients:
- 1 jar (8-ounce) pesto
- ⅓ cup Parmesan cheese, grated
- 1 package (16-ounce) shelf-stable gnocchi
- 1 onion, finely chopped
- 3 cloves garlic, sliced
- 1 tablespoon olive oil

Directions:
1. Mix the oil, onion, garlic, and gnocchi in a 6×6×2-inch baking pan. Place the pan into the air fryer basket.
2. Put the air fryer lid on and bake in the preheated instant pot at 400°F for 16 minutes, or until the gnocchi starts to brown. Stir once halfway through cooking time.
3. Transfer the gnocchi to a serving dish. Sprinkle with the Parmesan cheese and pesto. Stir well and serve warm.

Nutrition: Calories: 1382 Total Fat: 48.35g Saturated Fat: 15.423g Total Carbs: 83.21g Fiber: 6.6g Protein: 46.26g Sugar: 14.5g Sodium: 1435mg

40. Ham in a Cup

Preparation Time: 10 minutes
Cooking Time: 15 minutes
Servings: 18
Ingredients:
- 5 whole eggs
- 2 1/4 oz. Ham
- 1 cup milk
- 1/8 tsp. Pepper
- 1 1/2 cups swiss cheese
- 1/4 tsp. Salt
- 1/4 cup green onion
- 1/2 tsp. Thyme

Directions:
1. In the fryer preheat to 350F.
2. Beat Eggs
3. Add thyme onion, salt, swiss cheese pepper, milk to the beaten eggs.
4. Prepare your baking forms for muffins and place ham slices in each cooking way. Cover the ham with egg mixture.
5. Transfer to air fryer and bake for 15 minutes.

Nutrition: Calories: 80 Fat: 5 g Protein: 7 g Carbs: 0 g Fiber: 2 g

41. Cheese Sticks

Preparation Time: 22 minutes
Cooking Time: 7 minutes
Servings: 8
Ingredients:
- 6 cheese sticks, snake-sized
- 1/4 cup parmesan cheese, grated
- 2 eggs
- 1 tbsp. Italian seasoning
- 1/4 cup flour, whole wheat
- 1/4 tbsp. Rosemary, grounded
- 1 tbsp. Garlic powder

Directions:
1. Take cheese sticks and set aside.
2. Take a shallow bowl and beat eggs into the container.
3. Mix cheese, flour, and seasonings in another bowl.
4. Roll the cheese sticks in the eggs and then in the batter.
5. Now do the process again till the sticks as well coated.
6. Place them in the basket of the air fryer.
7. Cook for 6-7 minutes at 370 f.

Nutrition: Calories: 50 Fat: 2 g Protein: 3 g Carbs: 3 g Fiber: 1.8 g

42. Broccoli Cheese Quiche

Preparation Time: 20 minutes
Cooking Time: 30 minutes
Servings: 2
Ingredients:
- 4 eggs
- 1 cup whole milk
- 2 medium broccolis, cut into florets
- 2 medium tomatoes, diced
- 4 medium carrots, diced
- 1/4 cup feta cheese, crumbled
- 1 cup grated cheddar cheese
- Salt and pepper, to taste
- 1 tsp. Chopped parsley
- 1 tsp. Dried thyme

Directions:
1. Put the broccoli and carrots in a food steamer and cook until soft, about 10 minutes.
2. In a jug, crack in the eggs, add the parsley, salt, pepper, and thyme.
3. Using a whisk, beat the eggs while adding the milk gradually until a pale mixture is attained.
4. Once the broccoli and carrots are ready, strain them through a sieve, and set aside.
5. In a 3 x 3 cm quiche dish, add the carrots and broccoli. Put the tomatoes on top, then the feta and cheddar cheese following. Leave a little bit of cheddar cheese.
6. Pour the egg mixture over the layering and top with the remaining cheddar cheese.
7. Place the dish in the air fryer and cook at 350 f for 20 minutes.

Nutrition: Calories: 316 Fat: 23.8 g Protein: 9.9 g Carbs: 5 g Fiber: 1 g

43. Onion and Cheese Omelet

Preparation Time: 5 minutes
Cooking Time: 10 minutes
Servings: 2
Ingredients
- 2 eggs
- 2 tbsp. Grated cheddar cheese
- 1 tsp. Soy sauce
- 1/2 onion, sliced
- 1/4 tsp. Pepper
- 1 tbsp. Olive oil

Directions:
1. Whisk the eggs along with the pepper and soy sauce.
2. Three hundred fifty degrees preheat the air fryer.
3. Heat the olive oil and add the egg mixture and the onion.
4. Cook for 8 to 10 minutes.

5. Top with the grated cheddar cheese.

Nutrition: Calories: 347 Fat: 23.2 g Protein: 13.6 g Carbs: 6 g Fiber: 1.2 g

44. Air Fried Shirred Eggs

Preparation Time: 6 minutes
Cooking Time: 14 minutes
Servings: 2

Ingredients:
- 2 tsp. Butter, for greasing
- 4 eggs, divided
- 2 tbsp. Heavy cream
- 4 slices ham
- 3 tbsp. Parmesan cheese
- 1/4 tsp. Paprika
- 3/4 tsp. Salt
- 1/4 tsp. Pepper
- 2 tsp. Chopped chives

Directions:
1. The degrees 360 preheat the air fryer.
2. Grease a pie pan with the butter. Arrange the ham slices on the bottom of the pot to cover it completely.
3. Whisk one egg along with the heavy cream, salt, and pepper, in a small bowl.
4. Pour the mixture over the ham slices.
5. Crack the other eggs over the ham. Sprinkle with parmesan cheese.
6. Cook for 14 minutes.
7. Season with paprika, garnish with chives and serve with low carb bread.

Nutrition: Calories: 279 Fat: 20 g Protein: 20.8 g Carbs: 1.8 g Fiber: 0.2 g

45. Cheesy Hash Brown

Preparation Time: 30 minutes
Cooking Time: 7-10 minutes
Servings: 6

Ingredients:
- 1½ lbs. hash browns
- 6 bacon slices; chopped.
- 8 oz. cream cheese; softened
- 1 yellow onion; chopped.
- 6 eggs
- 6 spring onions; chopped.
- 1 cup cheddar cheese; shredded
- 1 cup almond milk
- A drizzle of olive oil
- Salt and black pepper to taste

Directions:
1. Heat up your air fryer with the oil at 350°F. In a bowl, mix all other Ingredients except the spring onions and whisk well
2. Add this mixture to your air fryer, cover and cook for 20 minutes
3. Divide between plates, sprinkle the spring onions on top and serve.

Nutrition: Saturated Fat 3.5g Sugar 2g Protein 8g Cholesterol 20mg Sodium 740mg Total Carbohydrate 16g Dietary Fiber 1g

46. Cream Bread

Preparation Time: 20 minutes
Cooking Time: 55 minutes
Servings: 12

Ingredients:
- 1 cup milk
- ¾ cup whipping cream
- 1 large egg
- 4½ cups bread flour
- ½ cup all-purpose flour
- 2 tablespoons milk powder
- 1 teaspoon salt
- ¼ cup fine sugar
- 3 teaspoons dry yeast

Directions:
1. In the baking pan of a bread machine, place all the Ingredients in the order recommended by the manufacturer.
2. Place the baking pan in bread machine and close with the lid.
3. Select the Dough cycle and press Start button.
4. Once the cycle is completed, remove the paddles from bread machine but keep the dough inside for about 45-50 minutes to proof.
5. Set the temperature of air fryer to 375 degrees F. Grease 2 loaf pans.
6. Remove the dough from pan and place onto a lightly floured surface.
7. Divide the dough into four equal-sized balls and then, roll each into a rectangle.
8. Tightly, roll each rectangle like a Swiss roll.
9. Place two rolls into each prepared loaf pan.
10. Set aside for about 1 hour.
11. Arrange the loaf pans into an air fryer basket.
12. Air fry for about 50-55 minutes or until a toothpick inserted in the center comes out clean.
13. Remove the pans from air fryer and place onto a wire rack for about 10-15 minutes.
14. Then, remove the bread rolls from pans and place onto a wire rack until they are completely cool before slicing.
15. Cut each roll into desired size slices and serve.

Nutrition: Calories: 215 Carbohydrate: 36.9g Protein: 6.5g Fat: 3.1g Sugar: 5.2g Sodium: 189mg

47. Sunflower Seeds Bread

Preparation Time: 15 minutes
Cooking Time: 18 minutes
Servings: 4

Ingredients:
- 2/3 cup whole-wheat flour
- 2/3 cup plain flour
- 1/3 cup sunflower seeds
- ½ sachet instant yeast
- 1 teaspoon salt
- 2/3-1 cup lukewarm water

Directions:
1. In a bowl, mix together the flours, sunflower seeds, yeast, and salt.
2. Slowly, add in the water, stirring continuously until a soft dough ball forms.
3. Now, move the dough onto a lightly floured surface and knead for about 5 minutes using your hands.
4. Make a ball from the dough and place into a bowl.
5. With a plastic wrap, cover the bowl and place at a warm place for about 30 minutes.
6. Set the temperature of air fryer to 390 degrees F. Grease a cake pan. (6"x 3")
7. Coat the top of dough with water and place into the prepared cake pan.
8. Arrange the cake pan into an air fryer basket.
9. Air fry for about 18 minutes or until a toothpick inserted in the center comes out clean.

BREAKFAST RECIPES

10. Remove from air fryer and place the pan onto a wire rack for about 10-15 minutes.
11. Carefully, take out the bread from pan and put onto a wire rack until it is completely cool before slicing.
12. Cut the bread into desired size slices and serve.

Nutrition: Calories: 177 Carbohydrate: 33g Protein: 5.5g Fat: 2.4g Sugar: 0.2g Sodium: 580mg

48. Date Bread

Preparation Time: 15 minutes
Cooking Time: 22 minutes
Servings: 10

Ingredients
- 2½ cup dates, pitted and chopped
- ¼ cup butter
- 1 cup hot water
- 1½ cups flour
- ½ cup brown sugar
- 1 teaspoon baking powder
- 1 teaspoon baking soda
- ½ teaspoon salt
- 1 egg

Directions:
1. In a large bowl, add the dates, butter and top with the hot water.
2. Set aside for about 5 minutes.
3. In a separate bowl, mix together the flour, brown sugar, baking powder, baking soda, and salt.
4. In the same bowl of dates, mix well the flour mixture, and egg.
5. Set the temperature of air fryer to 340 degrees F. Grease an air fryer non-stick pan.
6. Place the mixture into the prepared pan.
7. Arrange the pan into an air fryer basket.
8. Air fry for about 22 minutes or until a toothpick inserted in the center comes out clean.
9. Remove from air fryer and place the pan onto a wire rack for about 10-15 minutes.
10. Carefully, take out the bread from pan and put onto a wire rack until it is completely cool before slicing.
11. Cut the bread into desired size slices and serve.

Nutrition: Calories: 269 Carbohydrate: 55.1g Protein: 3.6g Fat: 5.4g Sugar: 35.3 Sodium: 585mg

49. Banana Bread

Preparation Time: 10 minutes
Cooking Time: 20 minutes
Servings: 8

Ingredients:
- 1 1/3 cups flour
- 2/3 cup sugar
- 1 teaspoon baking soda
- 1 teaspoon baking powder
- 1 teaspoon ground cinnamon
- 1 teaspoon salt
- ½ cup milk
- ½ cup olive oil
- 3 bananas, peeled and sliced

Directions:
1. Take the bowl of a stand mixer and mix well all the listed Ingredients.
2. Set the temperature of air fryer to 330 degrees F. Grease a loaf pan.
3. Place the mixture into the prepared pan.
4. Arrange the loaf pan into an air fryer basket.
5. Air fry for about 20 minutes or until a toothpick inserted in the center comes out clean.
6. Remove from air fryer and place the pan onto a wire rack for about 10-15 minutes.
7. Carefully, take out the bread from pan and put onto a wire rack until it is completely cool before slicing.
8. Cut the bread into desired size slices and serve.

Nutrition: Calories: 295 Carbohydrate: 44g Protein: 3.1g Fat: 13.3g Sugar: 22.8g Sodium: 458mg

50. Nutty Banana Bread

Preparation Time: 15 minutes
Cooking Time: 25 minutes
Servings: 10

Ingredients:
- 1½ cups self-rising flour
- ¼ teaspoon bicarbonate of soda
- 5 tablespoons plus 1 teaspoon butter
- 2/3 cup plus ½ tablespoon caster sugar
- 2 medium eggs
- 3½ ounces walnuts, chopped
- 2 cups bananas, peeled and mashed

Directions:
1. In a bowl, mix together the flour and bicarbonate of soda.
2. In another bowl, add the butter, and sugar. Beat until pale and fluffy.
3. Put the eggs, one at a time along with a little flour and mix them well.
4. Stir in the remaining flour and walnuts.
5. Now, add the bananas and mix until well combined.
6. Set the temperature of air fryer to 355 degrees F. Grease a loaf pan.
7. Place the mixture evenly into the prepared pan.
8. Arrange the loaf pan into an air fryer basket.
9. Air fry for 10 minutes on 355 degrees F, then 15 minutes for 338 degrees F.
10. Once done, remove from air fryer and place the pan onto a wire rack for about 10-15 minutes.
11. Carefully, take out the bread from pan and put onto a wire rack until it is completely cool before slicing.
12. Cut the bread into desired size slices and serve.

Nutrition: Calories: 337 Carbohydrate: 44.5g Protein: 7.3g Fat: 16g Sugar: 21.6g Sodium: 106mg

51. Yogurt Banana Bread

Preparation Time: 15 minutes
Cooking Time: 35 minutes
Servings: 5

Ingredients
- ½ cup all-purpose flour
- ¼ cup whole-wheat flour
- ¼ teaspoon baking soda
- ½ teaspoon salt
- 1 large egg
- ½ cup granulated sugar
- ¼ cup plain yogurt
- ¼ cup vegetable oil
- ½ teaspoon pure vanilla extract
- 2 ripe bananas, peeled and mashed
- 2 tablespoons turbinado sugar

Directions:
1. In a bowl, sift together the flours, baking soda, and salt.
2. In another large bowl, mix well the egg, granulated sugar, yogurt, oil, and vanilla extract.
3. Add in the bananas and beat until well combined.
4. Now, add the flour mixture and mix until just combined.

5. Set the temperature of Air Fryer to 310 degrees F.
6. Place the mixture evenly into a cake pan and sprinkle with the turbinado sugar.
7. Arrange the cake pan into an Air Fryer basket.
8. Air Fry for about 30-35 minutes or until a toothpick inserted in the center comes out clean, turning the pan once halfway through.
9. Carefully, take out the bread from pan and put onto a wire rack until it is completely cool before slicing.
10. Cut the bread into desired size slices and serve.

Nutrition: Calories: 317 Carbohydrate: 49.2g Protein: 7.3g Fat: 16g Sugar: 21.6g Sodium: 106mg

52. Peanut Butter Banana Bread

Preparation Time: 15 minutes
Cooking Time: 40 minutes
Servings: 6
Ingredients:
- 1 cup plus 1 tablespoon all-purpose flour
- 1 teaspoon baking powder
- ¼ teaspoon baking soda
- ¼ teaspoon salt
- 1 large egg
- 1/3 cup granulated sugar
- ¼ cup canola oil
- 2 tablespoons creamy peanut butter
- 2 tablespoons sour cream
- 1 teaspoon vanilla extract
- 2 medium ripe bananas, peeled and mashed
- ¾ cup walnuts, roughly chopped

Directions:
1. Take a bowl and mix together the flour, baking powder, baking soda, and salt.
2. In another large bowl, add the egg, sugar, oil, peanut butter, sour cream, and vanilla extract. Beat until well combined.
3. Add in the bananas and beat until well combined.
4. Now, add the flour mixture and mix until just combined.
5. Gently, fold in the walnuts.
6. Set the temperature of Air Fryer to 330 degrees F. Grease a non-stick baking dish.
7. Transfer the mixture evenly into the prepared baking dish.
8. Arrange the baking dish in an Air Fryer basket.
9. Air Fry for about 30-40 minutes or until a toothpick inserted in the center comes out clean.
10. Remove the dish from Air Fryer and place onto a wire rack for about 10-15 minutes.
11. Carefully, take out the bread from dish and place onto a wire rack until it is completely cool before slicing.
12. Cut the bread into desired size slices and serve.

Nutrition: Calories: 384 Carbohydrate: 39.3g Protein: 8.9g Fat: 2.6g Sugar: 16.6g Sodium: 189mg

53. Chocolate Banana Bread

Preparation Time: 6 minutes
Cooking Time: 20 minutes
Servings: 10
Ingredients:
- 2 cups flour
- ½ teaspoon baking soda
- ½ teaspoon baking powder
- ½ teaspoon salt
- ¾ cup sugar
- 1/3 cup butter, softened
- 3 eggs
- 1 tablespoon vanilla extract
- 1 cup milk
- ½ cup bananas, peeled and mashed
- 1 cup chocolate chips

Directions:
1. Take a bowl and mix together the flour, baking soda, baking powder, and salt.
2. In another large bowl, add the butter, and sugar. Beat until light and fluffy.
3. Now, add in the eggs, and vanilla extract. Beat until well combined.
4. Add the flour mixture and mix until well combined.
5. Add in the milk, and mashed bananas and mix them well.
6. Gently, fold in the chocolate chips.
7. Set the temperature of Air Fryer to 360 degrees F. Grease a loaf pan.
8. Place the mixture evenly into the prepared pan.
9. Arrange the loaf pan into an Air Fryer basket.
10. Air Fry for about 20 minutes or until a toothpick inserted in the center comes out clean.
11. Remove from Air Fryer and place the pan onto a wire rack for about 10-15 minutes.
12. Carefully, take out the bread from pan and put onto a wire rack until it is completely cool before slicing.
13. Cut the bread into desired size slices and serve.

Nutrition: Calories: 333 Carbohydrate: 47.4g Protein: 6.5g Fat: 13.2g Sugar: 26g Sodium: 267mg

54. Nutty Zucchini Bread

Preparation Time: 15 minutes
Cooking Time: 20 minutes
Servings: 16
Ingredients:
- 3 cups all-purpose flour
- 1 teaspoon baking powder
- 1 teaspoon baking soda
- 1 tablespoon ground cinnamon
- 1 teaspoon salt
- 2¼ cups white sugar
- 1 cup vegetable oil
- 3 eggs
- 3 teaspoons vanilla extract
- 2 cups zucchini, grated
- 1 cup walnuts, chopped

Directions:
1. Take a bowl and mix together the flour, baking powder, baking soda, cinnamon, and salt.
2. In another large bowl, add the sugar, oil, eggs, and vanilla extract. Beat until well combined.
3. Then, add in the flour mixture and stir until just combined.
4. Gently, fold in the zucchini and walnuts.
5. Set the temperature of Air Fryer to 320 degrees F. Grease and flour two (8x4-inch) loaf pans.
6. Place the mixture evenly into the prepared pans.
7. Arrange the loaf pans into an Air Fryer basket.
8. Air Fry for about 20 minutes or until a toothpick inserted in the center comes out clean.
9. Remove the pans from Air Fryer and place onto a wire rack for about 10-15 minutes.
10. Carefully, take out the bread from pans and put onto a wire rack until it is completely cool before slicing.
11. Cut the breads into desired size slices and serve.

Nutrition: Calories: 377 Carbohydrate: 47.9g Protein: 5.5g Fat: 19.3g Sugar: 28.7g Sodium: 241mg

55. Zucchini & Apple Bread

Preparation Time: 15 minutes
Cooking Time: 30 minutes
Servings: 8
Ingredients:
For Bread:
- 1 cup all-purpose flour
- ¾ teaspoon baking powder
- ¼ teaspoon baking soda
- 1¼ teaspoons ground cinnamon
- ¼ teaspoon salt
- 1/3 cup vegetable oil
- 1/3 cup sugar
- 1 egg
- 1 teaspoon vanilla extract
- ½ cup zucchini, shredded
- ½ cup apple, cored and shredded
- 5 tablespoons walnuts, chopped
- For Topping:
- 1 tablespoon walnuts, chopped
- 2 teaspoons brown sugar
- ¼ teaspoon ground cinnamon

Directions:
1. For bread: in a bowl, mix together the flour, baking powder, baking soda, cinnamon, and salt.
2. In another large bowl, mix well the oil, sugar, egg, and vanilla extract.
3. Then, add in the flour mixture and mix until just combined.
4. Gently, fold in the zucchini, apple and walnuts.
5. For the topping: in a small bowl, add all the Ingredients and whisk them well.
6. Preheat the Air Fryer to 325 degrees F. Grease and flour an 8 x 4-inch loaf pan.
7. Place the bread mixture evenly into the prepared pan and sprinkle with the topping mixture.
8. Arrange the loaf pan into an Air Fryer basket.
9. Air Fry for about 30 minutes or until a toothpick inserted in the center comes out clean.
10. Remove from Air Fryer and place the pan onto a wire rack for about 10-15 minutes.
11. Carefully, take out the bread from pan and put onto a wire rack until it is completely cool before slicing.
12. Cut the bread into desired size slices and serve.

Nutrition: Calories: 207 Carbohydrate: 24.4g Protein: 3.9g Fat: 13.3g Sugar: 10.9g Sodium: 140mg

56. Pumpkin & Yogurt Bread

Preparation Time: 10 minutes
Cooking Time: 15 minutes
Servings: 4
Ingredients:
- 2 large eggs
- 8 tablespoons pumpkin puree
- 6 tablespoons banana flour
- 4 tablespoons honey
- 4 tablespoons plain Greek yogurt
- 2 tablespoons vanilla essence
- Pinch of ground nutmeg
- 6 tablespoons oats

Directions:
1. Take a bowl, add in all the Ingredients except oats and with a hand mixer, mix until smooth.
2. Add the oats and mix them well using a fork.
3. Set the temperature of Air Fryer to 360 degrees F. Grease and flour a loaf pan.
4. Place the mixture evenly into the prepared pan.
5. Arrange the loaf pan into an Air Fryer basket.
6. Air Fry for about 15 minutes or until a toothpick inserted in the center comes out clean.
7. Remove the pans from Air Fryer and place onto a wire rack for about 5 minutes.
8. Carefully, take out the bread from pan and put onto a wire rack to cool for about 5-10 minutes before slicing.
9. Cut the bread into desired size slices and serve.

Nutrition: Calories: 212 Carbohydrate: 36g Protein: 6.6g Fat: 3.4g Sugar: 20.5g Sodium: 49mg

57. Spiced Pumpkin Bread

Preparation Time: 15 minutes
Cooking Time: 25 minutes
Serving: 4
Ingredients:
- ¼ cup coconut flour
- 2 tablespoons stevia blend
- 1 teaspoon baking powder
- ¾ teaspoon pumpkin pie spice
- ¼ teaspoon ground cinnamon
- 1/8 teaspoon salt
- ¼ cup canned pumpkin
- 2 large eggs
- 2 tablespoons unsweetened almond milk
- 1 teaspoon vanilla extract

Directions:
1. In a bowl, mix together the flour, stevia, baking powder, spices, and salt.
2. In another large bowl, add the pumpkin, eggs, almond milk, and vanilla extract. Beat until well combined.
3. Then, add in the flour mixture and mix until just combined
4. Set the temperature of air fryer to 350 degrees F. Line a cake pan with a greased parchment paper.
5. Place the mixture evenly into the prepared pan.
6. Arrange the pan into an air fryer basket.
7. Air fry for about 25 minutes or until a toothpick inserted in the center comes out clean.
8. Remove the pans from air fryer and place onto a wire rack for about 5 minutes.
9. Carefully, take out the bread from pan and put onto a wire rack to cool for about 5-10 minutes before slicing.
10. Cut the bread into desired size slices and serve.

Nutrition: Calories: 67 Carbohydrate: 9g Protein: 3.5g Fat: 2.8g Sugar: 6.9g Sodium: 118mg

58. Chocolate Peanut Butter Bread

Preparation Time: 15 minutes
Cooking Time: 30 minutes
Servings: 8
Ingredients:
- ¾ cup all-purpose flour
- ¼ cup cocoa powder
- ¼ cup sugar
- ½ teaspoon baking soda
- ½ teaspoon baking powder
- 1/8 teaspoon salt
- 1 egg
- 1/3 cup unsweetened applesauce
- ¼ cup plain Greek yogurt

- ½ teaspoon vanilla extract
- 1/3 cup creamy peanut butter
- 1/3 cup mini chocolate chips

Directions:
1. In a bowl, mix together the flour, cocoa powder, sugar, baking soda, baking powder, and salt.
2. In another bowl, add the egg, applesauce, yogurt, and vanilla extract. Beat until well combined.
3. Then, add in the flour mixture and mix until just combined.
4. Add the peanut butter and mix until smooth.
5. Gently, fold in the chocolate chips.
6. Set the temperature of Air Fryer to 350 degrees F. Grease a loaf pan.
7. Place the mixture evenly into the prepared pan.
8. Arrange the loaf pan into an Air Fryer basket.
9. Air Fry for about 30 minutes or until a toothpick inserted in the center comes out clean.
10. Remove from Air Fryer and place the pan onto a wire rack for about 10-15 minutes.
11. Carefully, take out the bread from pan and put onto a wire rack until it is completely cool before slicing.
12. Cut the bread into desired size slices and serve.

Nutrition: Calories: 191 Carbohydrate: 24.9g Protein: 6.1g Fat: 8.6g Sugar: 12.6g Sodium: 183mg

59. Simple Cornbread

Preparation Time: 15 minutes
Cooking Time: 25 minutes
Servings: 8

Ingredients:
- 1 cup cornmeal
- ¾ cup all-purpose flour
- 1 tablespoon sugar
- 1½ teaspoons baking powder
- ½ teaspoon baking soda
- ¼ teaspoon salt
- 1½ cups buttermilk
- 6 tablespoons unsalted butter, melted
- 2 large eggs, lightly beaten

Directions:
1. In a bowl, mix together the cornmeal, flour, sugar, baking soda, baking powder, and salt.
2. Take a separate bowl, mix well the buttermilk, butter, and eggs.
3. Then, add in the flour mixture and mix until just combined.
4. Set the temperature of Air Fryer to 360 degrees F. Lightly, grease an 8-inch baking dish.
5. Transfer the flour mixture evenly into the prepared baking dish.
6. Place the dish into an Air Fryer basket.
7. Air Fry for about 25 minutes or until a toothpick inserted in the center comes out clean, turning the dish once halfway through.
8. Remove from Air Fryer and place the dish onto a wire rack for about 10-15 minutes.
9. Carefully, take out the bread from dish and put onto a wire rack until it is completely cool before slicing.
10. Cut the bread into desired size slices and serve.

Nutrition: Calories: 217 Carbohydrate: 24.9g Protein: 5.6g Fat: 10.9g Sugar: 3.9g Sodium: 286mg

60. Pineapple Cornbread

Preparation Time: 10 minutes
Cooking Time: 15 minutes
Servings: 5

Ingredients:
- 1 (8½-ounces) package Jiffy corn muffin
- 7 ounces canned crushed pineapple
- 1/3 cup canned pineapple juice
- 1 egg

Directions:
1. In a bowl, mix together all the Ingredients.
2. Set the temperature of Air Fryer to 330 degrees F. Grease a round cake pan. (6"x 3")
3. Place the mixture evenly into the prepared pan.
4. Arrange the cake pan into an Air Fryer basket.
5. Air Fry for about 15 minutes or until a toothpick inserted in the center comes out clean.
6. Remove from Air Fryer and place the pan onto a wire rack for about 10-15 minutes.
7. Carefully, take out the bread from pan and put onto a wire rack until it is completely cool before slicing.
8. Cut the bread into desired size slices and serve.

Nutrition: Calories: 220 Carbohydrate: 40g Protein: 3.8g Fat: 6.4g Sugar: 14.1g Sodium: 423mg

61. Banana Oats

Preparation time: 5 minutes
Cooking time: 20 minutes
Servings: 4

Ingredients:
- 2 cups old fashioned oats
- 1/3 cup sugar
- 1 teaspoon vanilla extract
- 1 cup banana, peeled and mashed
- 2 cups almond milk
- 2 eggs, whisked
- Cooking spray

Directions:
1. In a bowl, combine the oats with the sugar and the other Ingredients except the cooking spray and whisk well.
2. Heat up your air fryer at 340 degrees F, grease with cooking spray, add oats mix, toss, cover and cook for 20 minutes.
3. Divide into bowls and serve for breakfast.

Nutrition: Calories 260 Fat 4 Fiber 7 Carbs 9 Protein 10

62. Cheesy Bread And Eggs Bowls

Preparation time: 10 minutes
Cooking time: 30 minutes
Servings: 4

Ingredients:
- 1 cup whole wheat bread, cubed
- 1 cup mozzarella, shredded
- 2 tablespoons olive oil
- 1 red onion, chopped
- 1 cup tomato sauce
- Salt and black pepper to the taste
- 8 eggs, whisked

Directions:
1. Add the oil to your air fryer, heat it up at 340 degrees F, add onion, bread and the other Ingredients, toss, cook for 20 minutes shaking halfway.
2. Divide between plates and serve for breakfast.

Nutrition: Calories 211 Fat 8 Fiber 7 Carbs 14 Protein 3

63. Creamy Carrots Hash Mix

Preparation time: 10 minutes
Cooking time: 20 minutes
Servings: 4

Ingredients:
- 1-pound carrots, peeled and cubed
- 4 eggs, whisked
- 1 cup coconut cream
- 1 tablespoon olive oil
- 1 red onion, chopped
- 1 cup mozzarella, shredded
- 1 tablespoon chives, chopped
- Salt and black pepper to the taste

Directions:
1. Heat up your air fryer with the oil at 350 degrees F, add the carrots hash and the other Ingredients, toss, cover, cook for 20 minutes, divide between plates and serve.

Nutrition: Calories 231 Fat 9 Fiber 9 Carbs 8 Protein 12

64. Tomato Frittata

Preparation time: 10 minutes
Cooking time: 20 minutes
Servings: 4

Ingredients:
- 1 cup cherry tomatoes, halved
- 8 eggs, whisked
- 1 red onion, chopped
- 1 tablespoon olive oil
- 1 tablespoon chives, chopped
- ½ cup mozzarella, shredded
- Salt and black pepper to the taste

Directions:
1. In a bowl, combine the eggs with the tomatoes and the other Ingredients except the oil and whisk well.
2. Heat up your air fryer at 300 degrees F, add the oil, heat it up, add the frittata mix, spread, and cook for 20 minutes.
3. Divide between plates and serve.

Nutrition: Calories 262 Fat 6 Fiber 9 Carbs 18 Protein 8

65. Strawberry Oatmeal

Preparation time: 4 minutes
Cooking time: 15 minutes
Servings: 4

Ingredients:
- 1 cup old fashioned oats
- ½ cup strawberries, chopped
- 2 cups almond milk
- 2 eggs, whisked
- ¼ teaspoon vanilla extract

Directions:
1. In a bowl, combine the oats with the milk and the other Ingredients and whisk well.
2. Heat up your air fryer at 350 degrees F, add berries mix, and cook for 15 minutes.
3. Divide into bowls and serve for breakfast.

Nutrition: Calories 180 Fat 5 Fiber 7 Carbs 12 Protein 5

66. Peppers and Tomato Eggs

Preparation time: 10 minutes
Cooking time: 20 minutes
Servings: 4

Ingredients:
- 8 eggs, whisked
- 1 cup roasted peppers, chopped
- 1 cup tomatoes, chopped
- Cooking spray
- 1 tablespoon chives, chopped
- ½ teaspoon sweet paprika
- Salt and black pepper to the taste

Directions:
1. In a bowl, combine the eggs with the peppers, tomatoes and the other Ingredients except the cooking spray and whisk well.
2. Heat up your air fryer at 320 degrees F, grease with the cooking spray, add the eggs mix, cover and cook for 20 minutes.
3. Divide between plates and serve for breakfast right away.

Nutrition: Calories 190 Fat 7 Fiber 7 Carbs 12 Protein 4

67. Mushroom Oatmeal

Preparation time: 5 minutes
Cooking time: 20 minutes
Servings: 4

Ingredients:
- 1 tablespoon avocado oil
- 1 cup white mushrooms, sliced
- 8 eggs, whisked
- 1 cup old fashioned oats
- 1 red onion, chopped
- ½ cup heavy cream
- Salt and black pepper to the taste
- 1 tablespoon dill, chopped

Directions:
1. In a bowl, mix the eggs with the oats, cream and the other Ingredients except the oil and the mushrooms and whisk.
2. Heat up the air fryer with the oil at 330 degrees F, add the mushrooms and cook them for 5 minutes.
3. Add the rest of the Ingredients, toss, and cook for 15 minutes more.
4. Divide into bowls and serve for breakfast.

Nutrition: Calories: 192 Fat: 6 Fiber: 6 Carbs: 14 Protein: 7

68. Cauliflower Hash

Preparation time: 10 minutes
Cooking time: 20 minutes
Servings: 4

Ingredients:
- 1-pound cauliflower florets
- 8 eggs, whisked
- 1 onion, chopped
- A drizzle of olive oil
- ½ teaspoon sweet paprika
- ½ teaspoon coriander, ground
- 1 cup mozzarella, shredded
- Salt and black pepper to the taste

Directions:
1. Heat up the air fryer at 350 degrees F with a drizzle of oil, add the cauliflower, eggs and the other Ingredients, whisk and cook for 20 minutes.
2. Divide the hash between plates and serve for breakfast.

Nutrition: Calories 194 Fat 4 Fiber 7 Carbs 11 Protein 6

69. Pesto Scramble

Preparation time: 3 minutes
Cooking time: 15 minutes
Servings: 4

Ingredients:
- 1 tablespoon butter, melted
- 8 eggs, whisked
- 1 tablespoon basil pesto
- ½ teaspoon sweet paprika
- 1 red onion, chopped
- Salt and black pepper to the taste
- 1 cup mozzarella cheese, grated

Directions:

BREAKFAST RECIPES

1. Heat up the air fryer at 350 degrees F with the butter, add the onion, eggs and the other Ingredients, whisk and cook for 15 minutes shaking the fryer halfway.
2. Divide the scramble between plates and serve.

Nutrition: Calories 187 Fat 6 Fiber 6 Carbs 13 Protein 5

70. Eggplant And Sausage Hash

Preparation time: 5 minutes
Cooking time: 20 minutes
Servings: 4

Ingredients:
- 1 eggplant, cubed
- 1 cup sausages, cubed
- ½ pound hash browns
- 2 eggs, whisked
- ½ teaspoon turmeric powder
- 1 tablespoon cilantro, chopped
- 1 tablespoon olive oil
- ½ cup mozzarella, shredded
- Salt and black pepper to the taste

Directions:
1. Heat up the air fryer with the oil at 360 degrees F, add the sausages and cook them for 5 minutes.
2. Add the hash browns, eggplant and the other Ingredients, cover and cook for 15 minutes more.
3. Divide everything between plates and serve.

Nutrition: Calories 270 Fat 14 Fiber 3 Carbs 23 Protein 16

71. Salmon Eggs

Preparation time: 10 minutes
Cooking time: 15 minutes
Servings: 4

Ingredients:
- 1 cup smoked salmon fillets, boneless and cubed
- 8 eggs, whisked
- 1 red onion, chopped
- Cooking spray
- ½ teaspoon sweet paprika
- ½ teaspoon turmeric powder
- ½ cup heavy cream
- 1 tablespoon chives, chopped
- Salt and black pepper to the taste

Directions:
1. Set the air fryer at 380 degrees F and grease it with the cooking spray.
2. In a bowl, mix the eggs with the salmon and the other Ingredients, whisk, pour into the fryer, cover and cook for 15 minutes.
3. Divide between plates and serve for breakfast.

Nutrition: Calories 170 Fat 2 Fiber 2 Carbs 12 Protein 4

72. Vanilla and Mango Bowls

Preparation Time: 5 minutes
Cooking Time: 10 minutes
Servings: 4

Ingredients:
- 1 cup mango, peeled and cubed
- 1 cup heavy cream
- 2 tablespoons sugar
- Juice of 1 lime
- 2 teaspoons vanilla extract

Directions:
1. In the air fryer's pan, combine the mango with the cream and the other Ingredients, cook at 370 degrees F for 10 minutes, divide into bowls and serve for breakfast.

Nutrition: Calories 170 Fat 6 Fiber 5 Carbs 11 Protein 2

73. Chili Bowls

Preparation Time: 5 minutes
Cooking Time: 20 minutes
Servings: 4

Ingredients:
- 1-pound beef stew meat, ground
- 1 red onion, chopped
- 1 teaspoon chili powder
- 8 eggs, whisked
- A drizzle of olive oil
- ½ cup canned tomatoes, crushed
- 1 red chili pepper, chopped
- 2 tablespoons parsley, chopped
- Salt and white pepper to the taste

Directions:
1. Heat up the air fryer at 400 degrees F, grease with the oil, add the meat and the onion and cook for 5 minutes.
2. Add the eggs and the other Ingredients, cover, cook for 15 minutes more, divide into bowls and serve for breakfast.

Nutrition: Calories 200 Fat 6 Fiber 1 Carbs 11 Protein 3

74. Mushroom, Potato and Beef Bowls

Preparation Time: 5 minutes
Cooking Time: 20 minutes
Servings: 4

Ingredients:
- 1-pound beef stew meat, ground
- 1 tablespoon olive oil
- ½ cup mushrooms, sliced
- 1 cup gold potatoes, cubed
- 1 red onion, chopped
- 1 garlic clove, minced
- ½ cup cherry tomatoes, halved
- 4 eggs, whisked
- Salt and black pepper to the taste

Directions:
1. Heat up the air fryer with the oil at 400 degrees F, add the meat, mushrooms and onion and cook for 5 minutes.
2. Add the potatoes and the other Ingredients, cook for 15 minutes more, divide between plates and serve for breakfast.

Nutrition: Calories 160 Fat 2 Fiber 5 Carbs 12 Protein 9

75. Carrot Muffins

Preparation Time: 5 minutes
Cooking Time: 20 minutes
Servings: 4

Ingredients:
- 3 eggs, whisked
- 1 tablespoon butter, melted
- 1 cup carrots, peeled and grated
- 1 cup heavy cream
- ½ cup almond flour
- 1 cup almond milk
- Cooking spray
- 1 tablespoon baking powder

Directions:
1. In a bowl, combine the eggs with the butter, carrots and the other Ingredients except the cooking spray, and whisk well.

2. Grease a muffin pan that fits your air fryer with the cooking spray, divide the carrots mix inside, put the pan in the air fryer and cook at 392 degrees F for 20 minutes.
3. Serve the muffins for breakfast.

Nutrition: Calories 190 Fat 12 Fiber 2 Carbs 11 Protein 5

76. Breakfast Peppers Frittata

Preparation Time: 10 minutes
Cooking Time: 10 minutes
Servings: 2

Ingredients:
- 2 large eggs
- 1 tbsp bell peppers, chopped
- 1 tbsp spring onions, chopped
- 1 sausage patty, chopped
- 1 tbsp butter, melted
- 2 tbsp cheddar cheese
- Pepper
- Salt

Directions:
1. Add sausage patty in air fryer baking dish and cook in air fryer 350 F for 5 minutes.
2. Meanwhile, in a bowl whisk together eggs, pepper, and salt.
3. Add bell peppers, onions and stir well.
4. Pour egg mixture over sausage patty and stir well.
5. Sprinkle with cheese and cook in the air fryer at 350 F for 5 minutes.
6. Serve and enjoy.

Nutrition: Calories 205 Fat 14.7g Cholesterol 5g Sugar 4g Protein 12g Cholesterol 221 mg

77. Scrambled Eggs

Preparation Time: 10 minutes
Cooking Time: 6 minutes
Servings: 2

Ingredients:
- 4 eggs
- 1/4 tsp garlic powder
- 1/4 tsp onion powder
- 1 tbsp parmesan cheese
- Pepper
- Salt

Directions:
1. Whisk eggs with garlic powder, onion powder, parmesan cheese, pepper, and salt.
2. Pour egg mixture into the air fryer baking dish.
3. Place dish in the air fryer and cook at 360 F for 2 minutes. Stir quickly and cook for 3-4 minutes more.
4. Stir well and serve.

Nutrition: Calories 149 Fat 9.1g Cholesterol 4.5g Sugar 1.1g Protein 11g Cholesterol 325 mg

78. Sausage Egg Cups

Preparation Time: 10 minutes
Cooking Time: 10 minutes
Servings: 2

Ingredients:
- 1/4 cup eggbeaters
- 1/4 sausage, cooked and crumbled
- 4 tsp jack cheese, shredded
- 1/4 tsp garlic powder
- 1/4 tsp onion powder
- 4 tbsp spinach, chopped
- Pepper
- Salt

Directions:
1. In a bowl, whisk together all Ingredients until well combined.
2. Pour batter into the silicone muffin molds and place in the air fryer basket.
3. Cook at 330 F for 10 minutes.
4. Serve and enjoy.

Nutrition: Calories 90 Fat 5g Cholesterol 1g Sugar 0.2g Protein 7g Cholesterol 14 mg

79. Cheese Stuff Peppers

Preparation Time: 5 minutes
Cooking Time: 8 minutes
Servings: 8

Ingredients:
- 8 small bell pepper, cut the top of peppers
- 3.5 oz. feta cheese, cubed
- 1 tbsp. olive oil
- 1 tsp Italian seasoning
- 1 tbsp. parsley, chopped
- ¼ tsp garlic powder
- Pepper
- Salt

Directions:
1. In a bowl, toss cheese with oil and seasoning.
2. Stuff cheese in each bell peppers and place into the air fryer basket.
3. Cook at 400 F for 8 minutes.
4. Serve and enjoy.

Nutrition: Calories 88 Fat 5g Cholesterol 9g Sugar 6g Protein 3g Cholesterol 10 mg

80. Roasted Pepper Salad

Preparation Time: 10 minutes
Cooking Time: 10 minutes
Servings: 4

Ingredients:
- 4 bell peppers
- 2 oz. rocket leaves
- 2 tbsp. olive oil
- 4 tbsp. heavy cream
- 1 lettuce head, torn
- 1 tbsp. fresh lime juice
- Pepper
- Salt

Directions:
1. Add bell peppers into the air fryer basket and cook for 10 minutes at 400 F.
2. Remove peppers from air fryer and let it cool for 5 minutes.
3. Peel cooked peppers and cut into strips and place into the large bowl.
4. Add remaining Ingredients into the bowl and toss well.
5. Serve and enjoy.

Nutrition: Calories 160 Fat 13g Cholesterol 11g Sugar 6g Protein 2g Cholesterol 20 mg

81. Crust-Less Quiche

Preparation Time: 5 minutes
Cooking Time: 30 minutes
Servings: 2

Ingredients:
- 4 eggs
- ¼ cup onion, chopped
- ½ cup tomatoes, chopped
- ½ cup milk

BREAKFAST RECIPES

- 1 cup gouda cheese, shredded
- Salt, to taste

Directions:
1. Preheat the Air fryer to 340 o F and grease 2 ramekins lightly.
2. Mix together all the ingredients in a ramekin until well combined.
3. Place in the Air fryer and cook for about 30 minutes.
4. Dish out and serve.

Nutrition: Calories: 312 Fat: 15g Saturated Fat: 4g Trans Fat: 0g Cholesterol: 14g Fiber: 2g Sodium: 403mg Protein: 25g

82. Milky Scrambled Eggs

Preparation Time: 10 minutes
Cooking Time: 9 minutes
Servings: 2

Ingredients:
- ¾ cup milk
- 4 eggs
- 8 grape tomatoes, halved
- ½ cup Parmesan cheese, grated
- 1 tablespoon butter
- Salt and black pepper, to taste

Directions:
1. Preheat the Air fryer to 360 o F and grease an Air fryer pan with butter.
2. Whisk together eggs with milk, salt and black pepper in a bowl.
3. Transfer the egg mixture into the prepared pan and place in the Air fryer.
4. Cook for about 6 minutes and stir in the grape tomatoes and cheese.
5. Cook for about 3 minutes and serve warm.

Nutrition: Calories: 312 Fat: 15g Saturated Fat: 4g Trans Fat: 0g Cholesterol: 14g Fiber: 2g Sodium: 403mg Protein: 25g

83. Toasties and Sausage In Egg Pond

Preparation Time: 10 minutes
Cooking Time: 22 minutes
Servings: 2

Ingredients:
- 3 eggs
- 2 cooked sausages, sliced
- 1 bread slice, cut into sticks
- 1/8 cup mozzarella cheese, grated
- 1/8 cup Parmesan cheese, grated
- ¼ cup cream

Directions:
1. Preheat the Air fryer to 365 o F and grease 2 ramekins lightly.
2. Whisk together eggs with cream in a bowl and place in the ramekins.
3. Stir in the bread and sausage slices in the egg mixture and top with cheese.
4. Transfer the ramekins in the Air fryer basket and cook for about 22 minutes.
5. Dish out and serve warm.

Nutrition: Calories: 261 Fat: 15g Saturated Fat: 4g Trans Fat: 0g Cholesterol: 14g Fiber: 2g Sodium: 403mg Protein: 25g

84. Flavorful Bacon Cups

Preparation Time: 10 minutes
Cooking Time: 15 minutes
Servings: 6

Ingredients:
- 6 bacon slices
- 6 bread slices
- 1 scallion, chopped
- 3 tablespoons green bell pepper, seeded and chopped
- 6 eggs
- 2 tablespoons low-fat mayonnaise

Directions:
1. Preheat the Air fryer to 375 o F and grease 6 cups muffin tin with cooking spray.
2. Place each bacon slice in a prepared muffin cup.
3. Cut the bread slices with round cookie cutter and place over the bacon slices.
4. Top with bell pepper, scallion and mayonnaise evenly and crack 1 egg in each muffin cup.
5. Place in the Air fryer and cook for about 15 minutes.
6. Dish out and serve warm.

Nutrition: Calories: 260 Fat: 15g Saturated Fat: 4g Trans Fat: 0g Cholesterol: 14g Fiber: 2g Sodium: 403mg Protein: 25g

85. Crispy Potato Rosti

Preparation Time: 10 minutes
Cooking Time: 15 minutes
Servings: 2

Ingredients:
- ½ pound russet potatoes, peeled and grated roughly
- 1 tablespoon chives, chopped finely
- 2 tablespoons shallots, minced
- 1/8 cup cheddar cheese
- 3.5 ounces smoked salmon, cut into slices
- 2 tablespoons sour cream
- 1 tablespoon olive oil
- Salt and black pepper, to taste

Directions:
1. Preheat the Air fryer to 365 o F and grease a pizza pan with the olive oil.
2. Mix together potatoes, shallots, chives, cheese, salt and black pepper in a large bowl until well combined.
3. Transfer the potato mixture into the prepared pizza pan and place in the Air fryer basket.
4. Cook for about 15 minutes and dish out in a platter.
5. Cut the potato rosti into wedges and top with smoked salmon slices and sour cream to serve.

Nutrition: Calories: 327 Fat: 15g Saturated Fat: 4g Trans Fat: 0g Cholesterol: 14g Fiber: 2g Sodium: 403mg Protein: 25g

86. Stylish Ham Omelet

Preparation Time: 10 minutes
Cooking Time: 30 minutes
Servings: 2

Ingredients:
- 4 small tomatoes, chopped
- 4 eggs
- 2 ham slices
- 1 onion, chopped
- 2 tablespoons cheddar cheese
- Salt and black pepper, to taste

Directions:
1. Preheat the Air fryer to 390 o F and grease an Air fryer pan.
2. Place the tomatoes in the Air fryer pan and cook for about 10 minutes.
3. Heat a nonstick skillet on medium heat and add onion and ham.
4. Stir fry for about 5 minutes and transfer into the Air fryer pan.

5. Whisk together eggs, salt and black pepper in a bowl and pour in the Air fryer pan.
6. Set the Air fryer to 335 °F and cook for about 15 minutes.
7. Dish out and serve warm.

Nutrition: Calories: 255 Fat: 15g Saturated Fat: 4g Trans Fat: 0g Cholesterol: 14g Fiber: 2g Sodium: 403mg Protein: 25g

87. Healthy Tofu Omelet

Preparation Time: 10 minutes
Cooking Time: 29 minutes
Servings: 2
Ingredients:
- ¼ of onion, chopped
- 12-ounce silken tofu, pressed and sliced
- 3 eggs, beaten
- 1 tablespoon chives, chopped
- 1 garlic clove, minced
- 2 teaspoons olive oil
- Salt and black pepper, to taste

Directions:
1. Preheat the Air fryer to 355 °F and grease an Air fryer pan with olive oil.
2. Add onion and garlic to the greased pan and cook for about 4 minutes.
3. Add tofu, mushrooms, chives, and season with salt and black pepper.
4. Beat the eggs and pour over the tofu mixture.
5. Cook for about 25 minutes, poking the eggs twice in between.
6. Dish out and serve warm.

Nutrition: Calories: 248 Fat: 29g Saturated Fat: 3g Trans Fat: 0g Cholesterol: 31g Fiber: 4g Sodium: 374mg Protein: 47g

88. Yummy Savory French Toasts

Preparation Time: 10 minutes
Cooking Time: 4 minutes
Servings: 2
Ingredients:
- ¼ cup chickpea flour
- 3 tablespoons onion, chopped finely
- 2 teaspoons green chili, seeded and chopped finely
- Water, as required
- 4 bread slices
- ½ teaspoon red chili powder
- ¼ teaspoon ground turmeric
- ¼ teaspoon ground cumin
- Salt, to taste

Directions:
1. Preheat the Air fryer to 375 °F and line an Air fryer pan with a foil paper.
2. Mix together all the ingredients in a large bowl except the bread slices.
3. Spread the mixture over both sides of the bread slices and transfer into the Air fryer pan.
4. Cook for about 4 minutes and remove from the Air fryer to serve.

Nutrition: Calories: 339 Fat: 12g Saturated Fat: 2g Trans Fat: 0g Cholesterol: 16g Fiber: 3.5g Sodium: 362mg Protein: 19g

89. Flaky Maple Donuts

Preparation Time: 10 minutes
Cooking Time: 15 minutes plus 1 hour to cool
Servings: 15
Ingredients:
- 1 frozen puff pastry sheet (15 by 10 inches), thawed
- 2 teaspoons all-purpose flour
- 2½ cups powdered sugar
- 3 tablespoons pure maple syrup
- 2 tablespoons 2% milk
- 2 tablespoons butter, melted
- ½ teaspoon vanilla extract
- ½ teaspoon ground cinnamon
- Pinch salt

Directions:
1. Put the puff pastry on a work surface dusted with the flour. Cut into 15 squares by cutting crosswise into five 3-inch-wide strips and then cutting each strip into thirds.
2. Set or preheat the air fryer to 325°F. Put a parchment paper round in the bottom of the basket and add as many pastry squares as will fit without touching or overlapping.
3. Bake for 14 to 19 minutes or until the donuts are browned and not doughy inside. Cool on a wire rack. Repeat with the remaining dough.
4. In a small bowl, combine the powdered sugar, maple syrup, milk, melted butter, vanilla, cinnamon, and salt and mix with a wire whisk until combined.
5. Let the donuts cool for about 1 hour, and then dip the top half of each in the glaze. Turn the donut over, glaze-side up, and put on wire racks. Let stand until set, then serve.

Nutrition: Calories: 109 Total fat: 3g Saturated fat: 1g Cholesterol: 4mg Sodium: 32mg Carbohydrates: 21g Fiber: 0g Protein: 0g

90. Coffee cake Muffins

Preparation Time: 20 minutes
Cooking Time: 15 minutes
Servings: 6
Ingredients:
- 1⅓ cups all-purpose flour, divided
- 5 tablespoons butter, melted, divided
- ¼ cup packed light brown sugar
- ½ teaspoon ground cinnamon
- ⅓ cup granulated sugar
- ¼ cup 2% milk
- 1 large egg
- 1 teaspoon vanilla extract
- 1 teaspoon baking powder
- Pinch salt
- Nonstick baking spray (containing flour)

Directions:
1. In a small bowl, combine ⅓ cup of flour, 2½ tablespoons of butter, the brown sugar, and cinnamon and mix until crumbly. Set the streusel topping aside.
2. In a medium bowl, combine the remaining 2½ tablespoons of butter, the granulated sugar, milk, egg, and vanilla and mix well.
3. Add the remaining 1 cup flour, baking powder, and salt and mix just until combined.
4. Spray 6 silicone muffin cups with baking spray.
5. Spoon half of the batter into the prepared muffin cups. Top each with about 1 teaspoon of the streusel, then add the remaining batter. Sprinkle each muffin with the remaining streusel and gently press into the batter.
6. Set or preheat the air fryer to 330°F. Place the muffin cups in the air fryer basket. Bake the muffins for 14 to 18 minutes or until a toothpick inserted into the center of a muffin comes out clean. Cool on a wire rack for 10 minutes, then remove the muffins from the silicone cups. Serve warm or cold.

Nutrition: Calories: 285 Total fat: 11g Saturated fat: 7g Cholesterol: 57mg Sodium: 122mg Carbohydrates: 42g Fiber: 1g Protein: 4g

91. Baked Oatmeal Apple Cups

Preparation Time: 15 minutes
Cooking Time: 15 minutes
Servings: 6
Ingredients:
- ½ cup unsweetened applesauce
- 1 large egg
- ⅓ cup packed light brown sugar
- 2 tablespoons butter, melted
- ½ cup 2% milk
- 1⅓ cups old-fashioned rolled oats
- 1 teaspoon ground cinnamon
- ½ teaspoon baking powder
- Pinch salt
- ½ cup diced peeled apple
- Nonstick baking spray (containing flour)

Directions:
1. In a medium bowl, combine the applesauce, egg, brown sugar, melted butter, and milk and mix until combined.
2. Add the oats, cinnamon, baking powder, and salt and stir until mixed. Stir in the apple.
3. Spray 6 silicone muffin cups with baking spray. Divide the batter among the muffin cups.
4. Set or preheat the air fryer to 350°F. Place the muffin cups in the air fryer basket. Bake the cups for 13 to 18 minutes or until they are set to the touch. Let cool for 15 minutes before serving.

Nutrition: Calories: 254 Total fat: 8g Saturated fat: 3g Cholesterol: 43mg Sodium: 82mg Carbohydrates: 40g Fiber: 4g Protein: 8g

92. Bacon-Roasted Fruit with Yogurt

Preparation Time: 15 minutes
Cooking Time: 20 minutes
Servings: 4
Ingredients:
- 3 bacon slices
- 1 Granny Smith apple, peeled and cubed
- 1 Bosc pear, peeled and cubed
- 1 cup canned cubed pineapple
- 2 tablespoons sugar
- ½ teaspoon ground cinnamon
- 2 cups plain Greek yogurt

Directions:
1. Put a rack inside a 7-inch cake pan. Cut the bacon slices in half crosswise and put them on the rack.
2. Set or preheat the air fryer to 350°F. Place the cake pan in the air fryer basket. Cook the bacon for 7 minutes, then check for doneness. Cook for another 2 to 3 minutes, if necessary, until crisp.
3. Remove the bacon from the rack and place on paper towels to drain. Remove the rack and scoop all but 2 teaspoons of bacon fat out of the pan.
4. Set or preheat the air fryer to 380°F. Add the apple, pear, and pineapple to the fat in the pan. Sprinkle with the sugar and cinnamon and toss.
5. Roast the fruit for 10 to 15 minutes, stirring the mixture every 5 minutes, until the fruit is tender and browned around the edges.
6. Crumble the bacon and add it to the fruit; serve over the yogurt.

Nutrition: Calories: 211 Total fat: 7g Saturated fat: 4g Cholesterol: 24mg Sodium: 203mg Carbohydrates: 30g Fiber: 3g Protein: 8g

93. Scrambled Eggs with Cheese

Preparation Time: 5 minutes
Cooking Time: 14 minutes
Servings: 4
Ingredients:
- 8 large eggs
- ¼ cup sour cream
- ¼ cup whole milk
- ¼ teaspoon salt
- Pinch freshly ground black pepper
- 3 tablespoons butter, divided
- 1 cup shredded Cheddar cheese
- 1 tablespoon minced fresh chives

Directions:
1. In a medium bowl, beat the eggs with the sour cream, milk, salt, and pepper until foamy.
2. Put 2 tablespoons of butter in a cake barrel, put it in the air fryer, and set or preheat to 350°F. The butter will melt while the air fryer preheats.
3. Remove the barrel from the air fryer basket. Add the egg mixture to the cake barrel and return to the air fryer.
4. Cook for 4 minutes, then stir the eggs with a heatproof spatula.
5. Cook for 3 minutes more minutes, then stir again.
6. Cook for 3 minutes more minutes, then add the remaining 1 tablespoon of butter and the Cheddar and stir gently.
7. Cook for 2 to 4 more minutes or until the eggs are just set.
8. Remove the cake barrel from the air fryer and put the eggs in a serving bowl. Sprinkle with the chives and serve.

Nutrition: Calories: 371; Total fat: 31g; Saturated fat: 16g; Cholesterol: 433mg; Sodium: 551mg; Carbohydrates: 2g; Fiber: 0g; Protein: 20g

94. Soda Bread Currant Muffins

Preparation Time: 15 minutes
Cooking Time: 15 minutes
Servings: 6
Ingredients:
- 1 cup all-purpose flour
- 2 tablespoons whole wheat flour
- 1 teaspoon baking powder
- ⅛ teaspoon baking soda
- Pinch salt
- 3 tablespoons light brown sugar
- ½ cup dried currants
- 1 large egg
- ⅓ cup buttermilk
- 3 tablespoons butter, melted
- Nonstick baking spray (containing flour)

Directions:
1. In a medium bowl, combine the flours, baking powder, baking soda, salt, and brown sugar and mix until combined. Stir in the currants.
2. In a small bowl, combine the egg, buttermilk, and melted butter and stir until blended.
3. Add the egg mixture to the flour mixture and stir just until combined.
4. Spray 6 silicone muffin cups with baking spray. Divide the batter among the muffin cups, filling each about two-thirds full.

5. Set or preheat the air fryer 350°F. Set the muffin cups in the air fryer basket. Bake the muffins for 14 to 18 minutes or until a toothpick inserted in the center comes out clean.
6. Cool on a wire rack for 10 minutes before serving.

Nutrition: Calories: 204 Total fat: 7g Saturated fat: 4g Cholesterol: 47mg Sodium: 140mg Carbohydrates: 32g Fiber: 2g Protein: 5g

95. Raspberry-Stuffed French toast

Preparation Time: 15 minutes
Cooking Time: 8 minutes
Servings: 4
Ingredients:
- 4 (1-inch-thick) slices French bread
- 2 tablespoons raspberry jam
- ⅓ cup fresh raspberries
- 2 egg yolks
- ⅓ cup 2% milk
- 1 tablespoon sugar
- ½ teaspoon vanilla extract
- 3 tablespoons sour cream

Directions:
1. Cut a pocket into the side of each bread slice, making sure you don't cut through to the other side.
2. In a small bowl, combine the raspberry jam and raspberries and crush the raspberries into the jam with a fork.
3. In a shallow bowl, beat the egg yolks with the milk, sugar, and vanilla until combined.
4. Spread some of the sour cream in the pocket you cut in the bread slices, then add the raspberry mixture. Squeeze the edges of the bread slightly to close the opening.
5. Dip the bread in the egg mixture, letting the bread stand in the egg for 3 minutes. Flip the bread over and let stand on the other side for 3 minutes.
6. Set or preheat the air fryer to 375°F. Arrange the stuffed bread in the air fryer basket in a single layer.
7. Air fry for 5 minutes, then carefully flip the bread slices and cook for another 3 to 6 minutes, until the French toast is golden brown.

Nutrition: Calories: 278 Total fat: 6g Saturated fat: 3g Cholesterol: 99mg Sodium: 406mg Carbohydrates: 46g Fiber: 2g Protein: 9g

96. Apple Roll-Ups

Preparation Time: 20 minutes
Cooking Time: 20 minutes
Servings: 8
Ingredients:
- 3 tablespoons ground cinnamon
- 3 tablespoons granulated sugar
- 2 teaspoons ground nutmeg
- 1 teaspoon ground cardamom
- ½ teaspoon ground allspice
- 2 large Granny Smith apples, peeled and cored
- 10 tablespoons butter, melted, divided
- 2 tablespoons light brown sugar
- 8 thin slices white sandwich bread, crusts cut off.

Directions:
1. In a 7-inch springform pan that has been wrapped in foil to prevent leaks, combine the olive oil, cherry tomatoes, plum tomatoes, tomato sauce, scallions, garlic, honey, salt, and cayenne.
2. Set or preheat the air fryer to 375°F. Set the pan in the air fryer basket. Cook the tomato mixture for 15 to 20 minutes, stirring twice during the cooking time, until the tomatoes are soft.
3. Use a fork to mash some of the tomatoes right in the pan, then stir the mashed tomatoes into the sauce.
4. Break the eggs into the sauce. Return the pan to the air fryer.
5. Cook for about 2 minutes or until the egg whites start to set. Remove the pan from the air fryer and gently stir the eggs into the sauce, marbling them through the sauce. Don't mix them in completely.
6. Continue cooking the mixture until the eggs are just set, 4 to 8 minutes more.
7. Cool for 10 minutes, then serve.

Nutrition: Calories: 232 Total fat: 15g Saturated fat: 9g Cholesterol: 38mg Sodium: 249mg Carbohydrates: 21g Fiber: 4g Protein: 4g

97. Pepper Egg Bites

Preparation Time: 15 minutes
Cooking Time: 15 minutes
Servings: 7
Ingredients:
- 5 large eggs, beaten
- 3 tablespoons 2% milk
- ½ teaspoon dried marjoram
- ⅛ teaspoon salt
- Pinch freshly ground black pepper
- ⅓ cup minced bell pepper, any color
- 3 tablespoons minced scallions
- ½ cup shredded Colby or Muenster cheese

Directions:
1. In a medium bowl, combine the eggs, milk, marjoram, salt, and black pepper; mix until combined.
2. Stir in the bell peppers, scallions, and cheese. Fill the 7 egg bite cups with the egg mixture, making sure you get some of the solids in each cup. Set or preheat the air fryer to 325°F.
3. Make a foil sling: Fold an 18-inch-long piece of heavy-duty aluminum foil lengthwise into thirds. Put the egg bite pan on this sling and lower it into the air fryer.
4. Leave the foil in the air fryer, but bend down the edges so they fit in the appliance.
5. Bake the egg bites for 10 to 15 minutes or until a toothpick inserted into the center comes out clean.
6. Use the foil sling to remove the egg bite pan. Let cool for 5 minutes, then invert the pan onto a plate to remove the egg bites. Serve warm.

Nutrition: Calories: 87 Total fat: 6g Saturated fat: 3g Cholesterol: 141mg Sodium: 149mg Carbohydrates: 1g Fiber: 0g Protein: 7g

98. Crunchy Nut Granola

Preparation Time: 10 minutes
Cooking Time: 15 minutes
Servings: 6
Ingredients:
- 2 cups old-fashioned rolled oats
- ¼ cup pistachios
- ¼ cup chopped pecans
- ¼ cup chopped cashews
- ¼ cup honey
- 2 tablespoons light brown sugar
- 3 tablespoons butter
- ½ teaspoon ground cinnamon
- Nonstick baking spray (containing flour)
- ½ cup dried cherries

Directions:

1. In a medium bowl, combine the oats, pistachios, pecans, and cashews and toss.
2. In a small saucepan, combine the honey, brown sugar, butter, and cinnamon. Cook over low heat, stirring frequently, until the butter melts and the mixture is smooth, about 4 minutes. Pour over the oat mixture and stir.
3. Spray a 7-inch springform pan with baking spray. Add the granola mixture.
4. Set or preheat the air fryer to 325°F. Set the pan in the air fryer basket. Cook for 7 minutes, then remove the pan and stir. Continue cooking for 6 to 9 minutes or until the granola is light golden brown. Stir in the dried cherries.
5. Remove the pan from the air fryer and let cool, stirring a couple of times as the granola cools. Store in a covered container at room temperature up to 4 days.

Nutrition: Calories: 446 Total fat: 18g Saturated fat: 5g Cholesterol: 15mg Sodium: 51mg Carbohydrates: 64g Fiber: 7g Protein: 11g

99. Breakfast Pizza

Preparation Time: 10 minutes
Cooking Time: 15 minutes
Servings: 4
Ingredients:
- 4 (½-inch-thick) slices French bread, cut on a diagonal
- 6 teaspoons butter, divided
- 4 large eggs
- 2 tablespoons light cream
- ½ teaspoon dried basil
- ¼ teaspoon sea salt
- ⅛ teaspoon freshly ground black pepper
- 4 bacon slices, cooked until crisp and crumbled
- ⅔ cup shredded Colby or Muenster cheese

Directions:
1. Spread each slice of bread with 1 teaspoon of butter and place in the air fryer basket.
2. Set or preheat the air fryer to 350°F. Toast the bread for 2 to 3 minutes or until it's light golden brown. Remove from the air fryer and set aside on a wire rack.
3. Melt the remaining 2 teaspoons of butter in a 6-inch cake pan in the air fryer for 1 minute. Remove the basket from the air fryer.
4. In a medium bowl, beat together the eggs, cream, basil, salt, and pepper and add to the melted butter in the pan. Return the basket to the air fryer. Cook for 3 minutes, then stir. Cook for another 3 to 5 minutes or until the eggs are just set. Remove the eggs from the pan and put them in a bowl.
5. Top the bread with the scrambled eggs mixture, bacon, and cheese. Put back in the air fryer basket. Cook for 4 to 8 minutes or until the cheese is melted and starting to turn brown in spots.
6. Let cool for 5 minutes and serve.

Nutrition: Calories: 425 Total fat: 23g Saturated fat: 11g Cholesterol: 233mg Sodium: 947mg Carbohydrates: 34g Fiber: 1g Protein: 21g

100. Veggie Frittata

Preparation Time: 15 minutes
Cooking Time: 25 minutes
Servings: 4
Ingredients:
- ¼ cup chopped red bell pepper
- ¼ cup chopped yellow summer squash
- 2 tablespoons chopped scallion
- 2 tablespoons butter
- 5 large eggs, beaten
- ¼ teaspoon sea salt
- ⅛ teaspoon freshly ground black pepper
- 1 cup shredded Cheddar cheese, divided

Directions:
1. In a 7-inch cake pan, combine the bell pepper, summer squash, and scallion. Add the butter.
2. Set or preheat the air fryer to 350°F. Set the cake pan in the air fryer basket. Cook the vegetables for 3 to 4 minutes or until they are crisp-tender. Remove the pan from the air fryer.
3. In a medium bowl, beat the eggs with the salt and pepper. Stir in half of the Cheddar. Pour into the pan with the vegetables.
4. Return the pan to the air fryer and cook for 10 to 15 minutes, then top the frittata with the remaining cheese. Cook for another 4 to 5 minutes or until the cheese is melted and the frittata is set. Cut into wedges to serve.

Nutrition: Calories: 260 Total fat: 21g Saturated fat: 11g Cholesterol: 277mg Sodium: 463mg Carbohydrates: 2g Fiber: 0g Protein: 15g

101. Spicy Hash Brown Potatoes

Preparation Time: 15 minutes
Cooking Time: 20 minutes
Servings: 4
Ingredients:
- 2 tablespoons chili powder
- 2 teaspoons ground cumin
- 2 teaspoons smoked paprika
- 1 teaspoon garlic powder
- 1 teaspoon cayenne pepper
- 1 teaspoon freshly ground black pepper
- 2 large russet potatoes, peeled
- 2 tablespoons olive oil
- ⅓ cup chopped onion
- 3 garlic cloves, minced
- ½ teaspoon sea salt

Directions:
1. For the spice mix: In a small bowl, combine the chili powder, cumin, smoked paprika, garlic powder, cayenne, and black pepper. Transfer to a screw-top glass jar and store in a cool, dry place. (Some of the spice mix is used in this recipe; save the rest for other uses.)
2. Grate the potatoes in a food processor or on the large holes of a box grater. Put the potatoes in a bowl filled with ice water, and let stand for 10 minutes.
3. When the potatoes have soaked, drain them, then dry them well with a kitchen towel.
4. Put the olive oil, onion, and garlic in a 7-inch cake pan.
5. Set or preheat the air fryer to 400°F. Put the onion mixture in the air fryer and cook for 3 minutes, then remove.
6. Put the grated potatoes in a medium bowl and sprinkle with 2 teaspoons of spice mixture and toss. Add to the cake pan with the onion mixture.
7. Cook in the air fryer for 10 minutes, then stir the potatoes gently but thoroughly. Cook for 8 to 12 minutes more or until the potatoes are crisp and light golden brown. Season with salt.

Nutrition: Calories: 235 Total fat: 8g Saturated fat: 1g Cholesterol: 0mg Sodium: 419mg Carbohydrates: 39g Fiber: 5g Protein: 5g

102. Sage and Pear Sausage Patties

Preparation Time: 15 minutes

Cooking Time: 20 minutes
Servings: 6
Ingredients:
- 1 pound ground pork
- ¼ cup diced fresh pear
- 1 tablespoon minced fresh sage leaves
- 1 garlic clove, minced
- ½ teaspoon sea salt
- ⅛ teaspoon freshly ground black pepper

Directions:
1. In a medium bowl, combine the pork, pear, sage, garlic, salt, and pepper, and mix gently but thoroughly with your hands.
2. Form the mixture into 8 equal patties about ½ inch thick.
3. Set or preheat the air fryer to 375°F. Arrange the patties in the air fryer basket in a single layer. You may have to cook the patties in batches.
4. Cook the sausages for 15 to 20 minutes, flipping them halfway through the cooking time, until a meat thermometer registers 160°F. Remove from the air fryer, drain on paper towels for a few minutes, and then serve.

Nutrition: Calories: 204 Total fat: 16g Saturated fat: 6g Cholesterol: 54mg Sodium: 236mg Carbohydrates: 1g Fiber: 0g Protein: 13g

103. Bacon Bombs
Preparation Time: 10 minutes
Cooking Time: 16 minutes
Servings: 4
Ingredients:
- 3 center-cut bacon slices
- 3 large eggs, lightly beaten
- 1 oz 1/3-less-fat cream cheese, softened
- 1 tbsp chopped fresh chives
- 4 oz fresh whole wheat pizza dough
- Cooking spray

Directions:
1. Sear the bacon slices in a skillet until brown and crispy then chop into fine crumbles. Add eggs to the same pan and cook for 1 minute then stir in cream cheese, chives and bacon. Mix well, then allow this egg filling to cool down. Spread the pizza dough and slice into four -5inches circles. Divide the egg filling on top of each circle and seal its edge to make dumplings. Place the bacon bombs in the Air Fryer basket and spray them with cooking oil. Set the Air Fryer basket inside the Air Fryer toaster oven and close the lid. Select the Air Fry mode at 350 degrees F temperature for 6 minutes. Serve warm.

Nutrition: Calories: 278 Protein: 7.9g Carbs: 23g Fat: 3.9g

104. Morning Potatoes
Preparation Time: 10 minutes
Cooking Time: 23 minutes
Servings: 4
Ingredients:
- 2 russet potatoes, washed & diced
- ½ tsp salt
- 1 tbsp. olive oil
- ¼ tsp garlic powder
- Chopped parsley, for garnish

Directions:
1. Soak the potatoes in cold water for 45 minutes, then drain and dry them. Toss potato cubes with garlic powder, salt, and olive oil in the Air Fryer basket. Set the Air Fryer basket inside the Air Fryer toaster oven and close the lid. Select the Air Fry mode at 400 degrees F temperature for 23 minutes. Toss them well when cooked halfway through then continue cooking. Garnish with chopped parsley to serve.

Nutrition: Calories: 146 Protein: 6.2g Carbs: 41.2g Fat: 5g

105. Breakfast Pockets
Preparation Time: 10 minutes
Cooking Time: 10 minutes
Servings: 6
Ingredients:
- 1 box puff pastry sheet
- 5 eggs
- ½ cup loose sausage, cooked
- ½ cup bacon, cooked
- ½ cup cheddar cheese, shredded

Directions:
1. Stir cook egg in a skillet for 1 minute then mix with sausages, cheddar cheese, and bacon. Spread the pastry sheet and cut it into four rectangles of equal size. Divide the egg mixture over each rectangle. Fold the edges around the filling and seal them. Place the pockets in the Air Fryer basket. Set the Air Fryer basket inside the Air Fryer toaster oven and close the lid. Select the Air Fry mode at 370 degrees F temperature for 10 minutes. Serve warm.

Nutrition: Calories: 387 Protein: 14.6g Carbs: 37.4g Fat: 6g

106. Avocado Flautas
Preparation Time: 10 minutes
Cooking Time: 24 minutes
Servings: 8
Ingredients:
- 1 tbsp butter
- 8 eggs, beaten
- ½ tsp salt
- ¼ tsp pepper
- 1 ½ tsp cumin
- 1 tsp chili powder
- 8 fajita-size tortillas
- 4 oz cream cheese, softened
- 8 slices cooked bacon
- Avocado Crème:
- 2 small avocados
- ½ cup sour cream
- 1 lime, juiced
- ½ tsp salt
- ¼ tsp pepper

Directions:
1. In a skillet, melt butter and stir in eggs, salt, cumin, pepper, and chili powder, then stir cook for 4 minutes. Spread all the tortillas and top them with cream cheese and bacon. Then divide the egg scramble on top and finally add cheese. Roll the tortillas to seal the filling inside. Place 4 rolls in the Air Fryer basket. Set the Air Fryer basket inside the Air Fryer toaster oven and close the lid. Select the Air Fry mode at 400 degrees F temperature for 12 minutes. Cook the remaining tortilla rolls in the same manner. Meanwhile, blend avocado crème ingredients in a blender then serves with warm flautas.

Nutrition: Calories: 212 Protein: 17.3g Carbs: 14.6g Fat: 11.8g

107. Cheese Sandwiches
Preparation Time: 10 minutes
Cooking Time: 10 minutes
Servings: 2
Ingredients:

BREAKFAST RECIPES

- 1 egg
- 3 tbsp half and half cream
- ¼ tsp vanilla extract
- 2 slices sourdough, white or multigrain bread
- 2½ oz sliced Swiss cheese
- 2 oz sliced deli ham
- 2 oz sliced deli turkey
- 1 tsp butter, melted
- Powdered sugar
- Raspberry jam, for serving

Directions:
1. Beat egg with half and half cream and vanilla extract in a bowl. Place one bread slice on the working surface and top it with ham and turkey slice and swiss cheese. Place the other bread slice on top, then dip the sandwich in the egg mixture, then place it in a suitable baking tray lined with butter. Set the baking tray inside the Air Fryer toaster oven and close the lid. Select the Air Fry mode at 350 degrees F temperature for 10 minutes. Flip the sandwich and continue cooking for 8 minutes. Slice and serve.

Nutrition: Calories: 412 Protein: 18.9g Carbs: 43.8g Fat: 24.8g

108. Sausage Cheese Wraps

Preparation Time: 10 minutes
Cooking Time: 3 minutes
Servings: 8

Ingredients:
- 8 sausages
- 2 pieces American cheese, shredded
- 8-count refrigerated crescent roll dough

Directions:
1. Roll out each crescent roll and top it with cheese and 1 sausage. Fold both the top and bottom edges of the crescent sheet to cover the sausage and roll it around the sausage. Place 4 rolls in the Air Fryer basket and spray them with cooking oil. Set the Air Fryer basket inside the Air Fryer toaster oven and close the lid. Select the Air Fry mode at 380 degrees F temperature for 3 minutes. Cook the remaining rolls in the same manner. Serve fresh.

Nutrition: Calories: 296 Protein: 34.2g Carbs: 17g Fat: 22.1g

109. Chicken Omelet

Preparation Time: 10 minutes
Cooking Time: 18 minutes
Servings: 4

Ingredients:
- 4 eggs
- ½ cup chicken breast, cooked and diced
- 2 tbsp. shredded cheese, divided
- ½ tsp salt, divided
- ¼ tsp pepper, divided
- ¼ tsp granulated garlic, divided
- ¼ tsp onion powder, divided

Directions:
1. Spray 2 ramekins with cooking oil and keep them aside. Crack two large eggs into each ramekin then add cheese and seasoning. Whisk well, then add ¼ cup chicken. Place the ramekins in a baking tray. Set the baking tray inside the Air Fryer toaster oven and close the lid. Select the Bake mode at 330 degrees F temperature for 18 minutes. Serve warm.

Nutrition: Calories: 322 Protein: 17.3g Carbs: 4.6g Fat: 21.8g

110. Sausage Burritos

Preparation Time: 10 minutes
Cooking Time: 10 minutes
Servings: 6

Ingredients:
- 6 medium flour tortillas
- 6 scrambled eggs
- ½ lb. ground sausage, browned
- ½ bell pepper, minced
- 1/3 cup bacon bits
- ½ cup shredded cheese
- Oil, for spraying

Directions:
1. Mix eggs with cheese, bell pepper, bacon, and sausage in a bowl. Spread each tortilla on the working surface and top it with ½ cup egg filling. Roll the tortilla like a burrito then place 3 burritos in the Air Fryer basket. Spray them with cooking oil. Set the Air Fryer basket inside the Air Fryer toaster oven and close the lid. Select the Air Fry mode at 330 degrees F temperature for 5 minutes. Cook the remaining burritos in the same manner. Serve fresh.

Nutrition: Calories: 197 Protein: 7.9g Carbs: 58.5g Fat: 15.4g

111. Sausage Patties

Preparation Time: 10 minutes
Cooking Time: 20 minutes
Servings: 4

Ingredients:
- 1.5 lbs. ground sausage
- 1 tsp chili flakes
- 1 tsp dried thyme
- 1 tsp onion powder
- ½ tsp each paprika and cayenne
- Sea salt and black pepper, to taste
- 2 tsp brown sugar
- 3 tsp minced garlic
- 2 tsp Tabasco
- Herbs for garnish

Directions:
1. Toss sausage ground with all the spices, herbs, sugar, garlic and tabasco sauce in a bowl. Make 1.5-inch-thick and 3-inch round patties out of this mixture. Place the sausage patties in the Air Fryer basket. Set the Air Fryer basket inside the Air Fryer toaster oven and close the lid. Select the Air Fry mode at 370 degrees F temperature for 20 minutes. Flip the patties when cooked halfway through then continue cooking.

Nutrition: Calories: 208 Protein: 24.3g Carbs: 9.5g Fat: 10.7g

112. Spicy Sweet Potato Hash

Preparation Time: 10 minutes
Cooking Time: 16 minutes
Servings: 4

Ingredients:
- 2 large sweet potato, diced
- 2 slices bacon, cooked and diced
- 2 tbsp olive oil
- 1 tbsp smoked paprika
- 1 tsp of sea salt
- 1 tsp ground black pepper
- 1 tsp dried dill weed

Directions:
1. Toss sweet potato with all the spices and olive oil in the Air Fry basket. Set the Air Fryer basket inside the Air Fryer toaster oven and close the lid. Select the Air Fry mode at 400 degrees F temperature for 16 minutes. Toss

the potatoes after every 5 minutes. Once done, toss in bacon and serve warm.

Nutrition: Calories: 134 Protein: 6.6g Carbs: 36.5g Fat: 6g

113. Cinnamon Cream Doughnuts

Preparation Time: 10 minutes
Cooking Time: 8 minutes
Servings: 4

Ingredients:
- 1/2 cup Sugar
- 2 1/2 tbsp butter
- 2 large egg yolks
- 2 1/4 cups all-purpose flour
- 1 1/2 tsp baking powder
- 1 tsp salt
- 1/2 cup sour cream
- To garnish
- 1/3 cup white Sugar
- 1 tsp cinnamon
- 2 tbsp butter, melted

Directions:
1. Beat egg with sugar and butter in a mixer until creamy, then whisk in flour, salt, baking powder, and sour cream. Mix well until smooth then refrigerate the dough for 1 hour. Spread this dough into ½ inch thick circle then cut 9 large circles out of it. Make the hole at the center of each circle. Place the doughnuts in the Air Fryer basket. Set the Air Fryer basket inside the Air Fryer toaster oven and close the lid. Select the Air Fry mode at 350 degrees F temperature for 8 minutes. Cook the doughnuts in two batches to avoid overcrowding. Mix sugar, cinnamon, and butter and glaze the doughnuts with this mixture. Serve.

Nutrition: Calories: 387 Protein: 10.6g Carbs: 26.4g Fat: 13g

114. Sausage Frittata

Preparation Time: 15 minutes
Cooking Time: 20 minutes
Servings: 4

Ingredients:
- 1/4-pound sausage, cooked and crumbled
- 4 eggs, beaten
- 1/2 cup shredded Cheddar cheese blend
- 2 tbsp. red bell pepper, diced
- 1 green onion, chopped
- 1 pinch cayenne pepper
- cooking spray

Directions:
1. Beat eggs with cheese, sausage, cayenne, onion, and bell pepper in a bowl. Spread the egg mixture in a 6x2 inch baking tray, greased with cooking spray. Set the baking tray inside the Air Fryer toaster oven and close the lid. Select the Bake mode at 360 degrees F temperature for 20 minutes. Slice and serve. Serve.

Nutrition: Calories: 212 Protein: 17.3 g Carbs: 14.6g Fat: 11.8g

115. Potato Jalapeno Hash

Preparation Time: 15 minutes
Cooking Time: 24 minutes
Servings: 4

Ingredients:
- 1 1/2 lbs. potatoes, peeled and diced
- 1 tbsp. olive oil
- 1 red bell pepper, seeded and diced
- 1 small onion, chopped
- 1 jalapeno, seeded and diced
- 1/2 tsp olive oil
- 1/2 tsp taco seasoning mix
- 1/2 tsp ground cumin
- Salt and black pepper to taste

Directions:
1. Soak the potato in cold water for 20 minutes then drain them. Toss the potatoes with 1 tbsp olive oil. Spread them in the Air Fryer basket. Set the Air Fryer basket inside the Air Fryer toaster oven and close the lid. Select the Air Fry mode at 370 degrees F temperature for 18 minutes. And Meanwhile, toss onion, pepper, olive oil, taco seasoning, and all other ingredients in a salad bowl. Add this vegetable mixture to the Air Fryer basket, and it return it to the oven. Continue cooking at 356 degrees F for 6 minutes. Serve warm

Nutrition: Calories: 242 Protein: 8.9g Carbs: 36.8g Fat: 14.4g

116. Bread Rolls

Preparation Time: 10 minutes
Cooking Time: 39 minutes
Servings: 8

Ingredients:
- 8 Bread Slices
- 2 Potatoes boiled and mashed
- 1 tsp Ginger grated
- 1 tbsp. Coriander powder
- 1 tsp Cumin powder
- 1/2 tsp Chili powder
- 1/2 tsp Garam Masala
- 1/2 tsp Dry Mango powder
- 1&1/2 tsp Salt
- 1 Large Bowl of Water
- Cooking Oil

Directions:
1. Mix mashed potatoes with ginger and all the spices. Divide this mixture into 16 balls and keep them aside. Slice the bread slices into half to get 16 rectangles. Dip each in water for 1 second, then place one potato ball at the center and wrap the slice around it. Place half of these wrapped balls in the Air Fryer basket and spray them with cooking oil. Set the Air Fryer basket inside the Air Fryer toaster oven and close the lid. Select the Air Fry mode at 390 degrees F temperature for 18 minutes. Flip the balls after 10 minutes of cooking then continue cooking. Cook the remaining balls in the same manner. Serve fresh.

Nutrition: Calories: 331 Protein: 14.8g Carbs: 46g Fat: 2.5g

LUNCH RECIPES

117. Vegetable Egg Rolls
Preparation Time: 15 minutes
Cooking Time: 10 minutes
Servings: 8
Ingredients:
- ½ cup chopped mushrooms
- ½ cup grated carrots
- ½ cup chopped zucchini
- 2 green onions, chopped
- 2 tablespoons low-sodium soy sauce
- 8 egg roll wrappers
- 1 tablespoon cornstarch
- 1 egg, beaten

Directions:
1. In a medium bowl, combine the mushrooms, carrots, zucchini, green onions, and soy sauce, and stir together.
2. Place the egg roll wrappers on a work surface. Top each with about 3 tablespoons of the vegetable mixture.
3. In a small bowl, combine the cornstarch and egg and mix well. Brush some of this mixture on the edges of the egg roll wrappers. Roll up the wrappers, enclosing the vegetable filling. Brush some of the egg mixture on the outside of the egg rolls to seal.
4. Air-fry for 7 to 10 minutes or until the egg rolls are brown and crunchy.

Nutrition: Calories: 112 Total Fat: 1g Saturated Fat: 0g Cholesterol: 23mg Sodium: 417mg Carbohydrates: 21g Fiber: 1g Protein: 4g

118. Veggies on Toast
Preparation Time: 12 minutes
Cooking Time: 11 minutes
Servings: 4
Ingredients:
- 1 red bell pepper, cut into ½-inch strips
- 1 cup sliced button or cremini mushrooms
- 1 small yellow squash, sliced
- 2 green onions, cut into ½-inch slices
- Extra light olive oil for misting
- 4 to 6 pieces sliced French or Italian bread
- 2 tablespoons softened butter
- ½ cup soft goat cheese

Directions:
1. Combine the red pepper, mushrooms, squash, and green onions in the air fryer and mist with oil. Roast for 7 to 9 minutes or until the vegetables are tender, shaking the basket once during cooking time.
2. Remove the vegetables from the basket and set aside.
3. Spread the bread with butter and place in the air fryer, butter-side up. Toast for 2 to 4 minutes or until golden brown.
4. Spread the goat cheese on the toasted bread and top with the vegetables; serve warm.
5. Variation tip: To add even more flavor, drizzle the finished toasts with extra-virgin olive oil and balsamic vinegar.

Nutrition: Calories: 162 Total Fat: 11g Saturated Fat: 7g Cholesterol: 30mg Sodium: 160mg Carbohydrates: 9g Fiber: 2g Protein: 7g

119. Jumbo Stuffed Mushrooms
Preparation Time: 10 minutes
Cooking Time: 20 minutes
Servings: 4
Ingredients:
- 4 jumbo portobello mushrooms
- 1 tablespoon olive oil
- ¼ cup ricotta cheese
- 5 tablespoons Parmesan cheese, divided
- 1 cup frozen chopped spinach, thawed and drained
- ⅓ cup bread crumbs
- ¼ teaspoon minced fresh rosemary

Directions:
1. Wipe the mushrooms with a damp cloth. Remove the stems and discard. Using a spoon, gently scrape out most of the gills.
2. Rub the mushrooms with the olive oil. Put in the air fryer basket, hollow side up, and bake for 3 minutes. Carefully remove the mushroom caps, because they will contain liquid. Drain the liquid out of the caps.
3. In a medium bowl, combine the ricotta, 3 tablespoons of Parmesan cheese, spinach, bread crumbs, and rosemary, and mix well.
4. Stuff this mixture into the drained mushroom caps. Sprinkle with the remaining 2 tablespoons of Parmesan cheese. Put the mushroom caps back into the basket.
5. Bake for 4 to 6 minutes or until the filling is hot and the mushroom caps are tender.

Nutrition: Calories: 117 Total Fat: 7g Saturated Fat: 3g Cholesterol: 10mg Sodium: 180mg Carbohydrates: 8g Fiber: 1g Protein: 7g

120. Mushroom Pita Pizzas
Preparation Time: 10 minutes
Cooking Time: 5 minutes
Servings: 4
Ingredients:
- 4 (3-inch) pitas
- 1 tablespoon olive oil
- ¾ cup pizza sauce
- 1 (4-ounce) jar sliced mushrooms, drained
- ½ teaspoon dried basil
- 2 green onions, minced
- 1 cup grated mozzarella or provolone cheese
- 1 cup sliced grape tomatoes

Directions:
1. Brush each piece of pita with oil and top with the pizza sauce.
2. Add the mushrooms and sprinkle with basil and green onions. Top with the grated cheese.
3. Bake for 3 to 6 minutes or until the cheese is melted and starts to brown. Top with the grape tomatoes and serve immediately.

Nutrition: Calories: 231 Total Fat: 9g Saturated Fat: 4g Cholesterol: 15mg Sodium: 500mg Carbohydrates: 25g Fiber: 2g Protein: 13g

121. Spinach Quiche
Preparation Time: 10 minutes
Cooking Time: 20 minutes
Servings: 3
Ingredients:
- 3 eggs
- 1 cup frozen chopped spinach, thawed and drained
- ⅓ cup heavy cream
- 2 tablespoons honey mustard
- ½ cup grated Swiss or Havarti cheese

- ½ teaspoon dried thyme
- Pinch salt
- Freshly ground black pepper
- Nonstick baking spray with flour

Directions:
1. In a medium bowl, beat the eggs until blended. Stir in the spinach, cream, honey mustard, cheese, thyme, salt, and pepper.
2. Spray a 6-by-6-by-2-inch pan baking pan with nonstick spray. Pour the egg mixture into the pan.
3. Bake for 18 to 22 minutes or until the egg mixture is puffed, light golden brown, and set.
4. Let cool for 5 minutes, then cut into wedges to serve.

Nutrition: Calories: 203 Total Fat: 15g Saturated Fat: 8g Cholesterol: 199mg Sodium: 211mg Carbohydrates: 6g Fiber: 0g Protein: 11g

122. Yellow Squash Fritters

Preparation Time: 15 minutes
Cooking Time: 7 minutes
Servings: 4

Ingredients:
- 1 (3-ounce) package cream cheese, softened
- 1 egg, beaten
- ½ teaspoon dried oregano
- Pinch salt
- Freshly ground black pepper
- 1 medium yellow summer squash, grated
- ⅓ cup grated carrot
- ⅔ cup bread crumbs
- 2 tablespoons olive oil

Directions:
1. In a medium bowl, combine the cream cheese, egg, oregano, and salt and pepper. Add the squash and carrot, and mix well. Stir in the breadcrumbs.
2. Form about 2 tablespoons of this mixture into a patty about ½ inch thick. Repeat with remaining mixture. Brush the fritters with olive oil.
3. Air-fry until crisp and golden, about 7 to 9 minutes.

Nutrition: Calories: 234 Total Fat: 17g Saturated Fat: 6g Cholesterol: 64mg Sodium: 261mg Carbohydrates: 16g Fiber: 2g Protein: 6g

123. Pesto Gnocchi

Preparation Time: 5 minutes
Cooking Time: 20 minutes
Servings: 4

Ingredients:
- 1 tablespoon olive oil
- 1 onion, finely chopped
- 3 cloves garlic, sliced
- 1 (16-ounce) package shelf-stable gnocchi
- 1 (8-ounce) jar pesto
- ⅓ cup grated Parmesan cheese

Directions:
1. Combine the oil, onion, garlic, and gnocchi in a 6-by-6-by-2-inch pan and put into the air fryer.
2. Bake for 10 minutes, then remove the pan and stir.
3. Return the pan to the air fryer and cook for 8 to 13 minutes or until the gnocchi are lightly browned and crisp.
4. Remove the pan from the air fryer. Stir in the pesto and Parmesan cheese, and serve immediately.

Nutrition: Calories: 646 Total Fat: 32g Saturated Fat: 7g Cholesterol: 103mg Sodium: 461mg Carbohydrates: 69g Fiber: 2g Protein: 22g

124. English Muffin Tuna Sandwiches

Preparation Time: 8 minutes
Cooking Time: 5 minutes
Servings: 4

Ingredients:
- 1 (6-ounce) can chunk light tuna, drained
- ¼ cup mayonnaise
- 2 tablespoons mustard
- 1 tablespoon lemon juice
- 2 green onions, minced
- 3 English muffins, split with a fork
- 3 tablespoons softened butter
- 6 thin slices provolone or Muenster cheese

Directions:
1. In a small bowl, combine the tuna, mayonnaise, mustard, lemon juice, and green onions.
2. Butter the cut side of the English muffins. Grill butter-side up in the air fryer for 2 to 4 minutes or until light golden brown. Remove the muffins from the air fryer basket.
3. Top each muffin with one slice of cheese and return to the air fryer. Grill for 2 to 4 minutes or until the cheese melts and starts to brown.
4. Remove the muffins from the air fryer, top with the tuna mixture, and serve.

Nutrition: Calories: 389 Total Fat: 23g Saturated Fat: 10g Cholesterol: 50mg Sodium: 495mg Carbohydrates: 25g Fiber: 3g Protein: 21g

125. Tuna Zucchini Melts

Preparation Time: 15 minutes
Cooking Time: 10 minutes
Servings: 4

Ingredients:
- 4 corn tortillas
- 3 tablespoons softened butter
- 1 (6-ounce) can chunk light tuna, drained
- 1 cup shredded zucchini, drained by squeezing in a kitchen towel
- ⅓ cup mayonnaise
- 2 tablespoons mustard
- 1 cup shredded Cheddar or Colby cheese

Directions:
1. Spread the tortillas with the softened butter. Place in the air fryer basket and grill for 2 to 3 minutes or until the tortillas are crisp. Remove from basket and set aside.
2. In a medium bowl, combine the tuna, zucchini, mayonnaise, and mustard, and mix well.
3. Divide the tuna mixture among the toasted tortillas. Top each with some of the shredded cheese.
4. Grill in the air fryer for 2 to 4 minutes or until the tuna mixture is hot, and the cheese melts and starts to brown. Serve.

Nutrition: Calories: 428 Total Fat: 30g Saturated Fat: 13g Cholesterol: 71mg Sodium: 410mg Carbohydrates: 19g Fiber: 3g Protein: 22g

126. Shrimp and Grilled Cheese Sandwiches

Preparation Time: 10 minutes
Cooking Time: 5 minutes
Servings: 4

Ingredients:
- 1¼ cups shredded Colby, Cheddar, or Havarti cheese

- 1 (6-ounce) can tiny shrimp, drained
- 3 tablespoons mayonnaise
- 2 tablespoons minced green onion
- 4 slices whole grain or whole-wheat bread
- 2 tablespoons softened butter

Directions:
1. In a medium bowl, combine the cheese, shrimp, mayonnaise, and green onion, and mix well.
2. Spread this mixture on two of the slices of bread. Top with the other slices of bread to make two sandwiches. Spread the sandwiches lightly with butter.
3. Grill in the air fryer for 5 to 7 minutes or until the bread is browned and crisp and the cheese is melted. Cut in half and serve warm.

Nutrition: Calories: 276 Total Fat: 14g Saturated Fat: 6g Cholesterol: 115mg Sodium: 573mg Carbohydrates: 16g Fiber: 2g Protein: 22g

127. Shrimp Croquettes

Preparation Time: 12 minutes
Cooking Time: 8 minutes
Servings: 3-4

Ingredients:
- ⅔ pound cooked shrimp, shelled and deveined
- 1½ cups bread crumbs, divided
- 1 egg, beaten
- 2 tablespoon lemon juice
- 2 green onions, finely chopped
- ½ teaspoon dried basil
- Pinch salt
- Freshly ground black pepper
- 2 tablespoons olive oil

Directions:
1. Finely chop the shrimp. Take about 1 tablespoon of the finely chopped shrimp and chop it further until it's almost a paste. Set aside.
2. In a medium bowl, combine ½ cup of the bread crumbs with the egg and lemon juice. Let stand for 5 minutes.
3. Stir the shrimp, green onions, basil, salt, and pepper into the bread crumb mixture.
4. Combine the remaining 1 cup of bread crumbs with the olive oil on a shallow plate; mix well.
5. Form the shrimp mixture into 1½-inch round balls and press firmly with your hands. Roll in the bread crumb mixture to coat.
6. Air-fry the little croquettes in batches for 6 to 8 minutes or until they are brown and crisp. Serve with cocktail sauce for dipping, if desired.

Nutrition: Calories: 330 Total Fat: 12g Saturated Fat: 2g Cholesterol: 201mg Sodium: 539mg Carbohydrates: 31g Fiber: 2g Protein: 24g

128. Dutch Pancake With Shrimp Salsa

Preparation Time: 5 minutes
Cooking Time: 10 minutes
Servings: 4

Ingredients:
- 1 tablespoon plus 2 teaspoons butter
- 3 eggs
- ½ cup flour
- ½ cup milk
- ⅛ teaspoon salt
- 1 cup salsa
- 1 cup frozen fully cooked small shrimp, thawed

Directions:
1. Preheat the air fryer with a 6-by-6-by-2-inch pan in the basket. Add the butter and heat until it melts.
2. Quickly combine the eggs, flour, milk, and salt in a medium bowl and beat well with an eggbeater until well mixed and frothy.
3. Carefully remove the basket with the pan from the air fryer and tilt so the butter covers the bottom of the pan. Immediately pour the batter into the hot pan and put it back in the fryer.
4. Bake for 12 to 16 minutes or until the pancake is puffed and golden brown.
5. Stir together the salsa and shrimp and top the pancake with this mixture.

Nutrition: Calories: 213 Total Fat: 9g Saturated Fat: 5g Cholesterol: 198mg Sodium: 593mg Carbohydrates: 18g Fiber: 2g Protein: 14g

129. Steamed Scallops With Dill

Preparation Time: 5 minutes
Cooking Time: 4 minutes
Servings: 4

Ingredients:
- 1-pound sea scallops
- 1 tablespoon lemon juice
- 2 teaspoons olive oil
- 1 teaspoon dried dill
- Pinch salt
- Freshly ground black pepper

Directions:
1. Check the scallops for a small muscle attached to the side, and pull it off and discard it.
2. Toss the scallops with the lemon juice, olive oil, dill, salt, and pepper. Put into the air fryer basket.
3. Steam for 4 to 5 minutes, tossing the basket once during cooking time, until the scallops are just firm when tested with your finger. The internal temperature should be 145°F at minimum.

Nutrition: Calories: 121 Total Fat: 3g Saturated Fat: 0g Cholesterol: 37mg Sodium: 223mg Carbohydrates: 3g Fiber: 0g Protein: 19g

130. Chicken Pita Sandwiches

Preparation Time: 10 minutes
Cooking Time: 10 minutes
Servings: 4

Ingredients:
- 2 boneless, skinless chicken breasts, cut into 1-inch cubes
- 1 small red onion, sliced
- 1 red bell pepper, sliced
- ⅓ cup Italian salad dressing, divided
- ½ teaspoon dried thyme
- 4 pita pockets, split
- 2 cups torn butter lettuce
- 1 cup chopped cherry tomatoes

Directions:
1. Place the chicken, onion, and bell pepper in the air fryer basket. Drizzle with 1 tablespoon of the Italian salad dressing, add the thyme, and toss.
2. Bake for 9 to 11 minutes or until the chicken is 165°F on a food thermometer, tossing once during cooking time.
3. Transfer the chicken and vegetables to a bowl and toss with the remaining salad dressing.
4. Assemble sandwiches with the pita pockets, butter lettuce, and cherry tomatoes.

Nutrition: Calories: 414 Total Fat: 19g Saturated Fat: 4g Cholesterol: 101mg Sodium: 253mg Carbohydrates: 22g Fiber: 2g Protein: 36g

131. Chicken À La King

Preparation Time: 10 minutes
Cooking Time: 17 minutes
Servings: 4
Ingredients:
- 2 boneless, skinless chicken breasts, cut into 1-inch cubes
- 8 button mushrooms, sliced
- 1 red bell pepper, chopped
- 1 tablespoon olive oil
- 1 (10-ounce) package refrigerated Alfredo sauce
- ½ teaspoon dried thyme
- 6 slices French bread
- 2 tablespoons softened butter

Directions:
1. Place the chicken, mushrooms, and bell pepper in the air fryer basket. Drizzle with the olive oil and toss to coat.
2. Roast for 10 to 15 minutes or until the chicken is 165°F on a food thermometer, tossing the food once during cooking time.
3. Remove the chicken and vegetables to a 6-inch metal bowl and stir in the Alfredo sauce and thyme. Return to the air fryer and cook for 3 to 4 minutes or until hot.
4. Meanwhile, spread the French bread slices with the butter. When the chicken is done, remove the pan from the basket and add the bread, butter-side up. Toast for 2 to 4 minutes or until light golden brown.
5. Place the toast on a serving plate and top with the chicken.

Nutrition: Calories: 744 Total Fat: 32g Saturated Fat: 15g Cholesterol: 142mg Sodium: 3,904mg Carbohydrates: 64g Fiber: 2g Protein: 50g

132. Sweet Sour Pork

Preparation Time: 1 hour and 10 minutes
Cooking Time: 20 minutes
Servings: 4
Ingredients:
- 1 tablespoon vegetable oil
- 1 lb. pork loin, sliced into cubes
- 1 teaspoon garlic, crushed and minced
- 2 teaspoons fresh ginger, grated or minced
- 2 tablespoons brown sugar
- ½ cup ketchup
- 1 ¼ cups water, divided
- ¼ cup pineapple juice
- ¼ cup rice vinegar
- 2 tablespoons reduced-sodium soy sauce
- 1 onion, sliced thinly
- 1 red bell pepper, sliced
- 1 green bell pepper, sliced
- 1 cup fresh pineapple, chopped
- 2 tablespoons cornstarch
- 1 tablespoon black sesame seeds, toasted

Directions:
1. Set your Instant Pot to sauté.
2. Pour in the oil.
3. Once hot, cook the pork cubes for 5 minutes or until brown on all sides.
4. Press cancel button.
5. In a bowl, mix the garlic, ginger, sugar, ketchup, 1 cup water, pineapple juice, vinegar, and soy sauce.
6. Add to the pot.
7. Mix to coat the pork evenly with the sauce.
8. Seal the pot.
9. Cook on high pressure for 5 minutes.
10. Release pressure naturally.
11. Release any remaining feature using the quick mode.
12. Carefully uncover the pot.
13. Transfer the pork to a plate.
14. Press sauté setting.
15. Add the onion, bell peppers and pineapple to the pot.
16. Cook for 6 minutes.
17. Mix the remaining water with cornstarch.
18. Add this mixture to the pot.
19. Simmer until the sauce has thickened.
20. Put the pork back to the pot.
21. Cook for 2 more minutes.
22. Garnish with the sesame seeds.

Nutrition: Calories: 328.7 Fat: 11.4 g Saturated fat: 3.1 g Carbohydrates: 36 g Fiber: 3.2 g Protein: 22.1 g Cholesterol: 54.3 mg Sugars: 24 g Sodium: 648.8 mg Potassium: 710.5 mg

133. Chicken Carnitas

Preparation Time: 1 hour
Cooking Time: 20 minutes
Servings: 10
Ingredients:
- Chicken
- Salt and pepper to taste
- 1 tablespoon ground cumin
- ½ teaspoon dried oregano
- ½ teaspoon chili powder
- 3 tablespoons olive oil, divided
- 2 lb. chicken breast fillet
- 1 onion, sliced into wedges
- 5 cloves garlic, crushed
- ¼ cup reduced-sodium chicken broth
- 1 chipotle pepper in adobo sauce
- ½ cup cilantro
- ¼ cup freshly squeezed lime juice
- 1 tablespoon orange juice
- 1 teaspoon orange zest
- 1 bay leaf
- Sauce
- 1 chipotle pepper in adobo sauce
- ½ cup mayonnaise
- 1 tablespoon milk
- Garlic powder to taste
- Salt to taste

Directions:
1. Mix the salt, pepper, cumin, oregano, and chili powder in a bowl.
2. Season both sides of the chicken with this mixture.
3. Press sauté setting in your Instant Pot.
4. Pour in 1 tablespoon olive oil.
5. Cook the chicken for 2 minutes per side.
6. Transfer to a plate.
7. Add the onion and garlic.
8. Cook for 2 minutes.
9. Put the chicken back to the pot.
10. Add the rest of the chicken ingredients.
11. Lock the lid in place.
12. Cook on high for 10 minutes.
13. Add the sauce ingredients to a food processor.
14. Pulse until smooth.
15. Use natural method for release pressure.
16. Transfer the chicken to a plate.
17. Shred the meat using forks.
18. Drizzle with the cooking liquid and remaining oil.

LUNCH RECIPES

19. Transfer to a baking pan.
20. Broil in the oven for 5 to 6 minutes.
21. Serve with the sauce.

Nutrition: Calories: 235.8 Fat: 15.3 g Saturated Fat: 2.5 g Carbohydrates: 4.7 g Fiber: 0.8 g Protein: 19.6 g Cholesterol: 56.1 mg Sugars: 1.6 g Sodium: 185.9 mg Potassium: 241.1 mg

134. Beef Stroganoff

Preparation Time: 1 hour
Cooking Time: 30 minutes
Servings: 8

Ingredients:
- 2 tablespoons oil
- 1/2 onion, diced
- Salt and pepper to taste
- 2 lb. beef stew meat, sliced into cubes
- ½ teaspoon dried thyme
- 3 cloves garlic, minced
- 2 tablespoons all-purpose flour
- 2 tablespoons soy sauce
- 3 cups low-sodium chicken broth
- 3 cups mushrooms, chopped
- 16 oz. egg noodles
- ¾ cup sour cream

Directions:
1. Select the sauté function in your Instant Pot.
2. Pour the oil into the pot.
3. Cook the onion and salt for 3 minutes.
4. Sprinkle all sides of the beef with the salt and pepper.
5. Add the beef to the pot.
6. Cook for 2 minutes.
7. Stir in the thyme and garlic.
8. Cook for 30 seconds.
9. Add the flour, soy sauce, broth, and mushrooms.
10. Seal the pot.
11. Cook on high for 15 minutes.
12. Release pressure quickly.
13. Uncover and add the egg noodles.
14. Cook on high for 5 minutes.
15. Release pressure naturally.
16. Stir in the sour cream before serving.

Nutrition: Calories: 535.9 Fat: 26.2 g Saturated Fat: 9.8 g Carbohydrates: 45.2 g Fiber: 2.4 g Protein: 29 g Cholesterol: 121.4 mg Sugars: 2.4 g Sodium: 1312.5 mg Potassium: 503.3 mg

135. Chicken Cacciatore

Preparation Time: 1 hour
Cooking Time: 15 minutes
Servings: 4

Ingredients:
- 4 chicken thighs
- 2 tablespoons olive oil
- ½ onion, minced
- 3 stalks celery, chopped
- 4 oz. mushrooms, sliced
- 2 cloves garlic, minced
- 2 tablespoons tomato paste
- 14 oz. canned stewed tomatoes
- 2 teaspoons herbes de Provence
- 3 cubes chicken bouillon, crushed
- ¾ cup water
- Pepper to taste
- Pinch red pepper flakes

Directions:
1. Set your Instant Pot to sauté.
2. Add the oil and cook the chicken for 5 to 6 minutes per side.
3. Transfer to a plate.
4. Add the onion, celery, and mushrooms to the pot.
5. Cook for 5 minutes.
6. Stir in the garlic and cook for 2 minutes.
7. Return chicken to the pot.
8. Stir in the tomato paste, tomatoes, herbs, bouillon, and water.
9. Seal the pot.
10. Cook on high for 12 minutes.
11. Release pressure quickly.
12. Sprinkle with the pepper and red pepper flakes before serving.

Nutrition: Calories: 392.4 Fat: 24.5 g Saturated Fat: 5.8 g Carbohydrates: 13.6 g Fiber: 2.7 g Protein: 29.9 g Cholesterol: 96.1 mg Sugars: 7.3 g Sodium: 1072.6mg Potassium: 714.8 mg

136. Salsa Chicken

Preparation Time: 40 minutes
Cooking Time: 15 minutes
Servings: 2

Ingredients:
- 1 lb. chicken breast fillet
- 1 oz. taco seasoning mix
- ½ cup salsa
- ½ cup reduced-sodium chicken broth

Directions:
1. Season the chicken breast fillet with taco seasoning mix.
2. Add the chicken to your Instant Pot.
3. Spread the salsa on top.
4. Pour in the chicken broth.
5. Lock the lid in place.
6. Choose the poultry setting.
7. Set it to 15 minutes.
8. Release pressure naturally.
9. Shred the chicken with fork.

Nutrition: Calories: 300.1 Fat: 4.8 g Saturated Fat: 1.4 g Carbohydrates: 13.9 g Fiber: 1 g Protein: 45.9 g Cholesterol: 118 mg Sugars: 4.6 g Sodium: 1045.5 mg Potassium: 476.5 mg

137. Corned Beef

Preparation Time: 1 hour and 40 minutes
Cooking Time: 90 minutes
Servings: 4

Ingredients:
- 12 oz. beer
- 2 cups water
- 4 cloves garlic, minced
- 3 lb. corned beef brisket
- 1 corned beef spice packet

Directions:
1. Pour the beer and water into your Instant Pot.
2. Stir in the garlic.
3. Add a steamer basket inside the pot.
4. Put the beef on top of the basket.
5. Season with the spice packet.
6. Seal the pot.
7. Cook on high for 90 minutes.
8. Release pressure quickly.
9. Let rest for 15 minutes.
10. Shred with a fork.

Nutrition: Calories: 416.7 Fat: 28.3 g Saturated Fat: 9.4 g Carbohydrates: 4.9 g Fiber: 0.1 g Protein: 27.7 g Cholesterol: 146 mg Sugars: 0 g Sodium: 1697.3 mg Potassium: 253.3 mg

138. Chicken Curry

Preparation Time: 1 hour and 10 minutes

LUNCH RECIPES

Cooking Time: 25 minutes
Servings: 4
Ingredients:
- 1 tablespoon coconut oil
- 1 onion, minced
- 2 cloves garlic, crushed and minced
- 3 tablespoons curry powder
- 2 tablespoons white sugar
- 8 oz. canned tomato sauce
- 14 oz. canned diced tomatoes
- ½ cup chicken broth
- 2 lb. chicken breast fillet
- Salt and pepper to taste
- 14 oz. coconut milk

Directions:
1. Choose the sauté function in your Instant Pot.
2. Pour in the coconut oil.
3. Cook the onion and garlic for 2 minutes.
4. Sprinkle with the curry powder and stir.
5. Press cancel button.
6. Add the sugar, tomato sauce, tomatoes, and chicken broth. Stir.
7. Season both sides of the chicken with the salt and pepper.
8. Place the chicken in the pot.
9. Secure the pot.
10. Cook on high for 10 minutes.
11. Release pressure naturally.
12. Shred the chicken and return to the pot.
13. Press sauté setting.
14. Cook for 3 minutes.
15. Pour in the coconut milk.
16. Cook for 10 more minutes.

Nutrition: Calories: 563.3 Fat: 30.6 g Saturated Fat: 23.1 g Carbohydrates: 21.5 g Fiber: 4.9 g Protein: 51.9 g Sugars: 12.5 g Cholesterol: 130 mg Sodium: 766.2 mg Potassium: 1038.3 mg

139. Pork Chops with Gravy

Preparation Time: 1 hour and 10 minutes
Cooking Time: 40 minutes
Servings: 5
Ingredients:
- 1 tablespoon avocado oil
- 5 pork chops
- Pepper to taste
- 1 clove garlic, minced
- ¼ cup dry white wine
- 10 oz. cream of mushroom soup
- 1 ½ cups water, divided
- 2 tablespoons all-purpose flour
- 1 teaspoon reduced-sodium soy sauce

Directions:
1. Pour the oil into your Instant Pot.
2. Set it to sauté.
3. Sprinkle both sides of the pork chops with pepper.
4. Cook the pork chops in oil for 4 to 5 minutes per side.
5. Transfer to a plate.
6. Cook the garlic in the pot for 30 seconds.
7. Add the wine and scrape bottom of the pot.
8. Simmer the sauce for 6 minutes.
9. Pour in the mushroom soup and 1 ¼ cups water.
10. Simmer for 3 minutes.
11. Put the pork chops to the pot.
12. Secure the lid.
13. Cook on high for 18 minutes.
14. Release pressure naturally.
15. Combine the flour and remaining water.
16. Choose the sauté setting.
17. Cook for 3 to 5 minutes.
18. Stir in the soy sauce.
19. Coat the pork chops evenly with the sauce.

Nutrition: Calories: 284.3 Fat: 14.7 g Saturated Fat: 4 g Carbohydrates: 7.3 g Fiber: 0.1 g Protein: 26.9 g Cholesterol: 65.2 mg Sugars: 1 g Sodium: 488.2 mg Potassium: 396.9 mg

140. Beef Stew

Preparation Time: 1 hour and 30 minutes
Cooking Time: 40 minutes
Servings: 4
Ingredients:
- 1 tablespoon butter
- 1 lb. beef chuck, sliced into cubes
- 1 onion, quartered
- 2 cloves garlic, crushed and minced
- 1 ½ cups mushrooms, sliced in half
- 4 potatoes, sliced into cubes
- 2 carrots, sliced
- 3 cups reduced-sodium beef broth
- 1 tablespoon Worcestershire sauce
- 1 tablespoon tomato paste
- Salt and pepper to taste
- ½ teaspoon dried rosemary

Directions:
1. Choose the sauté function in your Instant Pot.
2. Add the butter and cook the beef for 5 minutes.
3. Stir in the onion, garlic, mushrooms, potatoes, and carrots.
4. Lock the lid in place.
5. Press meat / stew function.
6. Set it to 35 minutes.
7. Release pressure naturally.
8. Serve in bowls.

Nutrition: Calories: 351.7 Fat: 16.4 g Saturated Fat: 7.2 g Carbohydrates: 32.2 g Fiber: 4 g Protein: 20 g Cholesterol: 59.1 mg Sugars: 4.6 g Sodium: 1020.5 mg Potassium: 541.8 mg

141. Salisbury Steak

Preparation Time: 2 hours and 40 minutes
Cooking Time: 40 minutes
Servings: 4
Ingredients:
- 1 lb. lean ground beef
- ½ lb. lean ground pork
- ¼ cup onion, diced
- 1 clove garlic, crushed and minced
- 1 egg, beaten
- 1 teaspoon Worcestershire sauce
- 1 teaspoon dried parsley
- ¼ cup breadcrumbs
- 2 tablespoons avocado oil
- 1 onion, sliced thinly
- 8 oz. mushrooms, sliced
- 2 cups reduced-sodium beef broth
- 1 tablespoon tomato paste
- ¼ cup dry red wine
- Salt and pepper to taste
- 4 tablespoons reduced-sodium beef broth mixed with 2 tablespoons cornstarch

Directions:

LUNCH RECIPES

1. In a bowl, combine ground beef, ground pork, onion, garlic, egg, Worcestershire sauce, dried parsley, and breadcrumbs.
2. Form patties from the mixture.
3. Wrap with plastic and place in the refrigerator for 1 hour.
4. Press sauté setting in your Instant Pot.
5. Pour in the oil and cook the patties for 2 to 3 minutes per side.
6. Transfer to a plate.
7. Add the onions and mushrooms and cook for 5 minutes.
8. Add the wine to the pot.
9. Scrape the browned bits.
10. Add the broth, tomato paste, red wine, salt, and pepper. Mix well.
11. Add the patties to the pot.
12. Seal the pot.
13. Cook on high for 15 minutes.
14. Release pressure naturally.
15. Add the cornstarch mixture to the pot.
16. Press sauté and simmer for 5 minutes or until the sauce has thickened.

Nutrition: Calories: 523.8 Fat: 34.5 g Saturated Fat: 11.3 g Fiber: 2.4 g Carbohydrates: 13.4 g Protein: 35.4 g Cholesterol: 152.8 mg Sugars: 3 g Sodium: 1227.1 mg Potassium: 620.3 mg

142. Pot Roast with Veggies

Preparation Time: 1 hour and 40 minutes
Cooking Time: 1 hour and 10 minutes
Servings: 8

Ingredients:
- 4 tablespoons olive oil, divided
- 3 lb. beef chuck roast
- 2 cups low-sodium beef broth
- 1 onion, sliced into wedges
- 1 packet dry onion soup mix
- 1 ½ cups baby carrots
- 1-pound baby potatoes
- 2 ½ tablespoons cornstarch mixed with ¼ cup water
- Pepper to taste
- 1 ½ teaspoons garlic salt

Directions:
1. Press sauté setting in your Instant Pot.
2. Add half of the oil to the pot.
3. Cook the chuck roast for 4 minutes per side.
4. Pour in the broth.
5. In a bowl, mix the oil, onion, onion soup mix, carrots, and potatoes.
6. Add the mixture to the pot.
7. Seal the pot.
8. Cook on high for 1 hour.
9. Release pressure quickly.
10. Transfer the roast to the plate.
11. Press sauté setting.
12. Add the cornstarch mixture to the pot.
13. Cook for 3 minutes.
14. Season the sauce with the pepper and garlic salt.
15. Serve the roast with veggies and sauce.

Nutrition: Calories: 323.2 Fat: 15.6 g Saturated Fat: 4.4 g Carbohydrates: 19 g Fiber: 2.6 g Protein: 25.7 g Cholesterol: 78.8 mg Sugars: 2.4 g Sodium: 1005.4 mg Potassium: 587.2 mg

143. Mexican Rice

Preparation Time: 40 minutes
Cooking Time: 20 minutes
Servings: 4

Ingredients:
- 1 tablespoon avocado oil
- ½ onion, chopped
- 2 cloves garlic, crushed and minced
- 1 cup rice
- 1 ½ cups reduced-sodium chicken broth
- ½ cup reduced-sodium tomato sauce
- Pinch cayenne pepper
- ¼ teaspoon ground cumin
- Salt to taste

Directions:
1. Select the sauté function in your Instant Pot.
2. Pour the avocado oil into the pot.
3. Cook the onion and garlic for 5 minutes, stirring frequently.
4. Stir in the rice.
5. Coat with the oil.
6. Add the chicken stock.
7. Stir in the cayenne pepper, cumin, and salt.
8. Seal the pot.
9. Cook on high for 15 minutes.
10. Release pressure quickly.
11. Stir the rice and serve.

Nutrition: Calories: 224.6 Protein: 5.2 g Carbohydrates: 41.1 g Fiber: 1.4 g Sugars: 2.2 g Fat: 4.1 g Saturated Fat: 0.7 g Cholesterol: 1.5 mg Potassium: 185.8 mg Sodium: 787.7 mg

144. Hamburger Soup

Preparation Time: 1 hour and 10 minutes
Cooking Time: 30 minutes
Servings: 8

Ingredients:
- 1 onion, chopped
- 1 ½ lb. ground beef
- 45 oz. canned beef consommé
- 10 oz. canned tomato soup
- 28 oz. canned diced tomatoes
- 2 cups water
- 3 stalks celery, chopped
- 4 carrots, chopped
- ½ teaspoon dried thyme
- 4 tablespoons pearl barley
- 1 bay leaf

Directions:
1. Press sauté setting in your Instant Pot.
2. Add the onion and beef.
3. Cook for 10 minutes, stirring frequently.
4. Stir in the rest of the ingredients.
5. Secure the lid.
6. Choose the soup setting.
7. Cook for 30 minutes.
8. Release pressure naturally.
9. Discard the bay leaf and serve.

Nutrition: Calories: 251.1 Fat: 11.2 g Saturated Fat: 4.3 g Carbohydrates: 17.8 g Fiber: 3.4 g Protein: 18.7 g Cholesterol: 51.7 mg Sugars: 7.7 g Sodium: 950.4 mg Potassium: 660.6 mg

145. Roasted Brussels sprouts

Preparation Time: 20 minutes
Cooking Time: 10 minutes
Servings: 4

Ingredients:
- 2 tablespoons olive oil
- 1 onion, chopped
- 1 lb. whole Brussels sprouts, sliced in half
- Salt and pepper
- ½ cup vegetable broth

Directions:
1. Set your Instant Pot to sauté.
2. Pour the olive oil into the pot.
3. Cook the onion for 2 minutes.
4. Stir in the Brussels sprouts.
5. Cook for 1 minute.
6. Season with the salt and pepper.
7. Add the vegetable broth to the pot.
8. Secure the lid.
9. Cook on high for 3 minutes.
10. Release pressure quickly.

Nutrition: Calories: 135.6 Fat: 7.2 g Saturated Fat: 1 g Carbohydrates: 16.3 g Fiber: 5.5 g Protein: 4.6 g Cholesterol: 0 mg Sugars: 5.3 g Sodium: 669.8 mg Potassium: 527.9 mg

DINNER RECIPES

146. Crispy Salt and Pepper Tofu
Preparation Time: 5 minutes
Cooking Time: 15 minutes
Servings: 4
Ingredients:
- ¼ cup chickpea flour
- ¼ cup arrowroot (or cornstarch)
- 1 teaspoon sea salt
- 1 teaspoon granulated garlic
- ½ teaspoon freshly grated black pepper
- 1 (15-ounce) package tofu, firm or extra-firm
- Cooking oil spray (sunflower, safflower, or refined coconut)
- Asian Spicy Sweet Sauce, optional

Directions:
1. In a medium bowl, combine the flour, arrowroot, salt, garlic, and pepper. Stir well to combine.
2. Cut the tofu into cubes (no need to press—if it's a bit watery, that's fine!). Place the cubes into the flour mixture. Toss well to coat. Spray the tofu with oil and toss again. (The spray will help the coating better stick to the tofu.)
3. Spray the air fryer basket with the oil. Place the tofu in a single layer in the air fryer basket (you may have to do this in 2 batches, depending on the size of your appliance) and spray the tops with oil. Fry for 8 minutes. Remove the air fryer basket and spray again with oil. Toss gently or turn the pieces over. Spray with oil again and fry for another 7 minutes, or until golden-browned and very crisp.
4. Serve immediately, either plain or with the Asian Spicy Sweet Sauce.

Nutrition: Calories: 148 Total fat: 5g Saturated fat: 0g Cholesterol: 0mg Sodium: 473mg Carbohydrates: 14g Fiber: 1g Protein: 11g

147. Crispy Indian Wrap
Preparation Time: 20 minutes
Cooking Time: 8 minutes
Servings: 4
Ingredients:
- Cilantro Chutney
- 2¾ cups diced potato, cooked until tender
- 2 teaspoons oil (coconut, sunflower, or safflower)
- 3 large garlic cloves, minced or pressed
- 1½ tablespoons fresh lime juice
- 1½ teaspoons cumin powder
- 1 teaspoon onion granules
- 1 teaspoon coriander powder
- ½ teaspoon sea salt
- ½ teaspoon turmeric
- ¼ teaspoon cayenne powder
- 4 large flour tortillas, preferably whole grain or sprouted
- 1 cup cooked garbanzo beans (canned are fine), rinsed and drained
- ½ cup finely chopped cabbage
- ¼ cup minced red onion or scallion
- Cooking oil spray (sunflower, safflower, or refined coconut)

Directions:
1. Make the Cilantro Chutney and set aside.
2. In a large bowl, mash the potatoes well, using a potato masher or large fork. Add the oil, garlic, lime, cumin, onion, coriander, salt, turmeric, and cayenne. Stir very well, until thoroughly combined. Set aside.
3. Lay the tortillas out flat on the counter. In the middle of each, evenly distribute the potato filling. Add some of the garbanzo beans, cabbage, and red onion to each, on top of the potatoes.
4. Spray the air fryer basket with oil and set aside. Enclose the Indian wraps by folding the bottom of the tortillas up and over the filling, then folding the sides in—and finally rolling the bottom up to form, essentially, an enclosed burrito.
5. Place the wraps in the air fryer basket, seam side down. They can touch each other a little bit, but if they're too crowded, you'll need to cook them in batches. Fry for 5 minutes. Spray with oil again, flip over, and cook an additional 2 or 3 minutes, until nicely browned and crisp. Serve topped with the Cilantro Chutney.

Nutrition: Calories: 288 Total fat: 7g Saturated fat: 1g Cholesterol: 0mg Sodium: 821mg Carbohydrates: 50g Fiber: 5g Protein: 9g

148. Easy Peasy Pizza
Preparation Time: 5 minutes
Cooking Time: 9 minutes
Servings: 1
Ingredients:
- Cooking oil spray (coconut, sunflower, or safflower)
- 1 flour tortilla, preferably sprouted or whole grain
- ¼ cup vegan pizza or marinara sauce
- ⅓ cup grated vegan mozzarella cheese or Cheesy Sauce
- Toppings of your choice

Directions:
1. Spray the air fryer basket with oil. Place the tortilla in the air fryer basket. If the tortilla is a little bigger than the base, no probs! Simply fold the edges up a bit to form a semblance of a "crust."
2. Pour the sauce in the center, and evenly distribute it around the tortilla "crust" (I like to use the back of a spoon for this purpose).
3. Sprinkle evenly with vegan cheese, and add your toppings. Bake for 9 minutes, or until nicely browned. Remove carefully, cut into four pieces, and enjoy.

Nutrition: Calories: 210 Total fat: 6g Saturated fat: 1g Cholesterol: 0mg Sodium: 700mg Carbohydrates: 33g Fiber: 2g Protein: 5g

149. Eggplant Parmigiana
Preparation Time: 15 minutes
Cooking Time: 40 minutes
Servings: 4
Ingredients:
- 1 medium eggplant (about 1-pound), sliced into ½-inch-thick rounds
- 2 tablespoons tamari or shoyu
- 3 tablespoons nondairy milk, plain and unsweetened
- 1 cup chickpea flour (see Substitution Tip)
- 1 tablespoon dried basil
- 1 tablespoon dried oregano
- 2 teaspoons garlic granules
- 2 teaspoons onion granules
- ½ teaspoon sea salt
- ½ teaspoon freshly ground black pepper

- Cooking oil spray (sunflower, safflower, or refined coconut)
- Vegan marinara sauce (your choice)
- Shredded vegan cheese (preferably mozzarella; see Ingredient Tip)

Directions:
1. Place the eggplant slices in a large bowl, and pour the tamari and milk over the top. Turn the pieces over to coat them as evenly as possible with the liquids. Set aside.
2. Make the coating: In a medium bowl, combine the flour, basil, oregano, garlic, onion, salt, and pepper and stir well. Set aside.
3. Spray the air fryer basket with oil and set aside.
4. Stir the eggplant slices again and transfer them to a plate (stacking is fine). Do not discard the liquid in the bowl.
5. Bread the eggplant by tossing an eggplant round in the flour mixture. Then, dip in the liquid again. Double up on the coating by placing the eggplant again in the flour mixture, making sure that all sides are nicely breaded. Place in the air fryer basket.
6. Repeat with enough eggplant rounds to make a (mostly) single layer in the air fryer basket. (You'll need to cook it in batches, so that you don't have too much overlap and it cooks perfectly.)
7. Spray the tops of the eggplant with enough oil so that you no longer see dry patches in the coating. Fry for 8 minutes. Remove the air fryer basket and spray the tops again. Turn each piece over, again taking care not to overlap the rounds too much. Spray the tops with oil, again making sure that no dry patches remain. Fry for another 8 minutes, or until nicely browned and crisp.
8. Repeat steps 5 to 7 one more time, or until all of the eggplant is crisp and browned.
9. Finally, place half of the eggplant in a 6-inch round, 2-inch deep baking pan and top with marinara sauce and a sprinkle of vegan cheese. Fry for 3 minutes, or until the sauce is hot and cheese is melted (be careful not to overcook, or the eggplant edges will burn). Serve immediately, plain or over pasta. Otherwise, you can store the eggplant in the fridge for several days and then make a fresh batch whenever the mood strikes by repeating this step!

Nutrition: Calories: 217 Total fat: 9g Saturated fat: 1g Cholesterol: 0mg Sodium: 903mg Carbohydrates: 38g Fiber: 10g Protein: 9g

150. <u>Luscious Lazy Lasagna</u>
Preparation Time: 15 minutes
Cooking Time: 15 minutes
Servings: 4
Ingredients:
- 8 ounces lasagna noodles, preferably bean-based, but any kind will do
- 1 tablespoon extra-virgin olive oil
- 2 cups crumbled extra-firm tofu, drained and water squeezed out
- 2 cups loosely packed fresh spinach
- 2 tablespoons Nutrition yeast
- 2 tablespoons fresh lemon juice
- 1 teaspoon onion granules
- 1 teaspoon sea salt
- ⅛ teaspoon freshly ground black pepper
- 4 large garlic cloves, minced or pressed
- 2 cups vegan pasta sauce, your choice
- ½ cup shredded vegan cheese (preferably mozzarella)

Directions:
1. Cook the noodles until a little firmer than al dente (they'll get a little softer after you air-fry them in the lasagna). Drain and set aside.
2. While the noodles are cooking, make the filling. In a large pan over medium-high heat, add the olive oil, tofu, and spinach. Stir-fry for a minute, then add the Nutrition yeast, lemon juice, onion, salt, pepper, and garlic. Stir well and cook just until the spinach is nicely wilted. Remove from heat.
3. To make half a batch (one 6-inch round, 2-inch deep baking pan) of lasagna: Spread a thin layer of pasta sauce in the baking pan. Layer 2 or 3 lasagna noodles on top of the sauce. Top with a little more sauce and some of the tofu mixture. Place another 2 or 3 noodles on top, and add another layer of sauce and then another layer of tofu. Finish with a layer of noodles, and then a final layer of sauce. Sprinkle about half of the vegan cheese on top (omit if you prefer; see the Ingredient Tip from the Eggplant Parmigiana).
4. Place the pan in the air fryer and bake for 15 minutes, or until the noodles are browning around the edges and the cheese is melted. Cut and serve.
5. If making the entire recipe now, repeat steps 3 and 4 (see Cooking Tip).

Nutrition: Calories: 317 Total fat: 8g Saturated fat: 1g Cholesterol: 0mg Sodium: 1203mg Carbohydrates: 46g Fiber: 4g Protein: 20g

151. <u>Pasta With Creamy Cauliflower Sauce</u>
Preparation Time: 10 minutes
Cooking Time: 18 minutes
Servings: 4
Ingredients:
- 4 cups cauliflower florets
- Cooking oil spray (sunflower,
- safflower, or refined coconut)
- 1 medium onion, chopped
- 8 ounces pasta, your choice (about 4 cups cooked; use gluten-free pasta if desired)
- Fresh chives or scallion tops, for garnish
- ½ cup raw cashew pieces (see Ingredient Tip)
- 1½ cups water
- 1 tablespoon Nutrition yeast
- 2 large garlic cloves, peeled
- 2 tablespoons fresh lemon juice
- 1½ teaspoons sea salt
- ¼ teaspoon freshly ground black pepper

Directions:
1. Place the cauliflower in the air fryer basket, spritz the tops with oil spray, and roast for 8 minutes. Remove the air fryer basket, stir, and add the onion. Spritz with oil again and roast for another 10 minutes, or until the cauliflower is browned and the onions are tender.
2. While the vegetables are roasting in the air fryer, cook the pasta according to the package directions and mince the chives or scallions. Set aside.
3. In a blender jar, place the roasted cauliflower and onions along with the cashews, water, Nutrition yeast, garlic, lemon, salt, and pepper. Blend well, until very smooth and creamy. Serve a generous portion of the sauce on top of the warm pasta, and top with the minced chives or scallions. The sauce will store, refrigerated in an airtight container, for about a week.

Nutrition: Calories: 341 Total fat: 9g Saturated fat: 1g Cholesterol: 0mg Sodium: 312mg Carbohydrates: 51g Fiber: 6g Protein: 14g

DINNER RECIPES

152. Lemony Lentils With "Fried" Onions

Preparation Time: 10 minutes
Cooking Time: 30 minutes
Servings: 4
Ingredients:
- 1 cup red lentils
- 4 cups water
- Cooking oil spray (coconut, sunflower, or safflower)
- 1 medium-size onion, peeled and cut into ¼-inch-thick rings
- Sea salt
- ½ cup kale, stems removed, thinly sliced
- 3 large garlic cloves, pressed or minced
- 2 tablespoons fresh lemon juice
- 2 teaspoons Nutrition yeast
- 1 teaspoon sea salt
- 1 teaspoon lemon zest (see Ingredient Tip)
- ¾ teaspoon freshly ground black pepper

Directions:
1. In a medium-large pot, bring the lentils and water to a boil over medium-high heat. Reduce the heat to low and simmer, uncovered, for about 30 minutes (or until the lentils have dissolved completely), making sure to stir every 5 minutes or so as they cook (so that the lentils don't stick to the bottom of the pot).
2. While the lentils are cooking, get the rest of your dish together. Spray the air fryer basket with oil and place the onion rings inside, separating them as much as possible. Spray them with the oil and sprinkle with a little salt. Fry for 5 minutes. Remove the air fryer basket, shake or stir, spray again with oil, and fry for another 5 minutes. (Note: You're aiming for all of the onion slices to be crisp and well browned, so if some of the pieces begin to do that, transfer them from the air fryer basket to a plate.)
3. Remove the air fryer basket, spray the onions again with oil, and fry for a final 5 minutes or until all the pieces are crisp and browned.
4. To finish the lentils: Add the kale to the hot lentils, and stir very well, as the heat from the lentils will steam the thinly sliced greens. Stir in the garlic, lemon juice, Nutrition yeast, salt, zest, and pepper. Stir very well and then distribute evenly in bowls. Top with the crisp onion rings and serve.

Nutrition: Calories: 220 Total fat: 1g Saturated fat: 0g Cholesterol: 0mg Sodium: 477mg Carbohydrates: 39g Fiber: 16g Protein: 15g

153. Our Daily Bean

Preparation Time: 5 minutes
Cooking Time: 8 minutes
Servings: 2
Ingredients:
- 1 (15-ounce) can pinto beans, drained
- ¼ cup tomato sauce
- 2 tablespoons Nutrition yeast
- 2 large garlic cloves, pressed or minced
- ½ teaspoon dried oregano
- ½ teaspoon cumin
- ¼ teaspoon sea salt
- ⅛ teaspoon freshly ground black pepper
- Cooking oil spray (sunflower, safflower, or refined coconut)

Directions:
1. In a medium bowl, stir together the beans, tomato sauce, Nutrition yeast, garlic, oregano, cumin, salt, and pepper until well combined.
2. Spray the 6-inch round, 2-inch deep baking pan with oil and pour the bean mixture into it. Bake for 4 minutes. Remove, stir well, and bake for another 4 minutes, or until the mixture has thickened and is heated through. It will most likely form a little crust on top and be lightly browned in spots. Serve hot. This will keep, refrigerated in an airtight container, for up to a week.

Nutrition: Calories: 284 Total fat: 4g Saturated fat: 1g Cholesterol: 0mg Sodium: 807mg Carbohydrates: 47g Fiber: 16g Protein: 20g

154. Taco Salad with Creamy Lime Sauce

Preparation Time: 7 minutes
Cooking Time: 20 minutes
Servings: 3
Ingredients:
- For the sauce
- 1 (12.3-ounce) package of silken-firm tofu
- ¼ cup plus 1 tablespoon fresh lime juice
- Zest of 1 large lime (1 teaspoon)
- 1½ tablespoons coconut sugar
- 3 large garlic cloves, peeled
- 1 teaspoon sea salt
- ½ teaspoon ground chipotle powder
- For the salad
- 6 cups romaine lettuce, chopped (1 large head)
- 1 (15-ounce) can vegan refried beans (or whole pinto or black beans if you prefer)
- 1 cup chopped red cabbage
- 2 medium tomatoes, chopped
- ½ cup chopped cilantro
- ¼ cup minced scallions
- Double batch of Garlic Lime Tortilla Chips

Directions:
1. To make the sauce
2. Drain the tofu (pour off any liquid) and place in a blender. Add the lime juice and zest, coconut sugar, garlic, salt, and chipotle powder. Blend until very smooth. Set aside.
3. To make the salad
4. Distribute the lettuce equally into three big bowls.
5. In a small pan over medium heat, warm the beans, stirring often, until hot (this should take less than a minute). Place on top of the lettuce. Top the beans with the cabbage, tomatoes, cilantro, and scallions. Drizzle generously with the Creamy Lime Sauce and serve with the double batch of air-fried chips. Enjoy immediately.

Nutrition: Calories: 422 Total fat: 7g Saturated fat: 1g Cholesterol: 0mg Sodium: 1186mg Carbohydrates: 71g Fiber: 15g; Protein: 22g

155. Bbq Jackfruit Nachos

Preparation Time: 30 minutes
Cooking Time: 20 minutes
Servings: 3
Ingredients:
- 1 (20-ounce) can jackfruit, drained
- ⅓ cup prepared vegan BBQ sauce
- ¼ cup water
- 2 tablespoons tamari or shoyu
- 1 tablespoon fresh lemon juice
- 4 large garlic cloves, pressed or minced
- 1 teaspoon onion granules

- ⅛ teaspoon cayenne powder
- ⅛ teaspoon liquid smoke
- Double batch Garlic Lime Tortilla Chips
- 2½ cups prepared Cheesy Sauce
- 3 medium-size tomatoes, chopped
- ¾ cup guacamole of your choice
- ¾ cup chopped cilantro
- ½ cup minced red onion
- 1 jalapeño, seeds removed and thinly sliced (optional)

Directions:
1. In a large skillet over high heat, place the jackfruit, BBQ sauce, water, tamari, lemon juice, garlic, onion granules, cayenne, and liquid smoke. Stir well and break up the jackfruit a bit with a spatula.
2. Once the mixture boils, reduce the heat to low. Continue to cook, stirring often (and breaking up the jackfruit as you stir), for about 20 minutes, or until all of the liquid has been absorbed. Remove from the heat and set aside.
3. Assemble the nachos: Distribute the chips onto three plates, and then top evenly with the jackfruit mixture, warmed Cheesy Sauce, tomatoes, guacamole, cilantro, onion, and jalapeño (if using). Enjoy immediately, because soggy chips are tragic.

Nutrition: Calories: 661 Total fat: 15g Saturated fat: 1g Cholesterol: 0mg Sodium: 1842mg Carbohydrates: 124g Fiber: 19g Protein: 22g

156. 10-Minute Chimichanga
Preparation Time: 2 minutes
Cooking Time: 8 minutes
Servings: 1
Ingredients:
- 1 whole-grain tortilla
- ½ cup vegan refried beans
- ¼ cup grated vegan cheese (optional)
- Cooking oil spray (sunflower, safflower, or refined coconut)
- ½ cup fresh salsa (or Green Chili Sauce)
- 2 cups chopped romaine lettuce (about ½ head)
- Guacamole (optional)
- Chopped cilantro (optional)
- Cheesy Sauce (optional)

Directions:
1. Lay the tortilla on a flat surface and place the beans in the center. Top with the cheese, if using. Wrap the bottom up over the filling, and then fold in the sides. Then roll it all up so as to enclose the beans inside the tortilla (you're making an enclosed burrito here).
2. Spray the air fryer basket with oil, place the tortilla wrap inside the basket, seam-side down, and spray the top of the chimichanga with oil. Fry for 5 minutes. Spray the top (and sides) again with oil, flip over, and spray the other side with oil. Fry for an additional 2 or 3 minutes, until nicely browned and crisp.
3. Transfer to a plate. Top with the salsa, lettuce, guacamole, cilantro, and/or Cheesy Sauce, if using. Serve immediately.

Nutrition: Calories: 317 Total fat: 6g Saturated fat: 2g Cholesterol: 0mg Sodium: 955mg Carbohydrates: 55g Fiber: 11g Protein: 13g

157. Mexican Stuffed Potatoes
Preparation Time: 15 minutes
Cooking Time: 40 minutes
Servings: 4
Ingredients:
- 4 large potatoes, any variety (I like Yukon Gold or russets for this dish; see Cooking Tip)
- Cooking oil spray (sunflower, safflower, or refined coconut)
- 1½ cups Cheesy Sauce
- 1 cup black or pinto beans (canned beans are fine; be sure to drain and rinse)
- 2 medium tomatoes, chopped
- 1 scallion, finely chopped
- ⅓ cup finely chopped cilantro
- 1 jalapeño, finely sliced or minced (optional)
- 1 avocado, diced (optional)

Directions:
1. Scrub the potatoes, prick with a fork, and spray the outsides with oil. Place in the air fryer (leaving room in between so the air can circulate) and bake for 30 minutes.
2. While the potatoes are cooking, prepare the Cheesy Sauce and additional items. Set aside.
3. Check the potatoes at the 30-minute mark by poking a fork into them. If they're very tender, they're done. If not, continue to cook until a fork inserted proves them to be well-done. (As potato sizes vary, so will your cook time—the average cook time is usually about 40 minutes.)
4. When the potatoes are getting very close to being tender, warm the Cheesy Sauce and the beans in separate pans.
5. To assemble: Plate the potatoes and cut them across the top. Then, pry them open with a fork—just enough to get all the goodies in there. Top each potato with the Cheesy Sauce, beans, tomatoes, scallions, cilantro, and jalapeño and avocado, if using. Enjoy immediately.

Nutrition: Calories: 420 Total fat: 5g Saturated fat: 0g Cholesterol: 0mg Sodium: 503mg Carbohydrates: 80g Fiber: 17g Protein: 15g

158. Kids' Taquitos
Preparation Time: 5 minutes
Cooking Time: 7 minutes
Servings: 4
Ingredients:
- 8 corn tortillas
- Cooking oil spray (coconut, sunflower, or safflower)
- 1 (15-ounce) can vegan refried beans
- 1 cup shredded vegan cheese
- Guacamole (optional)
- Cheesy Sauce (optional)
- Vegan sour cream (optional)
- Fresh salsa (optional)

Directions:
1. Warm the tortillas (so they don't break): Run them under water for a second, and then place in an oil-sprayed air fryer basket (stacking them is fine). Fry for 1 minute.
2. Remove to a flat surface, laying them out individually. Place an equal amount of the beans in a line down the center of each tortilla. Top with the vegan cheese.
3. Roll the tortilla sides up over the filling and place seam-side down in the air fryer basket (this will help them seal so the tortillas don't fly open). Add just enough to fill the basket without them touching too much (you may need to do another batch, depending on the size of your air fryer basket).
4. Spray the tops with oil. Fry for 7 minutes, or until the tortillas are golden-brown and lightly crisp. Serve immediately with your preferred toppings.

Nutrition: Calories: 286 Total fat: 9g Saturated fat: 4g Cholesterol: 0mg Sodium: 609mg Carbohydrates: 44g Fiber: 9g Protein: 9g

159. Immune-Boosting Grilled Cheese Sandwich
Preparation Time: 3 minutes

Cooking Time: 12 minutes
Servings: 1
Ingredients:
- 2 slices sprouted whole-grain bread (or substitute a gluten-free bread)
- 1 teaspoon vegan margarine or neutral-flavored oil (sunflower, safflower, or refined coconut)
- 2 slices vegan cheese (Violife cheddar or Chao creamy original) or Cheesy Sauce
- 1 teaspoon mellow white miso
- 1 medium-large garlic clove, pressed or finely minced
- 2 tablespoons fermented vegetables, kimchi, or sauerkraut
- Romaine or green leaf lettuce

Directions:
1. Spread the outsides of the bread with the vegan margarine. Place the sliced cheese inside and close the sandwich back up again (buttered sides facing out). Place the sandwich in the air fryer basket and fry for 6 minutes. Flip over and fry for another 6 minutes, or until nicely browned and crisp on the outside.
2. Transfer to a plate. Open the sandwich and evenly spread the miso and garlic clove over the inside of one of the bread slices. Top with the fermented vegetables and lettuce, close the sandwich back up, cut in half, and serve immediately.

Nutrition: Calories: 288 Total fat: 13g Saturated fat: 5g Cholesterol: 0mg Sodium: 1013mg Carbohydrates: 34g Fiber: 4g Protein: 8g

160. Tamale Pie With Cilantro Lime Cornmeal Crust

Preparation Time: 25 minutes
Cooking Time: 20 minutes
Servings: 4
Ingredients:
For the filling
- 1 medium zucchini, diced (1¼ cups)
- 2 teaspoons neutral-flavored oil (sunflower, safflower, or refined coconut)
- 1 cup cooked pinto beans, drained
- 1 cup canned diced tomatoes (unsalted) with juice
- 3 large garlic cloves, minced or pressed
- 1 tablespoon chickpea flour
- 1 teaspoon dried oregano
- 1 teaspoon onion granules
- ½ teaspoon salt
- ½ teaspoon crushed red chili flakes
- Cooking oil spray (sunflower, safflower, or refined coconut)

For the crust
- ½ cup yellow cornmeal, finely ground
- 1½ cups water
- ½ teaspoon salt
- 1 teaspoon Nutrition yeast
- 1 teaspoon neutral-flavored oil (sunflower, safflower, or refined coconut)
- 2 tablespoons finely chopped cilantro
- ½ teaspoon lime zest (see Cooking Tip)

Directions:
1. To make the filling
2. In a large skillet set to medium-high heat, sauté the zucchini and oil for 3 minutes, or until the zucchini begins to brown.
3. Add the beans, tomatoes, garlic, flour, oregano, onion, salt, and chili flakes to the mixture. Cook over medium heat, stirring often, for 5 minutes, or until the mixture is thickened and no liquid remains. Remove from the heat.
4. Spray a 6-inch round, 2-inch deep baking pan with oil and place the mixture in the bottom. Smooth out the top and set aside.
5. To make the crust
6. 1.In a medium pot over high heat, place the cornmeal, water, and salt. Whisk constantly as you bring the mixture to a boil. Once it boils, reduce the heat to very low. Add the Nutrition yeast and oil and continue to cook, stirring very often, for 10 minutes or until the mixture is very thick and hard to whisk. Remove from the heat.
7. 2.Stir the cilantro and lime zest into the cornmeal mixture until thoroughly combined. Using a rubber spatula, gently spread it evenly onto the filling in the baking pan to form a smooth crust topping. Place in the air fryer basket and bake for 20 minutes, or until the top is golden-brown. Let it cool for 5 to 10 minutes, then cut and serve.

Nutrition: Calories: 165 Total fat: 5g Saturated fat: 1g Cholesterol: 0mg Sodium: 831mg Carbohydrates: 26g Fiber: 6g Protein: 6g

161. Air Fryer Chicken Wings

Preparation Time: 5 minutes
Cooking Time: 20 minutes
Servings: 4
Ingredients:
- 4 (4-oz.) salmon fillets
- 1 tbsp. Grainy mustard
- 2 cloves garlic, finely minced
- 1 tbsp. finely minced shallots
- 2 tsp. fresh thyme leaves, chopped, plus more for garnish
- 2 tsp. fresh rosemary, chopped
- Juice of 1/2 lemon
- kosher salt
- Freshly ground black pepper
- Lemon slices, for serving

Directions:
1. Take the chicken wing parts out of the refrigerator and pat them dry (if you remove as much moisture as possible, you will get a crispy wing skin).
2. Mix sea salt, black pepper, smoked paprika, garlic powder, onion powder and baking powder in a small bowl or baking dish.
3. Sprinkle the spice mixture on the wings and throw it to cover.
4. Place the wings on the cooking basket. In Ninja Foodie this is known as the "Cook & Crisp" basket.
5. Drizzle the chicken wings with olive oil.
6. Use the Air Crisp setting at 400 degrees on air fryers to cook the wings for 14 minutes on each side.
7. Enjoy hot wings!

Nutrition: Calories: 32 kcal Protein: 2 g Fat: 1.73 g Carbohydrates: 2.56 g

162. Parmesan Chicken Wings

Preparation Time: 5 minutes
Cooking Time: 35 minutes
Servings: 5
Ingredients:
- 2 lemons, thinly sliced
- 1 large salmon fillet (about 3 lb.)
- Kosher salt
- Freshly ground black pepper
- 6 tbsp. butter, melted
- 2 tbsp. honey
- 3 cloves garlic, minced

DINNER RECIPES

- 1 tsp. chopped thyme leaves
- 1 tsp. dried oregano
- Chopped fresh parsley, for garnish

Directions:
1. Take the chicken wing parts out of the refrigerator and pat them dry.
2. Mix sea salt, black pepper, bell pepper, garlic powder, onion powder and baking powder in a small bowl.
3. Sprinkle the spice mixture on the wings and throw it to cover.
4. Place the wings on a flat layer in the air fryer.
5. Use the chicken air fryer (400 degrees) and cook for 30 minutes. To make the wings crispy quickly, you have to turn them about halfway.
6. Mix all the ingredients for the garlic parmesan sauce by stirring them in a small bowl.
7. Put the wings in the garlic-parmesan mixture and serve immediately.

Nutrition: Calories: 176 kcal Protein: 2.02 g Fat: 15.19 g Carbohydrates: 9.79 g

163. Buffalo Cauliflower Bites

Preparation Time: 5 minutes
Cooking Time: 25 minutes
Servings: 4

Ingredients:
- 3 tbsp. extra-virgin olive oil, divided
- 3 swordfish steaks
- kosher salt
- Freshly ground black pepper
- 2 pt. multicolored cherry tomatoes, halved
- 1/4 c. red onion, finely chopped
- 3 tbsp. Thinly sliced basil
- Juice of 1/2 a lemon

Directions:
1. Cut the cauliflower into florets of equal size and place in a large bowl.
2. Cut each clove of garlic into 3 pieces and smash them with the side of your knife. Don't be afraid to smash the garlic. You want to expose as much of the garlic surface as possible so that it cooks well. Add this to the cauliflower.
3. Pour over the oil and add salt. Mix well until the cauliflower is well covered with oil and salt.
4. Turn on the air fryer at 400 F for 20 minutes and add the cauliflower. Turn it in half once.
5. To make the Sauce:
6. While the cauliflower is cooking, make the sauce. Whisk the hot sauce, butter and Worcestershire sauce in a small bowl.
7. Once the cauliflower is cooked, place it in a large bowl. Pour the hot sauce over the cauliflower and mix well.
8. Put the cauliflower back in the air fryer. Set it to 400F for 3-4 minutes so the sauce becomes a little firm.
9. Serve with blue cheese dressing.

Nutrition: Calories: 69 kcal Protein: 1.87 g Fat: 6.06 g Carbohydrates: 1.99 g

164. Spicy Dry-Rubbed Chicken Wings

Preparation Time: 5 minutes
Cooking Time: 45 minutes
Servings: 6

Ingredients:
- 4 6-oz. skin-on salmon fillets
- Extra-virgin olive oil, for brushing
- kosher salt
- Freshly ground black pepper
- 2 lemons, sliced
- 2 tbsp. butter

Directions:
1. Marinating the wings:
2. Take the chicken out of the fridge and let it approach room temperature (30 minutes). Preheat the oven to 400 degrees.
3. Place the chicken in a Ziploc sachet with 1/4 cup of the spicy dry massage. You can keep the rest in a mason jar.
4. Shake the bag so that the mixture covers the chicken evenly.
5. Store in the refrigerator for at least four hours, ideally overnight.

Nutrition: Calories: 230 kcal Protein: 31.02 g Fat: 11.54 g Carbohydrates: 1.11 g

165. Air Fryer Steak Bites and Mushrooms

Preparation Time: 5 minutes
Cooking Time: 25 minutes
Servings: 4

Ingredients:
- 2 tbsp. extra-virgin olive oil
- 1 medium onion, chopped
- 1 bell pepper, chopped
- 3 cloves garlic, minced
- 1 tbsp. tomato paste
- 1 lb. Italian sausage
- 1 tbsp. chili powder
- 1 tsp. dried oregano
- 1/2 tsp. garlic powder
- 1/4 tsp. cayenne
- Kosher salt
- Freshly ground black pepper
- 4 large sweet potatoes, peeled and cubed into 1" pieces
- 3 c. low-sodium chicken broth
- 1 (14.5-oz.) can diced tomatoes
- Freshly chopped parsley, for serving

Directions:
1. Preheat the empty air fryer to 390 ° F with a crisp plate or basket for 4 minutes.
2. Pat the meat dry. As the air fryer heats up, throw beef cubes with olive oil and Montreal spices.
3. Halve or halve mushrooms. Pour beef cubes and mushrooms into the preheated air fryer and gently shake to combine.
4. Set the air fryer temperature to 390 ° F and the timer for 8 minutes.
5. Stop after 3 minutes and shake the basket. Repeat this process every 2 minutes until the beef cubes have reached the desired degree of cooking. Lift a large piece out and test it with a meat thermometer or cut and look in the middle to see the progress. Note that the meat will continue to cook as soon as it is removed from the air fryer and resting. Meat is medium at 145 ° F and has a warm pink center.
6. Let the meat rest for a few minutes before serving and then enjoy

Nutrition: Calories: 583 kcal Protein: 32.38 g Fat: 27.25 g Carbohydrates: 61.98 g

166. Pecan Crusted Chicken

Preparation Time: 10 minutes

DINNER RECIPES

Cooking Time: 25 minutes
Servings: 6
Ingredients:
- 3 breakfast sausage patties
- 1 avocado, mashed
- kosher salt
- Freshly ground black pepper
- 3 large eggs
- chives, for garnish
- Hot sauce, if desired

Directions:
1. Place the chicken tenders in a large bowl.
2. Add salt, pepper and smoked paprika and mix well until the chicken is covered with the spices.
3. Pour in honey and mustard and mix well.
4. Place the finely chopped pecans on a plate.
5. Roll the tender into the shredded pecans, one chicken tender at a time, until both sides are covered. Brush off excess material.
6. Place the offers in the air fryer basket and continue until all offers have been coated and are in the air fryer basket.
7. Set the air fryer to 350F for 12 minutes until the chicken is cooked through and the pecans are golden brown before serving.

Nutrition: Calories: 95 kcal Protein: 3.08 g Fat: 8.18 g Carbohydrates: 3.16 g

167. Chicken Tikka Kebab

Preparation Time: 10 minutes
Cooking Time: 30 minutes
Servings: 6
Ingredients:
- 1 bell pepper, sliced into 1/4" rings
- 6 eggs
- kosher salt
- Freshly ground black peppers
- 2 tbsp. Chopped chives
- 2 tbsp. chopped parsley

Directions:
1. Mix all the ingredients for the marinade in a bowl and mix well. Add chicken and spread the marinade on each side. Let it rest in the fridge for between 30 minutes and 8 hours.
2. Add oil, onions, green and red peppers to the marinade for cooking. Mix well.
3. Thread the marinated chicken, peppers and onions into the skewers in between.
4. Lightly grease the air fryer basket.
5. Arrange the chicken sticks in the Air fryer. Cook them at 180 degrees for 10 minutes.
6. Turn the chicken sticks and cook for another 7 minutes, then serve.

Nutrition: Calories: 147 kcal Protein: 10.25 g Fat: 10.68 g Carbohydrates: 1.85 g

168. Air Fryer Brussels sprouts

Preparation Time: 10 minutes
Cooking Time: 15 minutes
Servings: 2
Ingredients:
- 1/4 c. balsamic vinegar
- 3 tbsp. extra-virgin olive oil
- 2 tbsp. brown sugar
- 3 cloves garlic, minced
- 1 tsp. dried thyme
- 1 tsp. dried rosemary
- 4 chicken breasts
- Kosher salt
- Freshly ground black pepper
- Freshly chopped parsley, for garnish

Directions:
1. Preparation: remove the hard ends of the Brussels sprouts and remove any damaged outer leaves. Rinse under cold water and pat dry. If your sprouts are large, cut them in half. Add oil, salt and pepper.
2. Cooking: Arrange Brussels sprouts in a single layer in your air fryer and work in batches if not all fit. Cook for 8 to 12 minutes at 190 ° C and shake the pan halfway through the cooking process to brown it evenly. They are done when they are lightly browned and crispy at the edges.
3. Serving: Serve sprouts warm, optionally with balsamic reduction and parmesan

Nutrition: Calories: 1197 kcal Protein: 125.58 g Fat: 65.97 g Carbohydrates: 16.97 g

169. Crispy Air Fried Tofu

Preparation Time: 10 minutes
Cooking Time: 50 minutes
Servings: 8
Ingredients:
- 2 c. almond flour
- 1/2 tsp. baking soda
- 1/4 tsp. kosher salt
- 1/4 c. butter, room temperature
- 1/4 c. almond butter
- 3 tbsp. honey
- 1 large egg
- 1 tsp. pure vanilla extract
- 1 c. semisweet chocolate chips
- Flaky sea salt

Directions:
1. Squeeze: Squeeze the tofu for at least 15 minutes by placing either a heavy pan or a pan on top and letting the moisture drain. When you're done, cut the tofu into bite-sized blocks and put it in a bowl.
2. Taste: Mix all remaining ingredients in a small bowl. Drizzle over the tofu and toss to cover. Let the tofu marinate for another 15 minutes.
3. Air fryer: Preheat your air fryer to 190 ° C. Add tofu blocks to your air fryer basket in a single layer. Let cook for 10 to 15 minutes and shake the pan occasionally to promote even cooking.

Nutrition: Calories: 247 kcal Protein: 3.83 g Fat: 18.05 g Carbohydrates: 21.99 g

170. Buttermilk Fried Mushrooms

Preparation Time: 5 minutes
Cooking Time: 30 minutes
Servings: 2
Ingredients:
- 1 lb. shrimp
- 2 tbsp. olive oil
- 1 tsp. kosher salt
- 1 tsp. cayenne
- 1 tsp. paprika
- 1 tsp. garlic powder
- 1 tsp. onion powder
- 1 tsp. oregano
- 2 lemons, sliced thinly crosswise

Directions:

1. Marinate: Preheat the air fryer to 190 ° C. Clean the mushrooms and place in a large bowl with buttermilk. Let marinate for 15 minutes.
2. Breading: Mix the flour and spices in a large bowl. Put the mushrooms out of the buttermilk (keep the buttermilk). Dip each mushroom in the flour mixture, shake off excess flour, dip again in the buttermilk and then again in the flour (short: wet> dry> wet> dry).
3. Cooking: Grease the bottom of your air pan well and place the mushrooms in a layer, leaving space between the mushrooms. Let it cook for 5 minutes, then roughly coat all sides with a little oil to promote browning. Cook for another 5 to 10 minutes until golden brown and crispy.

Nutrition: Calories: 380 kcal Protein: 49.65 g Fat: 18.15 g Carbohydrates: 6.86 g

171. Crispy Baked Avocado Tacos

Preparation Time: 10 minutes
Cooking Time: 20 minutes
Servings: 5

Ingredients:
- 6 slices of ham (we used Applegate brand)
- 4 eggs
- 1/4 cup full-fat coconut milk
- 1/4 cup orange bell peppers, chopped
- 1/4 cup red bell peppers, chopped
- 1/4 cup yellow onions, chopped
- Salt & pepper, to taste
- Olive oil or coconut oil to sauté veggies

Directions:
1. Salsa: Combine all the salsa ingredients and put them in the fridge.
2. Prepare avocado: Halve the length of the avocado and remove the pit. Lay the avocado skin face down and cut each half into 4 equal pieces. Then gently peel off the skin.
3. Preparation station: Preheat the oven to 230 ° C or the air fryer to 190 ° C. Arrange your work area so that you have a bowl of flour, a bowl of whisk, a bowl of Panko with S&P, and a baking sheet lined with parchment at the end.
4. Coat: Dip each avocado slice first in the flour, then in the egg and then in the panko. Place on the prepared baking sheet and bake for 10 minutes or fry in the air. Lightly brown after half of the cooking process.
5. Sauce: While cooking avocados, combine all the sauce ingredients.
6. Serve: Put salsa on a tortilla, top with 2 pieces of avocado and drizzle with sauce. Serve immediately and enjoy!

Nutrition: Calories: 193 kcal Protein: 13.7 g Fat: 13.25 g Carbohydrates: 4.69 g

172. Buttery Cod

Preparation Time: 5 minutes
Cooking Time: 15 minutes
Servings: 4

Ingredients:
- 1 tbsp. Parsley, chopped
- 3 tbsp. Butter, melted
- 8 Cherry tomatoes, halved
- 0.25 cup Tomato sauce
- 2 Cod fillets, cubed

Directions:
1. Turn on the air fryer to 390 degrees.
2. Combine all of the ingredients and put them into a pan that works with the air fryer.
3. After 12 minutes of baking, you can divide this between the four bowls and enjoy.

Nutrition: Calories 232 Carbs 5g Protein 11g Fat 8g

173. Creamy Chicken

Preparation Time: 10 minutes
Cooking Time: 15 minutes
Servings: 4

Ingredients:
- Pepper and salt
- 1 tsp. Olive oil
- 0.5 tsp. Sweet paprika
- 0.25 cup Coconut cream
- 4 Chicken breasts, cubed

Directions:
1. Turn on the air fryer to 370 degrees.
2. Prepare a pan that fits into the machine with some oil before adding the ingredients inside.
3. Add this to the air fryer and let it bake. After 17 minutes, you can divide between the few plates and serve!

Nutrition: Calories 250 Carbs 5g Protein 11g Fat 12g

174. Mushroom and Turkey Stew

Preparation Time: 25 minutes
Cooking Time: 25 minutes
Servings: 4

Ingredients:
- Pepper and salt
- 1 tbsp. Parsley, chopped
- 0.25 cup Tomato sauce
- 1 Turkey breast, cubed
- 0.5 lb. Brown mushrooms, sliced

Directions:
1. Turn on the air fryer to 350 degrees.
2. Pick out a pan and mix the tomato sauce, pepper, salt, mushrooms, and turkey together. Add to the air fryer.
3. After 25 minutes, the stew is done—divide between four bowls and top with the parsley.

Nutrition: Calories 220 Carbs 5g Fat 12g Protein 12g

175. Basil Chicken

Preparation Time: 15 minutes
Cooking Time: 25 minutes
Servings: 4

Ingredients:
- Pepper and salt
- 2 tsp. Smoked paprika
- 0.5 tsp. Dried basil
- 0.5 cup Chicken stock
- 0.5 lb. Chicken breasts, cubed

Directions:
1. Turn on the air fryer to 390 degrees.
2. Bring out a pan and toss the ingredients inside before putting it into the air fryer.
3. After 25 minutes of baking, divide this between a few plates and serve with a side salad.

Nutrition: Calories 223 Carbs 5g Protein 13g Fat 12g

176. Eggplant Bake

Preparation Time: 20 minutes
Cooking Time: 15 minutes
Servings: 4

Ingredients:
- 2 tsp. Olive oil (2 tsp)
- Pepper and salt
- 4 Spring onions, chopped
- 1 Hot chili pepper, chopped

DINNER RECIPES

- 2 Eggplants, cubed
- 4 Garlic cloves, minced
- 0.5 cup Cilantro, chopped
- 0.5 lb. Cherry tomatoes, cubed

Directions:
1. Turn on the air fryer and let it heat up to 380 degrees.
2. Prepare a baking pan that will go into the air fryer and mix all of the ingredients onto it.
3. Place into the air fryer to cook. After 15 minutes, divide between four bowls and serve.

Nutrition: Calories 232 Carbs 5g Fat 12g Protein 10g

177. Meatball Casserole
Preparation Time: 15 minutes
Cooking Time: 15 minutes
Servings: 6
Ingredients:
- 1 tbsp. Thyme, chopped
- 0.25 cup Parsley, chopped
- 0.33 lb. Turkey sausage
- 1 Egg, beaten
- 0.66 lb. Ground beef
- 2 tbsp. Olive oil
- 1 Shallot, minced
- 1 tbsp. Dijon mustard
- 3 Garlic cloves, minced
- 2 tbsp. Whole milk
- 1 tbsp. Rosemary, chopped

Directions:
1. Turn on the air fryer to a High setting and then give it time to heat up with some oil inside.
2. Add the garlic and onions and cook for a few minutes to make soft.
3. Add the milk and bread crumbs to a bowl and then mix. Then add in the rest of the ingredients and set aside to soak.
4. Use this mixture, after five minutes, to prepare some small meatballs. Add these to the air fryer.
5. Turn the heat up to 400 degrees to cook. After 10 minutes, take the lid off and shake the basket. Cook another five minutes before serving.

Nutrition: Calories 168 Carbs 4g Protein 12g Fat 11g

178. Herbed Lamb Rack
Preparation Time: 10 minutes
Cooking Time: 10 minutes
Servings: 2
Ingredients:
- 4 tbsp. Olive oil
- 0.5 tsp. Pepper
- 1 tbsp. Dried thyme
- 2 tbsp. Dried rosemary
- 0.5 tsp. Salt
- 2 tsp. Garlic, minced
- 1 lb. Rack of lamb

Directions:
1. Turn on the air fryer to 400 degrees. In a bowl, combine the herbs and olive oil well.
2. Use this to coat the lamb before adding to the basket of the air fryer.
3. Close the lid, and then let this cook. Halfway through, you can shake the basket to make sure nothing sticks.
4. After ten minutes, take the lamb out and enjoy.

Nutrition: Calories 542 Carbs 3g Fat 37g Protein 45g

179. Baked Beef
Preparation Time: 1 hour
Cooking Time: 1 hour
Servings: 3
Ingredients:
- 1 bunch Garlic cloves
- 1 bunch Fresh herbs, mixed
- 2 Onions, sliced
- Olive oil
- 3 lbs. Beef
- 2 Celery sticks, chopped
- 2 Carrots, chopped

Directions:
1. Great up a pan and then add the herbs, olive oil, beef roast, and vegetables inside.
2. Turn the air fryer on to 400 degrees and place the pan inside. Let this heat up and close the lid.
3. After an hour of cooking, open the lid and then serve this right away.

Nutrition: Calories 306 Carbs 10g Fat 21g Protein 32g

180. Crispy Pork Chops
Preparation Time: 15 minutes
Cooking Time: 15 minutes
Servings: 6
Ingredients:
- Salt
- 0.5 tsp Onion powder
- 0.25 tsp. Chili powder
- 0.25 tsp. Pepper
- 1 tsp. Smoked paprika
- 1 cup Pork rind
- 3 tbsp. Parmesan, grated
- 5 Boneless pork chops
- 2 Beaten eggs

Directions:
1. Use the pepper and salt to season the pork chops. Blend the rind to make some crumbs.
2. In another bowl, beat the eggs and then coat this onto the pork chops with the crumbs.
3. Take out the air fryer and set it to 400 degrees to heat up.
4. When this is done, add the pork chops into the air fryer and let it heat up. When this is halfway done, flip the pork chops over and cook a little more.
5. After 15 minutes of cooking, turn off the air fryer and serve.

Nutrition: Calories 391 Carbs 17g Fat 18g Protein 38g

181. Turkey Pillows
Preparation Time: 15 minutes
Cooking Time: 15 minutes
Servings: 4
Ingredients:
- 15 slices Turkey breast
- 2 jars Cream cheese
- 1 Egg yolk
- 4 cup Flour
- 0.5 tbsp. Dried granular yeast
- 2 tbsp. Sugar
- 0.75 tsp. Salt
- 0.35 cup Olive oil
- 0.33 cup Water
- 1 cup Milk with an egg inside

Directions:

1. Mix the ingredients for the dough with your hands until smooth. Make it into small balls and put on a floured surface.
2. Open the dough balls with a roller to make it square. Cut into small pieces. Fill with the turkey breast and a bit of cream cheese. Close the points together.
3. Turn on the air fryer to 400 degrees. Place a few of the balls inside and let them cook.
4. After five minutes, take these out and repeat with the rest of the pillows until done.

Nutrition: Calories 528 Carbs 23g Fat 30g Protein 44g

182. Chicken Wings

Preparation Time: 20 minutes
Cooking Time: 25 minutes
Servings: 2
Ingredients:
- 2 tbsp. Chives
- 0.5 tbsp. Salt
- 1 tbsp. Lime
- 0.5 tbsp. Ginger, chopped
- 1 tbsp. Garlic, minced
- 1 tbsp. Chili paste
- 2 tbsp. Honey
- 0.5 tbsp. Cornstarch
- 1 tbsp. Soy sauce
- Oil
- 10 Chicken wings

Directions:
1. Dry the chicken and then cover it with spray. Add into the air fryer that is preheated to 400 degrees.
2. Let this cook for a bit. During that time, add the rest of the ingredients to a bowl and set aside.
3. After 25 minutes, the chicken is done. Add the chicken into a bowl and top with the sauce. Sprinkle the chives on top and serve.

Nutrition: Calories 81 Carbs 0g Fat 5g Protein 8g

183. Chicken Cordon Bleu

Preparation Time: 60 minutes
Cooking Time: 40 minutes
Servings: 6
Ingredients:
- 1 Garlic clove
- 2 Eggs
- 2 tsp. Butter, melted
- 1 cup Bread, ground
- 0.25 cup Flour
- 2 tsp. Fresh thyme
- 16 slices Swiss cheese
- 8 slices Ham
- 4 Chicken breasts

Directions:
1. Turn on the air fryer to heat to 350 degrees.
2. Flatten out the chicken and then fill with two slices of cheese, ham, and then cheese again. Roll up and use a toothpick to keep together.
3. Mix the garlic, thyme, and bread together with the butter. Beat the eggs and season the flour with pepper and salt.
4. Pass the chicken rolls through the flour, then the egg, and then the breadcrumbs. Add to the air fryer to cook.
5. After 20 minutes, take the chicken out and cool down before serving.

Nutrition: Calories 387 Carbs 18g Fat 20g Protein 33g

184. Fried Chicken

Preparation Time: 20 minutes
Cooking Time: 25 minutes
Servings: 4
Ingredients:
- 1 Lemon
- 1 Ginger, grated
- Ground pepper, salt, and garlic powder
- 1 lb. Chopped chicken

Directions:
1. Add the chicken to a bowl with the rest of the ingredients. Let it set for a bit to marinate.
2. After 15 minutes, add some oil to the air fryer and let it heat up to 320 degrees.
3. Add the chicken inside to cook for 25 minutes, shaking it a few times to cook through. Serve warm.

Nutrition: Calories 345 Carbs 23g Fat 3g Protein 3g

185. Sesame Chicken

Preparation Time: 1 hour
Cooking Time: 50 minutes
Servings: 4
Ingredients:
- Soy sauce
- Pepper
- Salt
- Olive oil
- Breadcrumbs
- Egg
- 1 lb. Chicken breast

Directions:
1. Slice the chicken into fillets and add to the bowl with the sesame and soy sauce. Let this marinate for half an hour.
2. Beat the eggs and then pass the chicken through it.
3. Add to the grill of the air fryer at 350 degrees. Let it grill for a bit.
4. After 20 minutes, take the chicken off and let it cool down before serving.

Nutrition: Calories 375 Carbs 6g Fat 18g Protein 35g

186. Chicken and Potatoes

Preparation Time: 1 hour
Cooking Time: 55 minutes
Servings: 2
Ingredients:
- Pepper and salt
- Provencal herbs
- 2 Chicken pieces
- 4 Potatoes
- Olive oil

Directions:
1. Peel the skin from the potatoes and cut into slices. Add some pepper and place into the air fryer.
2. Preheat to 340 degrees. Cover the chicken with the herbs, pepper, salt, and oil and add it in with the potatoes.
3. Cook this until well done. After forty minutes, turn the chicken around and let it cook another 15 minutes before serving.

Nutrition: Calories 200 Carbs 18g Fat 4g Protein 22g

187. Coconut-Crusted Chicken Tenders

Preparation Time: 15 minutes
Cooking Time: 8 minutes
Servings: 4
Ingredients:
- 3 Eggs

- 1 lb. Chicken tenders
- 1 cup Cornstarch
- 2 cups. Sweetened shredded coconut
- 1 tsp. Cayenne pepper

Directions:
1. Set the Air Fryer temperature at 360° Fahrenheit.
2. Prepare three dishes. In the first one, add the cornstarch and cayenne with any other desired seasonings. In the second bowl, add the eggs. Lastly, add the coconut in the third dish.
3. Dredge the chicken through the cornstarch, egg, and coconut.
4. Lightly spritz the fryer basket with a cooking oil spray as needed.
5. Set the timer for 8 minutes and air-fry until it's golden brown before serving.

Nutrition: Calories: 390 kcal Protein: 32.38 g Fat: 12.14 g Carbohydrates: 34.67 g

188. Crispy Chicken Sliders

Preparation Time: 10 minutes
Cooking Time: 8 minutes
Servings: 6

Ingredients:
- 1 pkg. Tyson Crispy Chicken Strips
- 1 pkg. Sweet Hawaiian Rolls
- Optional Ingredients:
- Spinach leaves
- Tomatoes
- Honey mustard

Directions:
1. Place the six chicken strips in the Air Fryer basket with a coating of olive oil spray. Cook at 390° Fahrenheit for 8 minutes.
2. Slice the rolls in half and top them with honey mustard, spinach, and tomatoes or other toppings of your choice.
3. Slice the chicken strips into chunks and place them on the rolls.

Nutrition: Calories: 53 kcal Protein: 3.9 g Fat: 3.27 g Carbohydrates: 1.87 g

189. Garlic Herb Turkey Breast

Preparation Time: 1 hour
Cooking Time: 40 minutes
Servings: 6

Ingredients:
- 2 lb. Turkey breast
- 4 tbsp. Melted butter
- 3 cloves Garlic
- 1 tsp. Thyme
- 1 tsp. Rosemary

Directions:
1. Warm the Air Fryer to reach 375° Fahrenheit.
2. Pat the turkey breast dry. Mince the garlic and chop the rosemary and thyme.
3. Melt the butter and mix with the garlic, thyme, and rosemary in a small mixing bowl. Brush the butter over turkey breast.
4. Place in the Air Fryer basket, skin side up, and cook for 40 minutes or until internal temperature reaches 160° Fahrenheit, flipping halfway through.
5. Wait for five minutes before slicing.

Nutrition: Calories: 321 kcal Protein: 34.35 g Fat: 19.32 g Carbohydrates: 0.56 g

190. Honey-Lime Chicken Wings

Preparation Time: 20 minutes
Cooking Time: 30 minutes
Servings: 4

Ingredients:
- 2 lb. Chicken wings
- 2 tbsp. Lime juice
- .25 cup Honey
- 1 tbsp. Lime zest
- 1 pressed Garlic clove

Directions:
1. Warm the Air Fryer at 360° Fahrenheit.
2. Whisk the garlic, honey, and lime juice and zest. Toss in the wings and cover with the mixture.
3. Prepare the wings in batches. Cook for 25-30 minutes until they're crispy. Shake the basket at 8-minute intervals.
4. Serve and garnish as desired.

Nutrition: Calories: 375 kcal Protein: 51.59 g Fat: 9.56 g Carbohydrates: 18.67 g

191. Rotisserie-Style, Whole Chicken

Preparation Time: 50 minutes
Cooking Time: 30 minutes
Servings: 4

Ingredients:
- 2 tsp. Olive oil, as needed
- 6-7 lb. Whole chicken
- 1 tbsp. Seasoned salt

Directions:
1. Set the Air Fryer at 350° Fahrenheit.
2. Coat the chicken with oil and a sprinkle of salt.
3. Arrange the chicken in the Air Fryer – skin-side down.
4. Cook for 30 minutes. Flip the chicken over and air-fry for another 30 minutes.
5. Wait for ten minutes before slicing.

Note: This recipe is for chickens under 6 lb. for a 3.7-quart Air Fryer.

Nutrition: Calories: 859 kcal Protein: 151.45 g Fat: 23.67 g Carbohydrates: 0 g

192. Tarragon Chicken

Preparation Time: 15 minutes
Cooking Time: 12 minutes
Servings: 1

Ingredients:
- 1 Skinless/boneless chicken breast
- .125 tsp. freshly cracked ground black pepper
- .5 tsp. Unsalted butter
- .125 tsp. kosher salt
- .25 cup dried tarragon
- Also Needed: Aluminum foil (12x14-inch piece)

Directions:
1. Warm the oven in advance to reach 390° Fahrenheit.
2. Arrange the chicken in the foil with the tarragon, butter, salt, and pepper.
3. Loosely wrap the foil for minimal airflow.
4. Air-fry the chicken packs for 12 minutes in the basket.

Nutrition: Calories: 101 kcal Protein: 6.53 g Fat: 8.02 g Carbohydrates: 0.53 g

193. Beef and Potato

Preparation Time: 5 minutes
Cooking Time: 2 minutes
Servings: 4

Ingredients:
- 3 cups Mashed potatoes
- 1 lb. Ground beef

- 2 Eggs
- 2 tbsp. Garlic powder
- 1 cup Sour cream

Directions:
1. Set the Air Fryer to reach 390º Fahrenheit.
2. Combine all of the fixings in a mixing container. Scoop it into a heat-safe dish.
3. Arrange in the fryer to cook for two minutes.
4. Serve for lunch or a quick dinner.

Nutrition: Calories: 509 kcal Protein: 41.36 g Fat: 25.15 g Carbohydrates: 27.77 g

194. Beef Roll-Ups
Preparation Time: 20 minutes
Cooking Time: 25 minutes
Servings: 4

Ingredients:
- 6 slices Provolone cheese
- 2 lbs. Beef flank steak
- 3 tbsp. Pesto
- .75 cup Baby spinach
- 3 oz. roasted red bell peppers

Directions:
1. Heat the Air Fryer at 400º Fahrenheit.
2. Slice the steak. Add the pesto and butter evenly on the meat.
3. Layer in the spinach, peppers, and cheese about ¾ of the way down through the roll-up. Roll the mixture. Secure it with skewers or toothpicks.
4. Air-fry for 14 minutes. Turn the beef halfway through the cooking process.
5. Wait for at least ten minutes before slicing to serve.

Nutrition: Calories: 550 kcal Protein: 62.48 g Fat: 30.7 g Carbohydrates: 2.88 g

195. Breaded Beef Schnitzel
Preparation Time: 15 minutes
Cooking Time: 12 minutes
Servings: 1

Ingredients:
- 2 tbsp. Olive oil
- 1 Thin beef schnitzel
- .5 cup Gluten-free breadcrumbs
- 1 Egg

Directions:
1. Heat the Air Fryer a couple of minutes (356º Fahrenheit).
2. Combine the breadcrumbs and oil in a shallow bowl. Whisk the egg in another mixing container.
3. Dip the beef into the egg, and then the breadcrumbs. Arrange in the basket of the Air Fryer.
4. Air-fry 12 minutes and serve.

Nutrition: Calories: 126 kcal Protein: 4.13 g Fat: 10.76 g Carbohydrates: 3.34 g

196. Cheeseburger 'Mini' Sliders
Preparation Time: 15 minutes
Cooking Time: 10 minutes
Servings: 1

Ingredients:
- 6 slices Cheddar cheese
- 1 lb. Ground beef
- Freshly cracked black pepper and salt (as desired)
- 6 Dinner rolls

Directions:
1. Warm the Air Fryer ahead of fry time to 390º Fahrenheit.
2. Shape six (2.5-oz.) patties and dust with the pepper and salt
3. Arrange the burgers in the fryer basket and cook for ten minutes.
4. Take them out of the cooker and add the cheese.
5. Return them to the basket for another minute until the cheese melts.

Nutrition: Calories: 382 kcal Protein: 35.62 g Fat: 16.77 g Carbohydrates: 20.38 g

197. Quick and Easy Rib Eye Steak
Preparation Time: 40 minutes
Cooking Time: 35 minutes
Servings: 2

Ingredients:
- 2 lb. Unchilled steak
- 1 tbsp. Olive oil
- Steak Rub: Salt and pepper mix (desired)
- Baking pan also needed to fit into the basket

Directions:
1. Press the "M" button for the French Fries icon. Adjust the time to four minutes at 400º Fahrenheit.
2. Rub the steak with the oil and seasonings. Arrange the steak in the basket and air-fry for 14 minutes. (Flip it over after seven minutes.)
3. Place the rib eye on a platter, and let it rest for ten minutes.
4. Slice it and garnish the way you like it.

Nutrition: Calories: 1017 kcal Protein: 129.44 g Fat: 55.78 g Carbohydrates: 0 g

198. Roast Beef
Preparation Time: 1 hour
Cooking Time: 55 minutes
Servings: 6

Ingredients:
- .5 tsp. Garlic powder
- .5 tsp. Oregano
- 1 tsp. Dried thyme
- 1 tbsp. Olive oil
- 2 lb. Round roast

Directions:
1. Heat the Air Fryer at 330º Fahrenheit.
2. Combine the spices. Brush the oil over the beef, and rub it using the spice mixture.
3. Add to a baking dish and arrange it in the Air Fryer basket for 30 minutes. Turn it over and continue cooking 25 more minutes.
4. Wait for a few minutes before slicing.
5. Serve on your choice of bread or plain with a delicious side dish.

Nutrition: Calories: 287 kcal Protein: 45.97 g Fat: 10.01 g Carbohydrates: 0.28 g

199. Sweet and Spicy Montreal Steak
Preparation Time: 30 minutes
Cooking Time: 6 minutes
Servings: 2

Ingredients:
- 2 boneless Sirloin steaks
- 1 tbsp. Brown sugar
- 1 tbsp. Montreal steak seasoning
- 1 tsp. Crushed red pepper
- 1 tbsp. Olive oil

Directions:
1. Set the temperature of the Air Fryer at 390º Fahrenheit.

2. Prepare the steaks with oil. Rub them with the desired seasonings.
3. Arrange the steaks in the basket and set the timer for three minutes.
4. Flip the steak over and air-fry for another three minutes.
5. Cool and slice it into strips before serving.

Nutrition: Calories: 1253 kcal Protein: 126.25 g Fat: 75.9 g Carbohydrates: 6.58 g

200. Bacon-Wrapped Pork Tenderloin

Preparation Time: 1 hour
Cooking Time:
Servings: 4 to 6
Ingredients:
- 1 lb. Pork tenderloin
- 1-2 tbsp. Dijon mustard
- 3-4 strips Bacon

Directions:
1. Set the Air Fryer temperature at 360° Fahrenheit.
2. Coat the tenderloin with the mustard and wrap with the bacon.
3. Air-fry them for 15 minutes. Flip and cook 10 to 15 more minutes.
4. Serve with your favorite sides.

Nutrition: Calories: 133 kcal Protein: 21.31 g Fat: 4.65 g Carbohydrates: 0.41 g

201. Bratwurst and Veggies

Preparation Time: 10 minutes
Cooking Time: 20 minutes
Servings: 2
Ingredients:
- 1 pkg. Bratwurst
- 1 each Red and green bell pepper
- .25 cup Onion - red or purple
- 5 tbsp. Gluten-free Cajun seasoning

Directions:
1. Warm the unit to reach 390° Fahrenheit.
2. Line the Air Fryer with foil, if preferred.
3. Slice and add in the vegetables.
4. Slice the bratwurst into about 0.5-inch size rounds, and place on top of the veggies.
5. Evenly sprinkle the seasoning on top.
6. Air-fry for 10 minutes. Carefully open and stir or mix.
7. Air-fry for another 10 minutes before serving.

Nutrition: Calories: 84 kcal Protein: 1.57 g Fat: 0.06 g Carbohydrates: 15.89 g

202. Crispy Dumplings

Preparation Time: 10 minutes
Cooking Time: 8 minutes
Servings: 2
Ingredients:
- .5 lb. Ground pork
- 1 tbsp. Olive oil
- .5 tsp. each Black pepper and salt
- Half of 1 pkg. Dumpling wrappers

Directions:
1. Set the Air Fryer temperature setting at 390° Fahrenheit.
2. Mix the fixings together.
3. Prepare each dumpling using two teaspoons of the pork mixture.
4. Seal the edges with a portion of water to make the triangle form.
5. Lightly spritz the Air Fryer basket using a cooking oil spray as needed. Add the dumplings to air-fry for eight minutes.
6. Serve when they're ready.

Nutrition: Calories: 442 kcal Protein: 32.56 g Fat: 33.36 g Carbohydrates: 1.06 g

203. Spicy Green Crusted Chicken

Preparation Time: 10 minutes
Cooking Time: 40 minutes
Servings: 4
Ingredients:
- 4 whole eggs, beaten
- 4 teaspoons parsley
- 3 teaspoons thyme
- 3 teaspoons paprika
- ¾ pound chicken pieces
- Salt and pepper, to taste
- 4 teaspoons oregano

Directions:
1. Preheat your air fryer to 360 degrees F.
2. Grease the air fryer cooking basket.
3. Crack eggs in a bowl and whisk well, take another bowl and mix all of the ingredients except chicken pieces.
4. Dip chicken in eggs and then into the dry mixture.
5. Transfer half of the chicken pieces to your air fryer and cook for 20 minutes.
6. Keep repeating until all ingredients are used up.
7. Enjoy!

Nutrition: Calories: 393 Total Fat: 22g Total Carbs: 7g Fiber: 1g Net Carbs: 4g Protein: 39g

204. Cheesy Chicken Drumsticks

Preparation Time: 18 minutes
Cooking Time: 15 minutes
Servings: 2
Ingredients:
- 1-pound small chicken drumsticks, bone-in
- 2 tablespoons almond flour
- 1 cup mixed cheese, grated
- 1 teaspoon dried rosemary
- 1 teaspoon dried oregano
- ½ teaspoon chili flakes
- ½ teaspoon salt
- ½ teaspoon pepper
- Chopped green onion for garnish

Directions:
1. Rinse drumsticks thoroughly and pat them dry.
2. Take a medium-sized bowl and add flour, mixed cheese, herbs, chili flakes, salt, and pepper.
3. Dip drumsticks in the mixture and turn them well, keep in the freezer for 5 minutes.
4. Spray air fryer cooking basket with cooking spray and preheat your fryer to 370 degrees F.
5. Transfer drumsticks to your fryer and cook for 15 minutes, making sure to shake the basket halfway through.
6. Transfer to a serving plate, and enjoy with your garnish!

Nutrition: Calories: 226 Total Fat: 10g Total Carbs: 4g Fiber: 1g Net Carbs: 2g Protein: 16g

205. Jamaican Pork Roast

Preparation Time: 10 minutes
Cooking Time: 50 minutes
Servings: 8
Ingredients:
- 2 tablespoons olive oil

- 2 pounds pork shoulder
- ¼ cup beef broth
- ¼ cup Jamaican jerk spice blend

Directions:
1. Marinate pork using the Jamaican jerk spice blend and olive oil, let it sit for 10 minutes.
2. Preheat your air fryer to 440 degrees F.
3. Add marinated pork to air fryer and cook for 2 minutes.
4. Add beef broth, cook for 45 minutes more.
5. Serve and enjoy!

Nutrition: Calories: 362 Total Fat: 27g Total Carbs: 10g Fiber: 2g Net Carbs: 6g Protein: 26g

206. Lime Chicken

Preparation Time: 5 minutes
Cooking Time: 15-20 minutes
Servings: 3

Ingredients:
- 16 chicken wings
- 2 tablespoons light coconut aminos
- 2 tablespoons agave nectar
- 2 tablespoons lemon juice
- Pinch of salt
- Pinch of pepper
- Sesame seeds for garnish

Directions:
1. Wash the chicken thoroughly under cold water.
2. Take a large bowl and add coconut aminos, agave, lemon juice, salt, pepper, and stir.
3. Pour the mixture into a Ziploc bag and add the wings, massage gently.
4. Let it refrigerate for 2 hours.
5. Preheat your air fryer to 350 degrees F, lightly spray the cooking basket with Keto-Friendly cooking oil and add the chicken to the basket.
6. Cook for 6 minutes, flip and cook for 6 minutes more.
7. Cook for 3 minutes more at 390 degrees F.
8. Serve with a garnish of sesame seeds, enjoy!

Nutrition: Calories: 42 Total Fat: 72g Total Carbs: 13g Fiber: 2g Net Carbs: 4g Protein: 38g

207. Swiss Bacon Pork Chops

Preparation Time: 5 minutes
Cooking Time: 40 minutes
Servings: 8

Ingredients:
- 2 tablespoons butter
- Salt and pepper to taste
- 12 bacon strips, cut in half
- 8 pork chops, bone-in
- 1 cup Swiss cheese, shredded

Directions:
1. Preheat your air fryer to 450 degrees F.
2. Grease air fryer cooking basket.
3. Season pork chops with salt and pepper, top with bacon strips and Swiss cheese.
4. Transfer to air fryer cooking basket and cook for 40 minutes.
5. Serve and enjoy!

Nutrition: Calories: 483 Total Fat: 40g Total Carbs: 4g Fiber: 1g, Net Carbs: 2g, Protein: 28g

208. Mustard Pork Chops

Preparation Time: 10 minutes
Cooking Time: 40 minutes
Servings: 6

Ingredients:
- 3 tablespoons Dijon mustard
- Salt and pepper to taste
- 6 pork chops
- 1½ tablespoons fresh rosemary, coarsely chopped
- 3 tablespoons butter

Directions:
1. Preheat your air fryer to 450 degrees F.
2. Grease air fryer cooking basket with butter.
3. Marinate pork chops with Dijon mustard, fresh rosemary, salt, pepper and let it marinate for 3 hours.
4. Transfer the chops to the air fryer cooking basket and cook for 40 minutes.
5. Serve and enjoy!

Nutrition: Calories: 315 Total Fat: 26g Total Carbs: 4g Fiber: 1g Net Carbs: 1g Protein: 20g

209. Buttery Scallops

Preparation Time: 10 minutes
Cooking Time: 10 minutes
Servings: 6

Ingredients:
- 2 pounds sea scallops
- 3 tablespoons butter, melted
- 2 tablespoons fresh thyme, minced
- Salt and pepper, to taste

Directions:
1. Preheat your air fryer to 390 degrees F, grease air fryer cooking basket with butter.
2. Take a bowl, mix in all of the remaining ingredients, and toss well to coat the scallops.
3. Transfer scallops to the air fryer cooking basket and cook for 5 minutes.
4. Repeat if any ingredients are left, serve and enjoy!

Nutrition: Calories: 186 Total Fat: 24g Total Carbs: 4g Fiber: 1g Net Carbs: 2g Protein: 20g

210. Herbed Buttery Chicken

Preparation Time: 5 minutes
Cooking Time: 25 minutes
Servings: 6

Ingredients:
- 1 cup butter
- 1 teaspoon black pepper
- 4 garlic cloves, minced
- 2 pounds chicken breasts
- 1 teaspoon salt
- ½ cup parsley chopped
- 1 teaspoon ginger powder
- 4 tablespoons lemon juice
- 1 cup baby spinach

Directions:
1. Preheat your air fryer to 450 degrees F.
2. Grease the air fryer cooking basket.
3. Take a bowl and mix in butter, garlic, parsley, ginger powder, lemon juice.
4. Season chicken breasts thoroughly with salt and pepper; transfer them to the air fryer cooking basket.
5. Top with baby spinach and butter mixture.
6. Cook for 25 minutes, serve and enjoy!

Nutrition: Calories: 427 Total Fat: 31g Total Carbs: 3g Fiber: 1g Net Carbs: 1g Protein: 35g

211. Coconut Crusted Prawns

Preparation Time: 5 minutes
Cooking Time: 6 minutes
Servings: 3

DINNER RECIPES

Ingredients:
- 12 large raw prawns, peeled and deveined
- Salt and pepper, to taste
- 1 cup egg white
- 1 cup dried unsweetened coconut
- ½ cup almond flour
- 4 tablespoons butter

Directions:
1. Preheat your air fryer to 400 degrees F for 5 minutes.
2. Season prawns with salt and pepper.
3. Transfer all ingredients to Ziploc bag and shake until combined well.
4. Transfer the ingredients to your air fryer cooking basket.
5. Cook for 6 minutes at 400 degrees F.
6. Serve and enjoy!

Nutrition: Calories: 497 Total Fat: 43g Total Carbs: 11g Fiber: 2g Net Carbs: 4g Protein: 19g

212. Turmeric Beef

Preparation Time: 10 minutes
Cooking Time: 30 minutes
Servings: 4

Ingredients:
- 2 pounds beef, steak pieces
- 2 cups yogurt
- 4 tablespoons salt
- 6 tablespoons olive oil
- 4 tablespoons turmeric powder
- 4 tablespoons coriander powder
- 4 tablespoons cumin powder
- 4 tablespoons red chili powder
- 4 tablespoons lemon juice

Directions:
1. Marinate beef pieces overnight in a mixture of cumin, yogurt, red chili powder, salt, lemon juice, coriander, vinegar, turmeric, and oil.
2. Preheat your air fryer to 450 degrees F.
3. Transfer marinated beefsteaks to air fryer.
4. Cook for 30 minutes.
5. Serve and enjoy!

Nutrition: Calories: 362 Total Fat: 28g Total Carbs: 8g Fiber: 1g Net Carbs: 6g Protein: 40g

213. Beef Tongue

Preparation Time: 10 minutes
Cooking Time: 20 minutes
Servings: 3

Ingredients:
- 1-pound beef tongue
- 1 teaspoon paprika
- 1 tablespoon butter
- Pinch of salt
- Pinch of pepper

Directions:
1. Rinse the beef tongues thoroughly under cold water.
2. Take a pot and add 4 cups of water, place it over a stove and add the tongues.
3. Simmer over low heat for 30 minutes.
4. Remove tongues from water and let them cool, slice into strips.
5. Take a microwave proof bowl and melt butter, add the tongues to the butter.
6. Season with salt, paprika, and pepper.
7. Preheat your air fryer to 350 degrees F.
8. Transfer beef tongues to the air fryer and cook for 20 minutes.
9. Transfer to a platter, serve and enjoy!

Nutrition: Calories: 234 Total Fat: 18g Total Carbs: 6g Fiber: 2g Net Carbs: 3g Protein: 16g

214. Crispy Parmesan Crusted Pork Chops

Preparation Time: 10 minutes
Cooking Time: 20 minutes
Servings: 4

Ingredients:
- ½ teaspoon salt
- ½ teaspoon onion powder
- 4 thick pork chops, center-cut boneless
- ¼ teaspoon pepper
- 1 teaspoon smoked paprika
- ¼ teaspoon chili powder
- 1 cup pork rind crumbs
- 2 large eggs, beaten
- 3 tablespoons Parmesan cheese, grated

Directions:
1. Preheat your air fryer to 400 degrees F.
2. Season pork chops with salt and pepper.
3. Take a bowl and mix in pork rind crumbs, Parmesan cheese, seasoning.
4. Place beaten eggs in another bowl.
5. Dip each pork chop into the egg mix, then in crumb mix.
6. Transfer to air fryer and cook for 20 minutes.
7. Serve and enjoy!

Nutrition: Calories: 271 Total Fat: 12g Total Carbs: 4g Fiber: 1g Net Carbs: 2g Protein: 28g

215. Easy Air Fried Catfish

Preparation Time: 5 minutes
Cooking Time: 15 minutes
Servings: 4

Ingredients:
- 4 catfish fillets
- Salt and pepper to taste
- 1 large egg, beaten
- 1/4 cup almond flour
- 4 tablespoons olive oil

Directions:
1. Preheat your air fryer to 350 degrees F.
2. Season catfish fillets generously with salt and pepper.
3. Soak the fillets in beaten eggs and dredge in almond flour.
4. Brush surface with olive oil, transfer fillets to the Ari Fryer cooking basket and cook for 15 minutes.
5. Serve and enjoy!

Nutrition: Calories: 382 Total Fat: 28g Total Carbs: 4g Fiber: 1g Net Carbs: 2g Protein: 29g

216. Lemon Fish Fillet

Preparation Time: 5 minutes
Cooking Time: 15 minutes
Servings: 4

Ingredients:
- 4 salmon fish fillets
- 1 lemon
- Salt and pepper, to taste
- 2 tablespoons olive oil
- 1 large egg, beaten
- ½ cup almond flour

Directions:
1. Preheat your air fryer to 400 degrees F for 5 minutes.
2. Season salmon fillets with oil, lemon, salt, and pepper.

3. Soak the fillets in beaten egg and dredge them in almond flour.
4. Transfer fillets to the air fryer cooking basket and cook for 15 minutes.
5. Serve and enjoy!

Nutrition: Calories: 628 Total Fat: 23g Total Carbs: 11g Fiber: 1g Net Carbs: 7g Protein: 43g

217. Pork Carnitas

Preparation Time: 10 minutes
Cooking Time: 40 minutes
Servings: 6

Ingredients:
- 2 oranges, juiced
- 2 pounds pork shoulder
- 1 teaspoon garlic powder
- Salt and pepper, to taste
- 2 tablespoons butter

Directions:
1. Preheat your air fryer to 450 degrees F.
2. Grease the air fryer cooking basket with butter.
3. Season pork with garlic powder, pepper, and salt.
4. Transfer to air fryer cooking basket and top with orange juice
5. Cook for 40 minutes.
6. Serve by shredding with forks, serve and enjoy!

Nutrition: Calories: 506 Total Fat: 36g Total Carbs: 7g Fiber: 1g Net Carbs: 5g Protein: 18g

218. Garlic Pork Roast

Preparation Time: 10 minutes
Cooking Time: 45 minutes
Servings: 8

Ingredients:
- 2 pounds pork shoulder
- 1½ tablespoons olive oil
- 2 teaspoons dried thyme
- 8 garlic cloves, minced
- Salt and pepper, to taste

Directions:
1. Preheat your air fryer to 470 degrees F.
2. Take a bowl and mix in olive oil, salt, pepper, thyme, and garlic.
3. Marinate pork with oil mixture for about 30 minutes.
4. Transfer pork to the air fryer cooking basket and cook for 40 minutes.
5. Serve and enjoy!

Nutrition: Calories: 359 Total Fat: 26g Total Carbs: 7g Fiber: 2g Net Carbs: 3g Protein: 26g

219. Grilled Skirt Steak with Sauce

Preparation Time: 45 minutes
Cooking Time: 10 minutes
Servings: 4

Ingredients:
- 1-pound skirt steak, cut into 4 pieces
- ⅛ teaspoon crushed red pepper flakes
- 2 tablespoons adobo sauce
- 1 chipotle pepper in adobo sauce, minced
- ⅛ teaspoon pepper

Directions:
1. In a bowl, mix together the salt, pepper, minced chipotle pepper, red pepper flakes, and adobo sauce. Rub both sides of the steaks with the marinade.
2. Let the steaks sit for at least 20 minutes at room temperature or refrigerate up to 12 hours.
3. Arrange the steaks in the air fryer basket. Put the air fryer lid on and grill in batches in the preheated instant pot at 400°F for 10 minutes, or until the steaks are cooked to medium doneness.
4. Transfer to a serving dish and slice to serve.

Nutrition: Calories: 794 Total Fat: 55.24g Saturated Fat: 23.564g Total Carbs: 24.79g Fiber: 5.3g Protein: 10.28g Sugar: 18.67g Sodium: 2934mg

220. Cheesy Beef and Mushroom Calzones with Sauce

Preparation Time: 30 minutes
Cooking Time: 15 minutes
Servings: 6

Ingredients:
- 1-pound 93% lean ground beef
- ¼ cup chopped mushrooms
- ½ cup chopped onion
- 2 garlic cloves, minced
- 1 tablespoon Italian seasoning
- 1½ cups pizza sauce
- 1 teaspoon all-purpose flour
- 1 can (13-ounce) refrigerated pizza dough
- 1 cup shredded Cheddar cheese
- Salt and pepper to taste
- Cooking spray

Directions:
1. Spray a skillet with cooking spray and place it over medium-high heat. Add the garlic, mushrooms and onion to the skillet. Sauté them for 2 to 3 minutes or until the onion is translucent.
2. Add the ground beef, salt, pepper, and Italian seasoning to the skillet. Divide the ground beef into smaller pieces with a spatula or spoon. Sauté for 2 to 4 minutes or until the meat is thoroughly browned. Pour in the pizza sauce into the skillet and stir well.
3. On a lightly floured (1 teaspoon flour) work surface, unroll the pizza dough and cut evenly into 6 dough rectangles.
4. To make the calzones, evenly spread the beef mixture onto each dough rectangle. Top with the cheddar cheese. Brush the edges of the dough rectangles with water. Fold the dough over the filling, making sure not to pull the dough too tightly. Crimp the open edges to seal.
5. Arrange the calzones in the air fryer basket and spritz with cooking spray.
6. Put the air fryer lid on and cook in batches in the preheated instant pot at 375°F for 10 minutes.
7. Transfer the fried calzones to a plate lined with paper towels. Serve warm.

Nutrition: Calories: 202 Total Fat: 14g Saturated Fat: 6g Cholesterol: 36mg Sodium: 689mg Carbohydrates: 1g Fiber: 2g Protein: 21g

221. Mexican Stuffed Beef Fajitas

Preparation Time: 20 minutes
Cooking Time: 10 minutes
Servings: 4

Ingredients:
- 1-pound beef flank steak, cut into strips
- 1 red bell pepper, cut into strips
- 1 green bell pepper, cut into strips
- ½ red onion, cut into strips
- 2 tablespoons fajita seasoning
- 2 tablespoons extra-virgin olive oil

- 8 medium (8-inch) flour tortillas
- Salt and pepper to taste

Directions:
1. In a large bowl, combine the beef strips, bell peppers, fajita seasoning, onion, salt, pepper and olive oil. Toss well to coat the beef steak evenly.
2. Transfer the coated beef-vegetable mixture to the air fryer basket. Put the air fryer lid on and cook in the preheated instant pot at 375°F for 5 minutes. Shake the basket when the lid screen indicates 'TURN FOOD' during cooking time. Cook for an additional 4 to 5 minutes.
3. Transfer to a large dish. Evenly divide the mixture onto each tortilla and serve with parsley, if desired.

Nutrition: Calories: 491 Total Fat: 16g Saturated Fat: 4g Cholesterol: 50mg Sodium: 389mg Carbohydrates: 52g Fiber: 4g Protein: 33g

222. Pork Chops With Ranch Dressing

Preparation Time: 25 minutes
Cooking Time: 8 minutes
Servings: 4

Ingredients:
- 4 boneless, center-cut pork chops, 1-inch thick
- 2 teaspoons dry ranch salad dressing mix (such as Hidden Valley Ranch)
- Cooking spray

Directions:
1. Arrange the pork chops on a large platter. Spritz the cooking spray all over the chops and sprinkle with ranch salad dressing mix. Let stand for 10 minutes.
2. Spritz the air fryer basket with cooking spray. Arrange the chops in the basket.
3. Put the air fryer lid on and cook in batches in the preheated instant pot at 400°F for 8 minutes or until cooked through. Turn the chops over when the lid screen indicates 'TURN FOOD' halfway through the cooking.
4. Remove the pork chops from the basket to a platter. Let stand for 5 minutes, then serve.

Nutrition: Calories: 260 Total Fat: 9.1g Cholesterol: 107mg Sodium: 148mg Carbohydrates: 0.6g Protein: 40.8g

223. Beef Sirloin Steak with Mushrooms

Preparation Time: 20 minutes
Cooking Time: 15 minutes
Servings: 4

Ingredients:
- 1-pound beef sirloin steak, cut into 1-inch cubes
- 8 ounces button mushrooms, sliced
- ¼ cup Worcestershire sauce
- 1 tablespoon olive oil
- 1 teaspoon paprika
- 1 teaspoon chile flakes, crushed
- 1 teaspoon parsley flakes

Directions:
1. In a large bowl, put the steak and mushrooms. Pour the Worcestershire sauce and olive oil over them. Sprinkle with paprika, chile flakes, and parsley. Toss the steak and mushrooms to coat well.
2. Wrap the bowl in plastic and refrigerate to marinate for at least 4 hours, or overnight.
3. Remove the bowl from the refrigerator and let stand at room temperature for 30 minutes before cooking.
4. Discard the marinade and transfer the steak and mushrooms to a clean work surface. Pat dry, then place them into the air fryer basket.
5. Put the air fryer lid on and cook in the preheated instant pot at 400°F for 10 minutes. Give the basket a shake when the lid indicates 'TURN FOOD' halfway through the cooking.
6. Remove the steak and mushrooms from the basket to a large serving platter. Let them cool for 5 minutes and serve with cilantro, if desired.

Nutrition: Calories: 225 Total Fat: 13.2g Cholesterol: 60mg Sodium: 213mg Carbohydrates: 5.8g Protein: 20.8g

SEAFOOD RECIPES

224. Air Fried Cod with Basil Vinaigrette

Preparation Time: 20 minutes
Cooking Time: 15 minutes
Servings: 4
Ingredients:
- ¼ cup olive oil
- 4 cod fillets
- A bunch of basil, torn
- Juice from 1 lemon, freshly squeezed
- Salt and pepper to taste

Directions:
1. Preheat the air fryer for 5 minutes.
2. Season the cod fillets with salt and pepper to taste.
3. Place in the air fryer and cook for 15 minutes at 3500F.
4. Meanwhile, mix the rest of the ingredients in a bowl and toss to combine.
5. Serve the air fried cod with the basil vinaigrette.

Nutrition: Calories: 235 Carbohydrates: 1.9g Protein: 14.3g Fat: 18.9g

225. Almond Flour Coated Crispy Shrimps

Preparation Time: 15 minutes
Cooking Time: 10 minutes
Servings: 4
Ingredients:
- ½ cup almond flour
- 1 tablespoon yellow mustard
- 1-pound raw shrimps, peeled and deveined
- 3 tablespoons olive oil
- Salt and pepper to taste

Directions:
1. Place all ingredients in a Ziploc bag and give a good shake.
2. Place in the air fryer and cook for 10 minutes at 4000F.

Nutrition: Calories: 206 Carbohydrates: 1.3g Protein: 23.5g Fat: 11.9g

226. Another Crispy Coconut Shrimp Recipe

Preparation Time: 20 minutes
Cooking Time: 20 minutes
Servings: 4
Ingredients:
- ½ cup flour
- ½ stick cold butter, cut into cubes
- ½ tablespoon lemon juice
- 1 egg yolk, beaten
- 1 green onion, chopped
- 1-pound salmon fillets, cut into small cubes
- 3 tablespoons whipping cream
- 4 eggs, beaten
- Salt and pepper to taste

Directions:
1. Preheat the air fryer to 3900F.
2. Season salmon fillets with lemon juice, salt and pepper.
3. In another bowl, combine the flour and butter. Add cold water gradually to form a dough. Knead the dough on a flat surface to form a sheet.
4. Place the dough on the baking dish and press firmly on the dish.
5. Beat the eggs and egg yolk and season with salt and pepper to taste.
6. Place the salmon cubes on the pan lined with dough and pour the egg over.
7. Cook for 15 to 20 minutes.
8. Garnish with green onions once cooked.

Nutrition: Calories per serving: 483 Carbs: 5.2g Protein: 45.2 Fat: 31.2g

227. Apple Slaw Topped Alaskan Cod Filet

Preparation Time: 10 minutes
Cooking Time: 15 minutes
Servings: 3
Ingredients:
- ¼ cup mayonnaise
- ½ red onion, diced
- 1 ½ pounds frozen Alaskan cod
- 1 box whole wheat panko bread crumbs
- 1 granny smith apple, julienned
- 1 tablespoon vegetable oil
- 1 teaspoon paprika
- 2 cups Napa cabbage, shredded
- Salt and pepper to taste

Directions:
1. Preheat the air fryer to 3900F.
2. Place the grill pan accessory in the air fryer.
3. Brush the fish with oil and dredge in the breadcrumbs.
4. Place the fish on the grill pan and cook for 15 minutes. Make sure to flip the fish halfway through the cooking time.
5. Meanwhile, prepare the slaw by mixing the remaining ingredients in a bowl.
6. Serve the fish with the slaw.

Nutrition: Calories per serving: 316 Carbs: 13.5g Protein: 37.8g Fat: 12.2g

228. Baked Cod Fillet Recipe From Thailand

Preparation Time: 15 minutes
Cooking Time: 20 minutes
Servings: 4
Ingredients:
- ¼ cup coconut milk, freshly squeezed
- 1 tablespoon lime juice, freshly squeezed
- 1-pound cod fillet, cut into bite-sized pieces
- Salt and pepper to taste

Directions:
1. Preheat the air fryer for 5 minutes.
2. Place all ingredients in a baking dish that will fit in the air fryer.
3. Place in the air fryer.
4. Cook for 20 minutes at 3250F.

Nutrition: Calories per serving: 844 Carbohydrates: 2.3g Protein: 21.6g Fat: 83.1g

229. Baked Scallops With Garlic Aioli

Preparation Time: 15 minutes
Cooking Time: 10 minutes

SEAFOOD RECIPES

Servings: 4

Ingredients:
- 1 cup bread crumbs
- 1/4 cup chopped parsley
- 16 sea scallops, rinsed and drained
- 2 shallots, chopped
- 3 pinches ground nutmeg
- 4 tablespoons olive oil
- 5 cloves garlic, minced
- 5 tablespoons butter, melted
- Salt and pepper to taste

Directions:
1. Lightly grease baking pan of air fryer with cooking spray.
2. Mix in shallots, garlic, melted butter, and scallops. Season with pepper, salt, and nutmeg.
3. In a small bowl, whisk well olive oil and bread crumbs. Sprinkle over scallops.
4. For 10 minutes, cook on 390oF until tops are lightly browned.
5. Serve and enjoy with a sprinkle of parsley.

Nutrition: Calories per Serving: 452 Carbs: 29.8g Protein: 15.2g Fat: 30.2g

230. Basil 'N Lime-Chili Clams

Preparation Time: 10 minutes
Cooking Time: 15 minutes
Servings: 3

Ingredients:
- ½ cup basil leaves
- ½ cup tomatoes, chopped
- 1 tablespoon fresh lime juice
- 25 littleneck clams
- 4 cloves of garlic, minced
- 6 tablespoons unsalted butter
- Salt and pepper to taste

Directions:
1. Preheat the air fryer to 3900F.
2. Place the grill pan accessory in the air fryer.
3. On a large foil, place all ingredients. Fold over the foil and close by crimping the edges.
4. Place on the grill pan and cook for 15 minutes.
5. Serve with bread.

Nutrition: Calories per serving: 163 Carbs: 4.1g Protein: 1.7g Fat: 15.5g

231. Bass Filet In Coconut Sauce

Preparation Time: 20 minutes
Cooking Time: 15 minutes
Servings: 4

Ingredients:
- ¼ cup coconut milk
- ½ pound bass fillet
- 1 tablespoon olive oil
- 2 tablespoons jalapeno, chopped
- 2 tablespoons lime juice, freshly squeezed
- 3 tablespoons parsley, chopped
- Salt and pepper to taste

Directions:
1. Preheat the air fryer for 5 minutes
2. Season the bass with salt and pepper to taste
3. Brush the surface with olive oil.
4. Place in the air fryer and cook for 15 minutes at 3500F.
5. Meanwhile, place in a saucepan, the coconut milk, lime juice, jalapeno and parsley.
6. Heat over medium flame.
7. Serve the fish with the coconut sauce.

Nutrition: Calories per serving: 139 Carbohydrates: 2.7g Protein: 8.7g Fat: 10.3

232. Beer Battered Cod Filet

Preparation Time: 10 minutes
Cooking Time: 15 minutes
Servings: 2

Ingredients:
- ½ cup all-purpose flour
- ¾ teaspoon baking powder
- 1 ¼ cup lager beer
- 2 cod fillets
- 2 eggs, beaten
- Salt and pepper to taste

Directions:
1. Preheat the air fryer to 3900F.
2. Pat the fish fillets dry then set aside.
3. In a bowl, combine the rest of the ingredients to create a batter.
4. Dip the fillets on the batter and place on the double layer rack.
5. Cook for 15 minutes.

Nutrition: Calories per serving: 229 Carbs: 33.2g Protein: 31.1g Fat: 10.2g

233. Buttered Baked Cod with Wine

Preparation Time: 15 minutes
Cooking Time: 12 minutes
Servings: 2

Ingredients:
- 1 tablespoon butter
- 1 tablespoon butter
- 2 tablespoons dry white wine
- 1/2 pound thick-cut cod loin
- 1-1/2 teaspoons chopped fresh parsley
- 1-1/2 teaspoons chopped green onion
- 1/2 lemon, cut into wedges
- 1/4 sleeve buttery round crackers (such as Ritz®), crushed
- 1/4 lemon, juiced

Directions:
1. In a small bowl, melt butter in microwave. Whisk in crackers.
2. Lightly grease baking pan of air fryer with remaining butter. And melt for 2 minutes at 390oF.
3. In a small bowl whisk well lemon juice, white wine, parsley, and green onion.
4. Coat cod filets in melted butter. Pour dressing. Top with butter-cracker mixture.
5. Cook for 10 minutes at 390oF.
6. Serve and enjoy with a slice of lemon.

Nutrition: Calories per Serving: 266 Carbs: 9.3g Protein: 20.9g Fat: 16.1g

234. Buttered Garlic-Oregano On Clams

Preparation Time: 10 minutes
Cooking Time: 5 minutes
Servings: 4

Ingredients:
- ¼ cup parmesan cheese, grated
- ¼ cup parsley, chopped
- 1 cup breadcrumbs

- 1 teaspoon dried oregano
- 2 dozen clams, shucked
- 3 cloves of garlic, minced
- 4 tablespoons butter, melted

Directions:
1. In a medium bowl, mix together the breadcrumbs, parmesan cheese, parsley, oregano, and garlic. Stir in the melted butter.
2. Preheat the air fryer to 3900F.
3. Place the baking dish accessory in the air fryer and place the clams.
4. Sprinkle the crumb mixture over the clams.
5. Cook for 5 minutes.

Nutrition: Calories per serving: 160 Carbs: 6.3g Protein: 2.9g Fat: 13.6g

235. Butterflied Prawns with Garlic-Sriracha

Preparation Time: 10 minutes
Cooking Time: 15 minutes
Servings: 2

Ingredients:
- 1 tablespoon lime juice
- 1 tablespoon sriracha
- 1-pound large prawns, shells removed and cut lengthwise or butterflied
- 1teaspoon fish sauce
- 2 tablespoons melted butter
- 2 tablespoons minced garlic
- Salt and pepper to taste

Directions:
1. Preheat the air fryer to 3900F.
2. Place the grill pan accessory in the air fryer.
3. Season the prawns with the rest of the ingredients.
4. Place on the grill pan and cook for 15 minutes. Make sure to flip the prawns halfway through the cooking time.

Nutrition: Calories per serving: 443 Carbs:9.7 g Protein: 62.8g Fat: 16.9g

236. Cajun Seasoned Salmon Filet

Preparation Time: 10 minutes
Cooking Time: 15 minutes
Servings: 1

Ingredients:
- 1 salmon fillet
- 1 teaspoon juice from lemon, freshly squeezed
- 3 tablespoons extra virgin olive oil
- A dash of Cajun seasoning mix
- Salt and pepper to taste

Directions:
1. Preheat the air fryer for 5 minutes.
2. Place all ingredients in a bowl and toss to coat.
3. Place the fish fillet in the air fryer basket.
4. Bake for 15 minutes at 3250F.
5. Once cooked drizzle with olive oil

Nutrition: Calories per serving: 523 Carbohydrates: 4.6g Protein: 47.9g Fat: 34.8g

237. Cajun Spiced Lemon-Shrimp Kebabs

Preparation Time: 15 minutes
Cooking Time: 10 minutes
Servings: 2

Ingredients:
- 1 tsp cayenne
- 1 tsp garlic powder
- 1 tsp kosher salt
- 1 tsp onion powder
- 1 tsp oregano
- 1 tsp paprika
- 12 pcs XL shrimp
- 2 lemons, sliced thinly crosswise
- 2 tbsp olive oil

Directions:
1. In a bowl, mix all ingredients except for sliced lemons. Marinate for 10 minutes.
2. Thread 3 shrimps per steel skewer.
3. Place in skewer rack.
4. Cook for 5 minutes at 390oF.
5. Serve and enjoy with freshly squeezed lemon.

Nutrition: Calories per Serving: 232 Carbs: 7.9g Protein: 15.9g Fat: 15.1g

238. Cajun Spiced Veggie-Shrimp Bake

Preparation Time: 15 minutes
Cooking Time: 20 minutes
Servings: 4

Ingredients:
- 1 Bag of Frozen Mixed Vegetables
- 1 Tbsp Gluten Free Cajun Seasoning
- Olive Oil Spray
- Season with salt and pepper
- Small Shrimp Peeled & Deveined (Regular Size Bag about 50-80 Small Shrimp)

Directions:
1. Lightly grease baking pan of air fryer with cooking spray. Add all ingredients and toss well to coat. Season with pepper and salt, generously.
2. For 10 minutes, cook on 330oF. Halfway through cooking time, stir.
3. Cook for 10 minutes at 330oF.
4. Serve and enjoy.

Nutrition: Calories per Serving: 78 Carbs: 13.2g Protein: 2.8g Fat: 1.5g

239. Tempura Shrimp

Preparation Time: 15 minutes
Cooking Time: 10 minutes
Servings: 4

Ingredients:
- 1 package frozen shrimp tempura

Directions:
1. Spread shrimp tempura on the air fryer basket or tray; don't let them overlap to allow even cooking
2. Put them in air fryer and air fry at 380f for 10 minutes, check and flip halfway through cooking
3. Serve and enjoy

Nutrition: Calories: 21 kcal Protein: 1.6 g Fat: 1.52 g Carbohydrates: 0 g

240. Tuna Patties

Preparation Time:15 minutes
Cooking Time: 10 minutes
Servings: 4

Ingredients:
- 1 egg
- 5–6 ounces of tuna
- 1 tsp. lemon zest
- 1 tbsp. Italian seasoning
- 1/2 cup bread crumbs
- 1 tsp. Dijon mustard

- 1 tbsp. of lemon juice

Directions:
1. Combine together egg, Dijon mustard, lemon zest, tuna, lemon juice, Italian seasoning and bread crumbs in a bowl
2. Spray olive oil in the air fryer basket
3. Form patties with about 1/4 cup of tuna mixture
4. Then place them in the air fryer basket and softly spray with olive oil to make the tuna patties crispy
5. Place the basket in the air fryer and set to 360 F for 5 minutes
6. Flip tuna patties and air fry for more 5 minutes
7. Serve and enjoy

Nutrition: Calories: 104 kcal Protein: 11.28 g Fat: 4.47 g Carbohydrates: 4.09 g

241. Crusted Tilapia Coconut Flavour

Preparation Time: 10 minutes
Cooking Time: 10 minutes
Servings: 4

Ingredients:
- 4 (4 ounces filets) tilapia fillets
- 3/4 cup unsweetened flaked coconut
- 1/2 cup coconut flour
- 1 tsp. sea salt
- 3 eggs, beaten

Directions:
1. Mix coconut flour, unsweetened flaked, coconut and sea salt together.
2. Crack egg into a bowl
3. Then sink the fillets into the cracked egg and then into the coconut mixture
4. Grease the air fryer pan with oil
5. Put the fish in the pan and spray with olive oil
6. Place the pan into the air fryer and set to cook at 400 F for 4 minutes
7. Check and flip the fish after 4 minutes and continue cooking for another 4 minutes
8. Serve and enjoy

Nutrition: Calories: 243 kcal Protein: 32.16 g Fat: 10.87 g Carbohydrates: 3.54 g

242. Fried French Mussels

Preparation Time: 20 minutes
Cooking Time: 15 minutes
Servings: 4

Ingredients:
- 1-pound mussels
- 2 tbsp. minced garlic
- 4 tbsps. melted butter
- 2 tbsp. dry white wine
- 2 tbsp. heavy cream

Directions:
1. Put in a bowl the mussels, garlic, butter, white wine, and heavy cream and mix together
2. Pour the mussels mixture into the air fryer basket
3. Set the air fryer to 400f for 5 minutes, shake after 5 minutes and set for more 5 minutes
4. Serve and enjoy

Nutrition: Calories: 172 kcal Protein: 15.95 g Fat: 6.91 g Carbohydrates: 10.47 g

243. Crab Cakes

Preparation Time: 25 minutes
Cooking Time: 15 minutes
Servings: 3

Ingredients:
- 1 egg
- 2 tbsps. Mayonnaise
- 1 tsp. Old Bay Seasoning.
- 1/2 tsp. salt
- 2 tbsps. Fresh parsley (diced)
- 1 cup fresh crab meat
- 1 cup saltines (crushed)
- 1/2 cup panko
- 1 onion (peeled and diced)
- 1/2 tsp. Dijon mustard
- 1 tsp. Worcestershire sauce

Directions:
1. Mix together mayonnaise, onion, Dijon mustard, egg, old Bay seasoning, Worcestershire, saltines, salt and parsley in a bowl
2. Pour the crab in the mixture and mix properly.
3. Make the crab mixture into patties, then soak them into the panko allowing the both side to coat well
4. Put it in the fridge for about 1 hour
5. Spray the crab cake on both sides with oil
6. Set into the air fryer and cook at 350 F for 15 minutes. Enjoy!

Nutrition: Calories: 298 kcal Protein: 19.44 g Fat: 8.25 g Carbohydrates: 37.76 g

244. Lobster Tails

Preparation Time: 10 minutes
Cooking Time: 7 minutes
Servings: 3

Ingredients:
- 4 lobster tails (thawed)
- 1 tsp. of pepper
- 2 tbsp. of melted butter
- 1/2 tsp. of salt

Directions:
1. Melt the butter
2. With kitchen scissors, cut lobster right through the tail part
3. Then break the shell and pull backwards with your fingers
4. Rub the lobster tail with butter and add salt and pepper
5. Place it in the air fryer and cook at 380f for 4 minutes
6. Add melted butter and cook for another 3 minutes
7. Serve with more butter

Nutrition: Calories: 255 kcal Protein: 35.55 g Fat: 11.23 g Carbohydrates: 1.42 g

245. Breaded Shrimp

Preparation Time: 15 minutes
Cooking Time: 11 minutes
Servings: 3

Ingredients:
- 1-pound of shrimp, peeled and deveined
- 2 eggs
- 1/2 cup of panko
- 1/2 cup of onion, peeled and diced
- 1 tsp. of ginger
- 1 tsp. of garlic powder
- 1 tsp. of black pepper

Directions:
1. Preheat air fryer to 350 F
2. Crack the eggs in a bowl
3. Then combine onion, panko and spices in another bowl
4. Sink the shrimps in the eggs and then in the panko bowl
5. Air fry for about 6 minutes, turn over the shrimps and cook for another 5 minutes

6. Serve and enjoy

Nutrition: Calories: : 279 kcal Protein: 39.48 g Fat: 10.57 g Carbohydrates: 3.96 g

246. Salmon with Mustard Sauce

Preparation Time: 10 minutes
Cooking Time: 8 minutes
Servings: 2-4

Ingredients:
- 1/4 cup honey
- 1/4 cup Dijon mustard
- 2–4 pieces salmon
- 1/2 cup mayonnaise

Directions:
1. Make a salmon fillet
2. Cut the salmon into desired pieces
3. Then combine together mayo, honey, Dijon mustard, salt, and pepper in a bowl then leave the rest for dipping sauce
4. Spread the mixture on the salmon fillets
5. Spray the air fryer basket and put the salmon in it
6. Cook at 400f for about 8 minutes
7. Remove from air fryer and serve with remaining side sauce

Nutrition: Calories: 191 kcal Protein: 4.03 g Fat: 11.57 g Carbohydrates: 19.29 g

247. Sweet And Sour Shrimp

Preparation Time: 5 minutes
Cooking Time: 5 minutes
Servings: 3

Ingredients:
- 1-pound shrimp, peeled and deveined
- 1/2 cup sweet and sour sauce

Directions:
1. Combine the shrimps, sweet and sour sauce together in a bowl
2. Then spread on the air fryer tray and put it in air fryer
3. Cook at 400f for 5 minutes and serve

Nutrition: Calories: 226 kcal Protein: 32.65 g Fat: 2.8 g Carbohydrates: 17.84 g

248. Fish Cakes

Preparation Time: 15 minutes
Cooking Time: 12 minutes
Servings: 3

Ingredients:
- Nonstick cooking spray
- 10 ounces finely chopped white fish
- ⅔ Cup whole-wheat panko breadcrumbs
- 3 tsp. finely chopped fresh cilantro
- 2 tsp. Thai sweet chili sauce
- 2 tsp. canola mayonnaise
- 1 large eggs
- ⅛ Tsp. salt
- ¼ teaspoon ground pepper
- 2 lime wedges

Directions:
1. Oil the air fryer basket with cooking spray
2. Mix together egg, chili sauce, fish, panko, cilantro, mayonnaise, salt and pepper in a bowl
3. Mold the mixture into 3-inch size cake
4. Spray the cake with cooking spray and put it in the air fryer basket
5. Cook at 380f for about 12 minutes or till the cakes are brown and the inner temperature reads 140f
6. Serve with lime wedges and enjoy

Nutrition: Calories: 196 kcal Protein: 21.04 g Fat: 7.07 g Carbohydrates: 12.21 g

249. Cod

Preparation Time: 15 minutes
Cooking Time: 11 minutes
Servings: 4

Ingredients:
- 1-pound of cod
- 1 egg
- 1/2 tsp. salt
- 1/8 tsp. black pepper
- 1/2 cup all-purpose flour
- 1 1/2 cups panko breadcrumbs or regular breadcrumbs
- 2 tsp. taco seasoning (optional)
- 1 teaspoon Italian seasoning or old bay seasoning

Directions:
1. Preheat your air fryer to 400F
2. Pat the cod dry, place on cutting board set aside
3. Whisk the egg in a bowl.
4. Pour flour in another bowl
5. Then panko breadcrumbs, pepper, salt and taco seasoning in the third bowl and mix well.
6. Dip the cod into the egg and wet the 2 sides, and transfer to the bowl of flour and press into the flour on both sides.
7. Then Move the cod to the panko breadcrumbs and press both sides into the breadcrumbs.
8. Spray the air fryer with non-stick spray. Add the cod in batches to the air fryer and cook at 400°f for 11 minutes, gently turn around halfway through.

Nutrition: Calories: 264 kcal Protein: 30.37 g Fat: 9 g Carbohydrates: 14.93 g

250. Broiled Tilapia

Preparation Time: 15 minutes
Cooking Time: 7 minutes
Servings: 2

Ingredients:
- Tilapia fillets
- Light spritz of canola oil from an oil spritz
- Old bay seasoning
- Lemon pepper
- Salt
- Molly Mcbutter or butter buds

Directions:
1. Defrost fillets, if frozen then Spray air fryer basket with cooking spray.
2. Place fillets in the basket and season to taste with the spices. Spray little oil.
3. Set air fryer to 400f for 7 minutes. Check for doneness after the timer goes off, Fish should flake easily with a fork.
4. Serve and enjoy with your favorite veggies.

Nutrition: Calories: 106 kcal Protein: 15.3 g Fat: 4.06 g Carbohydrates: 2.13 g

251. Cod Nuggets

Preparation Time: 20 minutes
Cooking Time: 15 minutes
Servings: 5

Ingredients:
For the breaded Cod:
- 1 1/2 pounds cod fillets cut in about 8 chunks
- Salt and pepper to season
- 1/2 cup flour

SEAFOOD RECIPES

- 1 tbsp. Egg + 1 tbsp. Water
- 1/2 cup cracker crumbs, or cornflake crumbs
- 1 tsp. Vegetable oil

For the Lemon Honey Tartar Sauce:
- 1/2 cup low-fat or no-fat mayonnaise
- 1 tsp. honey
- Zest of half a lemon, finely minced
- Juice of half a lemon
- 1/2 tsp. Worcestershire sauce
- 1 tbsp. sweet pickle relish
- Pinch black pepper

Directions:
1. Crush crackers or corn flakes into fine crumbs in a food processor, about a cup. Put 1 tbsp. of vegetable oil into the crumbs.
2. Season the cod chunks with pepper and salt then dip them in the flour.
3. After that, dip into the egg wash and finally into the cracker crumbs. Press the crumbs onto all surfaces to mix all sides.
4. Preheat air fryer to 180 degrees C.
5. Put half of the cod nuggets in the basket and use the rack to cook half on the upper level.
6. Set air fryer to 15 minutes.
7. Remove from basket and serve.
8. To make the Honey Lemon Tartar Sauce:
9. Blend all of the ingredients together and refrigerate for the flavors to mix until ready to serve.

Nutrition: Calories: 221 kcal Protein: 27.32 g Fat: 5.78 g Carbohydrates: 13.68 g

252. Air Fryer Cajun Shrimp

Preparation Time: 5 minutes
Cooking Time: 6 minutes
Servings: 2

Ingredients:
- 12 ounces uncooked medium shrimp, peeled and deveined
- 1 teaspoon cayenne pepper
- 1 teaspoon Old Bay seasoning
- ½ teaspoon smoked paprika
- 2 tablespoons olive oil
- 1 teaspoon salt

Directions:
1. Preheat the Innsky air fryer to 390°F.
2. Meanwhile, in a medium mixing bowl, combine the shrimp, cayenne pepper, Old Bay, paprika, olive oil, and salt. Toss the shrimp in the oil and spices until the shrimp is thoroughly coated with both.
3. Place the shrimp in the air fryer basket. Set the timer and steam for 3 minutes. Remove the drawer and shake, so the shrimp redistribute in the basket for even cooking. Reset the timer and steam for another 3 minutes. Check that the shrimp are done. When they are cooked through, the flesh will be opaque. Add additional time if needed. Plate, serve, and enjoy!

Nutrition: Calories: 286 Fat: 16g Saturated fat: 2g Carbohydrate: 1g Fiber: 0g Sugar: 0g Protein: 37g Iron: 6mg Sodium: 1868mg

253. Grilled Salmon

Preparation Time: 5 minutes
Cooking Time: 10 minutes
Servings: 3

Ingredients:
- 2 Salmon Fillets
- 1/2 Tsp Lemon Pepper
- 1/2 Tsp Garlic Powder
- Salt and Pepper
- 1/3 Cup Soy Sauce
- 1/3 Cup Sugar
- 1 Tbsp. Olive Oil

Directions:
1. Season salmon fillets with lemon pepper, garlic powder and salt. In a shallow bowl, add a third cup of water and combine the olive oil, soy sauce and sugar. Place salmon the bowl and immerse in the sauce. Cover with cling film and allow to marinate in the refrigerator for at least an hour
2. Preheat the Innsky air fryer at 350 degrees.
3. Place salmon into the Air fryer and cook for 10 minutes or more until the fish is tender. Serve with lemon wedges

Nutrition: Calories: 185 kcal Protein: 5.16 g Fat: 11.74 g Carbohydrates: 16.06 g

254. Crispy Paprika Fish Fillets

Preparation Time: 5 minutes
Cooking Time: 15 minutes
Servings: 4

Ingredients:
- 1/2 cup seasoned breadcrumbs
- 1 tablespoon balsamic vinegar
- 1/2 teaspoon seasoned salt
- 1 teaspoon paprika
- 1/2 teaspoon ground black pepper
- 1 teaspoon celery seed
- 2 fish fillets, halved
- 1 egg, beaten

Directions:
1. Add the breadcrumbs, vinegar, salt, paprika, ground black pepper, and celery seeds to your food processor. Process for about 30 seconds.
2. Coat the fish fillets with the beaten egg; then, coat them with the breadcrumbs mixture.
3. Cook at 350 degrees F for about 15 minutes.

Nutrition: Calories: 208 kcal Protein: 15.19 g Fat: 9.44 g Carbohydrates: 11.61 g

255. Bacon Wrapped Shrimp

Preparation Time: 5 minutes
Cooking Time: 5 minutes
Servings: 4

Ingredients:
- 1¼ pound tiger shrimp, peeled and deveined
- 1-pound bacon

Directions:
1. Wrap each shrimp with a slice of bacon.
2. Refrigerate for about 20 minutes. Preheat the Innsky air fryer to 390 degrees F.
3. Arrange the shrimp in the Air fryer basket. Cook for about 5-7 minutes.

Nutrition: Calories: 514 kcal Protein: 42.66 g Fat: 36.92 g Carbohydrates: 7.17 g

256. Bacon-Wrapped Scallops

Preparation Time: 5 minutes
Cooking Time: 10 minutes
Servings: 4

Ingredients:
- 16 sea scallops
- 8 slices bacon, cut in half
- 8 toothpicks
- Salt

- Freshly ground black pepper

Directions:
1. Using a paper towel, pat dry the scallops.
2. Wrap each scallop with a half slice of bacon. Secure the bacon with a toothpick.
3. Place the scallops into the air fryer in a single layer. (You may need to cook your scallops in more than one batch.)
4. Spray the scallops with olive oil, and season them with salt and pepper.
5. Set the temperature of your Innsky AF to 370°F. Set the timer and fry for 5 minutes.
6. Flip the scallops.
7. Reset your timer and cook the scallops for 5 minutes more.
8. Using tongs, remove the scallops from the air fryer basket. Plate, serve, and enjoy!

Nutrition: Calories: 311 Fat: 17g Saturated fat: 5g Carbohydrate: 3g Fiber: 0g Sugar: 0g Protein: 34g Sodium: 1110mg

257. Air Fryer Salmon

Preparation Time: 5 minutes
Cooking Time: 10 minutes
Servings: 2

Ingredients:
- ½ tsp. salt
- ½ tsp. garlic powder
- ½ tsp. smoked paprika
- Salmon

Directions:
1. Mix spices together and sprinkle onto salmon. Place seasoned salmon into the Air fryer.
2. Close crisping lid. Set temperature to 400°F, and set time to 10 minutes.

Nutrition: Calories: 185 Fat: 11g; Protein: 21g Sugar: 0g

258. Lemon Pepper, Butter and Cajun Cod

Preparation Time: 5 minutes
Cooking Time: 12 minutes
Servings: 2

Ingredients:
- 2 (8-ounce) cod fillets, cut to fit into the air fryer basket
- 1 tablespoon Cajun seasoning
- ½ teaspoon lemon pepper
- 1 teaspoon salt
- ½ teaspoon freshly ground black pepper
- 2 tablespoons unsalted butter, melted
- 1 lemon, cut into 4 wedges

Directions:
1. Spray the Innsky air fryer basket with olive oil. Place the fillets on a plate. In a small mixing bowl, combine the Cajun seasoning, lemon pepper, salt, and pepper.
2. Rub the seasoning mix onto the fish.
3. Place the cod into the greased air fryer basket. Brush the top of each fillet with melted butter.
4. Set the temperature of your Innsky AF to 360°F. Set the timer and bake for 6 minutes. After 6 minutes, open up your air fryer drawer and flip the fish. Brush the top of each fillet with more melted butter.
5. Reset the timer and bake for 6 minutes more. Squeeze fresh lemon juice over the fillets.
6. Per Serving: Calories: 283; Fat: 14g; Saturated fat: 7g; Carbohydrate: 0g; Fiber: 0g; Sugar: 0g; Protein: 40g; Iron: 0mg; Sodium: 1460mg

Nutrition: Calories: 377 kcal Protein: 23.49 g Fat: 26.1g Carbohydrates: 11.8 g

259. Steamed Salmon & Sauce

Preparation Time: 5 minutes
Cooking Time: 10 minutes
Servings: 2

Ingredients:
- 1 cup Water
- 2 x 6 oz. Fresh Salmon
- 2 Tsp Vegetable Oil
- A Pinch of Salt for Each Fish
- ½ cup Plain Greek Yogurt
- ½ cup Sour Cream
- 2 tbsp. Finely Chopped Dill (Keep a bit for garnishing)
- A Pinch of Salt to Taste

Directions:
1. Pour the water into the bottom of the fryer and start heating to 285° F.
2. Drizzle oil over the fish and spread it. Salt the fish to taste.
3. Now pop it into the fryer for 10 min.
4. In the meantime, mix the yogurt, cream, dill and a bit of salt to make the sauce. When the fish is done, serve with the sauce and garnish with sprigs of dill.

Nutrition: Calories: 223 kcal Protein: 12.12 g Fat: 16.62 g Carbohydrates: 7.72 g

260. Salmon Patties

Preparation Time: 5 minutes
Cooking Time: 10 minutes
Servings: 4

Ingredients:
- 1 (14.75-ounce) can wild salmon, drained
- 1 large egg
- ¼ cup diced onion
- ½ cup bread crumbs
- 1 teaspoon dried dill
- ½ teaspoon freshly ground black pepper
- 1 teaspoon salt
- 1 teaspoon Old Bay seasoning

Directions:
1. Spray the Innsky air fryer basket with olive oil. Put the salmon in a medium bowl and remove any bones or skin. Add the egg, onion, bread crumbs, dill, pepper, salt, and Old Bay seasoning and mix well. Form the salmon mixture into 4 equal patties. Place the patties in the greased air fryer basket.
2. Set the temperature of your Innsky AF to 370°F. Set the timer and grill for 5 minutes. Flip the patties. Reset the timer and grill the patties for 5 minutes more. Plate, serve, and enjoy.

Nutrition: Calories: 239; Fat: 9g Saturated fat: 2g Carbohydrate: 11g Fiber: 1g Sugar: 1g Protein: 27g Iron: 2mg Sodium: 901mg

261. Sweet and Savory Breaded Shrimp

Preparation Time: 5 minutes
Cooking Time: 20 minutes
Servings: 2

Ingredients:
- ½ pound of fresh shrimp, peeled from their shells and rinsed
- 2 raw eggs
- ½ cup of breadcrumbs (we like Panko, but any brand or home recipe will do)
- ½ white onion, peeled and rinsed and finely chopped
- 1 teaspoon of ginger-garlic paste

SEAFOOD RECIPES

- ½ teaspoon of turmeric powder
- ½ teaspoon of red chili powder
- ½ teaspoon of cumin powder
- ½ teaspoon of black pepper powder
- ½ teaspoon of dry mango powder
- Pinch of salt

Directions:
1. Cover the basket of the Air fryer with a lining of tin foil, leaving the edges uncovered to allow air to circulate through the basket.
2. Preheat the Innsky air fryer to 350 degrees. In a large mixing bowl, beat the eggs until fluffy and until the yolks and whites are fully combined. Dunk all the shrimp in the egg mixture, fully submerging. In a separate mixing bowl, combine the bread crumbs with all the dry ingredients until evenly blended. One by one, coat the egg-covered shrimp in the mixed dry ingredients so that fully covered, and place on the foil-lined air-fryer basket.
3. Set the air-fryer timer to 20 minutes. Halfway through the cooking time, shake the handle of the air-fryer so that the breaded shrimp jostles inside and fry-coverage is even. After 20 minutes, when the fryer shuts off, the shrimp will be perfectly cooked and their breaded crust golden-brown and delicious! Using tongs, remove from the air fryer and set on a serving dish to cool.

Nutrition: Calories: 296 kcal Protein: 35.83 g Fat: 14.49 g Carbohydrates: 3.52 g

262. **Healthy Fish And Chips**
Preparation Time: 5 minutes
Cooking Time: 15 minutes
Servings: 3
Ingredients:
- Old Bay seasoning
- ½ C. panko breadcrumbs
- 1 egg
- 2 tbsp. almond flour
- 4-6-ounce tilapia fillets
- Frozen crinkle cut fries

Directions:
1. Add almond flour to one bowl, beat egg in another bowl, and add panko breadcrumbs to the third bowl, mixed with Old Bay seasoning. Dredge tilapia in flour, then egg, and then breadcrumbs. Place coated fish in Air fryer along with fries.
2. Set temperature to 390°F, and set time to 15 minutes.

Nutrition: Calories: 219 Fat: 5g Protein: 25g Sugar: 1g

263. **Indian Fish Fingers**
Preparation Time: 35 minutes
Cooking Time: 15 minutes
Servings: 4
Ingredients:
- 1/2 pound fish fillet
- 1 tablespoon finely chopped fresh mint leaves or any fresh herbs
- 1/3 cup bread crumbs
- 1 teaspoon ginger garlic paste or ginger and garlic powders
- 1 hot green chili finely chopped
- 1/2 teaspoon paprika
- Generous pinch of black pepper
- Salt to taste
- 3/4 tablespoons lemon juice
- 3/4 teaspoons garam masala powder
- 1/3 teaspoon rosemary
- 1 egg

Directions:
1. Start by removing any skin on the fish, washing, and patting dry. Cut the fish into fingers. In a medium bowl mix together all ingredients except for fish, mint, and bread crumbs. Bury the fingers in the mixture and refrigerate for 30 minutes. Remove from the bowl from the fridge and mix in mint leaves. In a separate bowl beat the egg, pour bread crumbs into a third bowl. Dip the fingers in the egg bowl then toss them in the bread crumbs bowl.
2. Cook at 360 degrees for 15 minutes, toss the fingers halfway through.

Nutrition: Calories: 187 Fat: 7g Protein: 11g Fiber: 1g

264. **Spicy Shrimp Kebab**
Preparation Time: 25 minutes
Cooking Time: 20 minutes
Servings: 4
Ingredients:
- ½ pounds jumbo shrimp, cleaned, shelled and deveined
- 1-pound cherry tomatoes
- tablespoons butter, melted
- 1 tablespoons sriracha sauce
- Sea salt and ground black pepper, to taste
- 1/2 teaspoon dried oregano
- 1/2 teaspoon dried basil
- 1 teaspoon dried parsley flakes
- 1/2 teaspoon marjoram
- 1/2 teaspoon mustard seeds

Directions:
1. Toss all ingredients in a mixing bowl until the shrimp and tomatoes are covered on all sides.
2. Soak the wooden skewers in water for 15 minutes.
3. Thread the jumbo shrimp and cherry tomatoes onto skewers. Cook in the preheated air fryer at 400 degrees f for 5 minutes, working with batches.

Nutrition: Calories: 247 Fat: 8.4g Carbs: 6g Protein: 36.4 Sugars: 3.5g Fiber: 1.8 g

265. **Crumbed Fish Fillets with Tarragon**
Preparation Time: 25 minutes
Cooking Time: 20 minutes
Servings: 4
Ingredients:
- 2 eggs, beaten
- 1/2 teaspoon tarragon
- 4 fish fillets, halved
- 2 tablespoons dry white wine
- 1/3 cup parmesan cheese, grated
- teaspoon seasoned salt
- 1/3 teaspoon mixed peppercorns
- 1/2 teaspoon fennel seed

Directions:
1. Add the parmesan cheese, salt, peppercorns, fennel seeds, and tarragon to your food processor; blitz for about 20 seconds.
2. Drizzle fish fillets with dry white wine. Dump the egg into a shallow dish.
3. Now, coat the fish fillets with the beaten egg on all sides; then, coat them with the seasoned cracker mix.
4. Air-fry at 345 degrees f for about 17 minutes.

Nutrition: 305 calories 17.7g fat 6.3g carbs 27.2g protein 0.3g sugars 0.1g fiber

266. Smoked And Creamed White Fish

Preparation time: 20 minutes
Cooking time: 15 minutes
Servings: 4
Ingredients:
- 1/2 tablespoon yogurt
- 1/3 cup spring garlic, finely chopped
- Fresh chopped chives, for garnish
- 3 eggs, beaten
- 1/2 teaspoon dried dill weed
- teaspoon dried rosemary
- 1/3 cup scallions, chopped
- 1/3 cup smoked whitefish, chopped
- 1 ½ tablespoon crème fraîche
- 1 teaspoon kosher salt
- 1 teaspoon dried marjoram
- 1/3 teaspoon ground black pepper, or more to taste
- Cooking spray

Directions
1. Firstly, spritz four oven-safe ramekins with cooking spray. Then, divide smoked whitefish, spring garlic, and scallions among greased ramekins.
2. Crack an egg into each ramekin; add the crème, yogurt, and all seasonings.
3. Now, air-fry approximately 13 minutes at 355 degrees f. Taste for doneness and eat warm garnished with fresh chives.

Nutrition: 249 calories 22.1g fat 7.6g carbs 5.3g protein 3.1g sugars 0.7g fiber

267. Parmesan and Paprika Baked Tilapia

Preparation time: 20 minutes
Cooking time: 15 minutes
Servings: 6
Ingredients:
- cup parmesan cheese, grated
- 1 teaspoon paprika
- 1 teaspoon dried dill weed
- pounds tilapia fillets
- 1/3 cup mayonnaise
- 1/2 tablespoon lime juice
- Salt and ground black pepper, to taste

Directions
1. Mix the mayonnaise, parmesan, paprika, salt, black pepper, and dill weed until everything is thoroughly combined.
2. Then, drizzle tilapia fillets with the lime juice.
3. Cover each fish fillet with parmesan/mayo mixture; roll them in parmesan/paprika mixture. Bake at 335 for about 10 minutes. Serve and eat warm.

Nutrition: 294 calories 16.1g fat 2.7g carbs 35.9g protein 0.1g sugars 0.2g fiber

268. Tangy Cod Fillets

Preparation time: 20 minutes
Cooking time: 15 minutes
Servings: 2
Ingredients:
- ½ tablespoons sesame oil
- 1/2 heaping teaspoon dried parsley flakes
- 1/3 teaspoon fresh lemon zest, finely grated
- medium-sized cod fillets
- 1 teaspoon sea salt flakes
- A pinch of salt and pepper
- 1/3 teaspoon ground black pepper, or more to savor
- 1/2 tablespoon fresh lemon juice

Directions
1. Set the air fryer to cook at 375 degrees f. Season each cod fillet with sea salt flakes, black pepper, and dried parsley flakes. Now, drizzle them with sesame oil.
2. Place the seasoned cod fillets in a single layer at the bottom of the cooking basket; air-fry approximately 10 minutes.
3. While the fillets are cooking, prepare the sauce by mixing the other ingredients. Serve cod fillets on four individual plates garnished with the creamy citrus sauce.

Nutrition: 291 calories 11.1g fat 2.7g carbs 41.6g protein 1.2g sugars 0.5g fiber

269. Fish and Cauliflower Cakes

Preparation Time: 2 hours 20 minutes
Cooking Time: 13 minutes
Servings: 4
Ingredients:
- 1/2-pound cauliflower florets
- 1/2 teaspoon English mustard
- 2 tablespoons butter, room temperature
- 1/2 tablespoon cilantro, minced
- 2 tablespoons sour cream
- 2 ½ cups cooked white fish
- Salt and freshly cracked black pepper, to savor

Directions:
1. Boil the cauliflower until tender. Then, purée the cauliflower in your blender. Transfer to a mixing dish.
2. Now, stir in the fish, cilantro, salt, and black pepper.
3. Add the sour cream, English mustard, and butter; mix until everything's well incorporated. Using your hands, shape into patties.
4. Place in the refrigerator for about 2 hours. Cook for 13 minutes at 395 degrees f. Serve with some extra English mustard.

Nutrition: 285 calories 15.1g fat 4.3g carbs 31.1g protein 1.6g sugars 1.3g fiber

270. Marinated Scallops with Butter And Beer

Preparation Time: 1 hour 10 minutes
Cooking Time: 7 minutes
Servings: 4
Ingredients:
- 2 pounds sea scallops
- 1/2 cup beer
- 4 tablespoons butter
- 2 sprigs rosemary, only leaves
- Sea salt and freshly cracked black pepper, to taste

Directions:
1. In a ceramic dish, mix the sea scallops with beer; let it marinate for 1 hour.
2. Meanwhile, preheat your air fryer to 400 degrees f. Melt the butter and add the rosemary leaves. Stir for a few minutes.
3. Discard the marinade and transfer the sea scallops to the air fryer basket. Season with salt and black pepper.

SEAFOOD RECIPES

4. Cook the scallops in the preheated air fryer for 7 minutes, shaking the basket halfway through the cooking time. Work in batches.

Nutrition: 471 calories 27.3g fat 1.9g carbs 54g protein 0.2g sugars; 0.1g fiber

271. **Cheesy Fish Gratin**

Preparation Time: 30 minutes
Cooking Time: 20 minutes
Servings: 4
Ingredients:
- tablespoon avocado oil
- 1-pound hake fillets
- 1 teaspoon garlic powder
- Sea salt and ground white pepper, to taste
- tablespoons shallots, chopped
- 1 bell pepper, seeded and chopped
- 1/2 cup cottage cheese
- 1/2 cup sour cream
- 1 egg, well whisked
- 1 teaspoon yellow mustard
- 1 tablespoon lime juice
- 1/2 cup swiss cheese, shredded

Directions:
1. Brush the bottom and sides of a casserole dish with avocado oil. Add the hake fillets to the casserole dish and sprinkle with garlic powder, salt, and pepper.
2. Add the chopped shallots and bell peppers.
3. In a mixing bowl, thoroughly combine the cottage cheese, sour cream, egg, mustard, and lime juice. Pour the mixture over fish and spread evenly.
4. Cook in the preheated air fryer at 370 degrees f for 10 minutes.
5. Top with the Swiss cheese and cook an additional 7 minutes. Let it rest for 10 minutes before slicing and serving.

Nutrition: 335 calories 18.1g fats 7.8g carbs 33.7g protein 2.6g sugars 0.6g fiber

272. **Fijian Coconut Fish**

Preparation Time: 20 minutes + marinating time
Cooking Time: 15 minutes
Servings: 2
Ingredients:
- cup coconut milk
- tablespoons lime juice
- tablespoons shoyu sauce
- Salt and white pepper, to taste
- 1 teaspoon turmeric powder
- 1/2 teaspoon ginger powder
- 1/2 thai bird's eye chili, seeded and finely chopped
- 1-pound tilapia
- 2 tablespoons olive oil

Directions:
1. In a mixing bowl, thoroughly combine the coconut milk with the lime juice, shoyu sauce, salt, pepper, turmeric, ginger, and chili pepper. Add tilapia and let it marinate for 1 hour.
2. Brush the air fryer basket with olive oil. Discard the marinade and place the tilapia fillets in the air fryer basket.
3. Cook the tilapia in the preheated air fryer at 400 degrees f for 6 minutes; turn them over and cook for 6 minutes more. Work in batches.
4. Serve with some extra lime wedges if desired.

Nutrition: 426 calories 21.5g fat 9.4g carbs 50.2g protein 5g sugars 3.4g fiber

273. **Sole Fish and Cauliflower Fritters**

Preparation Time: 30 minutes
Cooking Time: 25 minutes
Servings: 2
Ingredients:
- 1/2 pound sole fillets
- 1/2 pound mashed cauliflower
- egg, well beaten
- 1/2 cup red onion, chopped
- garlic cloves, minced
- tablespoons fresh parsley, chopped
- 1 bell pepper, finely chopped
- 1/2 teaspoon scotch bonnet pepper, minced
- 1 tablespoon olive oil
- 1 tablespoon coconut aminos
- 1/2 teaspoon paprika
- Salt and white pepper, to taste

Directions:
1. Start by preheating your air fryer to 395 degrees f. Spritz the sides and bottom of the cooking basket with cooking spray.
2. Cook the sole fillets in the preheated air fryer for 10 minutes, flipping them halfway through the cooking time.
3. In a mixing bowl, mash the sole fillets into flakes. Stir in the remaining ingredients. Shape the fish mixture into patties.
4. Bake in the preheated air fryer at 390 degrees f for 14 minutes, flipping them halfway through the cooking time.

Nutrition: 322 calories 14g fat 27.4g carbs 22.1g protein 4.2g sugars 3.5g fiber

274. **French-Style Sea Bass**

Preparation Time: 15 minutes
Cooking Time: 10 minutes
Servings: 2
Ingredients:
- tablespoon olive oil
- sea bass fillets
- Sauce:
- 1/2 cup mayonnaise
- tablespoon capers, drained and chopped
- 1 tablespoon gherkins, drained and chopped
- tablespoons scallions, finely chopped
- tablespoons lemon juice

Directions:
1. Start by preheating your air fryer to 395 degrees f. Drizzle olive oil all over the fish fillets.
2. Cook the sea bass in the preheated air fryer for 10 minutes, flipping them halfway through the cooking time.
3. Meanwhile, make the sauce by whisking the remaining ingredients until everything is well incorporated. Place in the refrigerator until ready to serve.

Nutrition: 384 calories 28.5g fat 3.5g carbs 27.6g protein 1g sugars 1g fiber

275. **Asian-Style Salmon Burgers**

Preparation Time: 15 minutes
Cooking Time: 10 minutes
Servings: 4
Ingredients:
- pound salmon

- 1 egg
- 1 garlic clove, minced
- green onions, minced
- 1 cup parmesan cheese
- Sauce:
- teaspoon rice wine
- 1 ½ tablespoons soy sauce
- A pinch of salt
- 1 teaspoon gochugaru (Korean red chili pepper flakes)

Directions:
1. Start by preheating your air fryer to 380 degrees f. Spritz the air fryer basket with cooking oil.
2. Mix the salmon, egg, garlic, green onions, and parmesan cheese in a bowl; knead with your hands until everything is well incorporated.
3. Shape the mixture into equally sized patties. Transfer your patties to the air fryer basket.
4. Cook the fish patties for 10 minutes, turning them over halfway through.
5. Meanwhile, make the sauce by whisking all ingredients. Serve the warm fish patties with the sauce on the side.

Nutrition: 301 calories 15.1g fat 5.6g carbs 33.1g protein 1.4g sugars 0.2g fiber

276. Crusted Flounder Fillets

Preparation Time: 20 minutes
Cooking Time: 12 minutes
Servings: 2

Ingredients:
- 2 flounder fillets
- egg
- 1/2 teaspoon Worcestershire sauce
- 1/4 cup coconut flour
- 1/4 cup almond flour
- 1/2 teaspoon lemon pepper
- 1/2 teaspoon coarse sea salt
- 1/4 teaspoon chili powder

Directions:
1. Rinse and pat dry the flounder fillets.
2. Whisk the egg and Worcestershire sauce in a shallow bowl. In a separate bowl, mix the coconut flour, almond flour, lemon pepper, salt, and chili powder.
3. Then, dip the fillets into the egg mixture. Lastly, coat the fish fillets with the coconut flour mixture until they are coated on all sides.
4. Spritz with cooking spray and transfer to the air fryer basket. Cook at 390 degrees for 7 minutes.
5. Turn them over, spritz with cooking spray on the other side, and cook another 5 minutes.

Nutrition: 325 calories 18.3g fat 6.1g carbs 34.4g protein 2.2g sugar 1.7g fiber

277. Pecan Crusted Tilapia

Preparation Time: 20 minutes
Cooking Time: 15 minutes
Servings: 5

Ingredients:
- 2 tablespoons ground flaxseeds
- teaspoon paprika
- Sea salt and white pepper, to taste
- 1 teaspoon garlic paste
- tablespoons extra-virgin olive oil
- 1/2 cup pecans, ground
- 5 tilapia fillets, slice into halves

Directions:
1. Combine the ground flaxseeds, paprika, salt, white pepper, garlic paste, olive oil, and ground pecans in a ziplock bag. Add the fish fillets and shake to coat well.
2. Spritz the air fryer basket with cooking spray. Cook in the preheated air fryer at 400 degrees f for 10 minutes; turn them over and cook for 6 minutes more. Work in batches.
3. Serve with lemon wedges, if desired.

Nutrition: 264 calories 17.1g fat 3.9g carbs 25.5g protein 1g sugars 2g fiber

278. Grilled Salmon with Butter And Wine

Preparation Time: 45 minutes
Cooking Time: 10 minutes
Servings: 4

Ingredients:
- 2 cloves garlic, minced
- 4 tablespoons butter, melted
- Sea salt and ground black pepper, to taste
- teaspoon smoked paprika
- 1/2 teaspoon onion powder
- 1 tablespoon lime juice
- 1/4 cup dry white wine
- 4 salmon steaks

Directions:
1. Place all ingredients in a large ceramic dish. Cover and let it marinate for 30 minutes in the refrigerator.
2. Arrange the salmon steaks on the grill pan. Bake at 390 degrees for 5 minutes, or until the salmon steaks are easily flaked with a fork.
3. Flip the fish steaks, baste with the reserved marinade, and cook another 5 minutes.

Nutrition: 516 calories 25.6g fat 2.4g carbs 65.7g protein 0.7g sugars 0.5g fiber

279. Ranch Flavored Tilapia

Preparation Time: 15 minutes
Cooking Time: 13 minutes
Servings: 4

Ingredients:
- ¾ cup cornflakes, crushed
- 1-ounce dry ranch mix
- 2 and ½ tablespoons vegetable oil
- 2 whole eggs
- 4 pieces 6 ounces each tilapia fillets

Directions:
1. Take a shallow bowl, crack in eggs and beat them well
2. Take another bowl and add cornflakes, ranch dressing, oil and mix well until you have a crumbly ix
3. Dip fish fillets into the egg, coat well with bread crumbs mixture
4. Press "Power Button" on your Air Fryer and select "Air Fry" mode
5. Press the Time Button and set time to 13 minutes
6. Push Temp Button and set temp to 356 degrees F
7. Press the "Start/Pause" button and start the device
8. Once the appliance beeps to indicated that it is pre-heated, arrange prepared tilapia into Air Fryer basket, insert into oven
9. Let it cook until done, serve, and enjoy!

Nutrition: Calories: 267 Fat: 12 g Saturated Fat: 3 g Carbohydrates: 5 g Fiber: 0.2 g Sodium: 168 mg Protein: 34 g

280. Butter Up Salmon

Preparation Time: 10 minutes
Cooking Time: 10 minutes

Servings: 2
Ingredients:
- 2 pieces 6 ounces salmon fillets
- Salt and pepper to taste
- tablespoon butter, melted

Directions:
1. Season salmon fillet well with salt and pepper, coat them with butter
2. Press "Power Button" on your Air Fryer and select "Air Fry" mode
3. Press the Time Button and set time to 20 minutes
4. Push Temp Button and set temp to 320 degrees F
5. Press the "Start/Pause" button and start the device
6. Once the appliance beeps to indicated that it is pre-heated, transfer fillets to a greased Air Fryer basket and push into oven
7. Serve and enjoy!

Nutrition: Calories: 270 Fat: 16 g Saturated Fat: 5.2 g Carbohydrates: 0 g Fiber: 0 g Sodium: 193 mg Protein: 33 g

281. Coconut Lime Shrimp
Preparation Time: 5 minutes
Cooking Time: 10 minutes
Servings: 4
Ingredients:
- 1-pound shrimp, cleaned and deveined
- 1 cup unsweetened, shredded coconut
- 1 tablespoon lime zest, grated
- ½ teaspoon cayenne powder
- 1 cup flour
- 1 tablespoon cornstarch
- 1 teaspoon salt
- 1 teaspoon pepper
- 1 egg white

Directions:
1. Set the air fryer to 350°F.
2. In a bowl, combine the unsweetened shredded coconut, lime zest, and cayenne powder.
3. In a second bowl, combine the flour, cornstarch, salt, and pepper.
4. Place the egg white in a third bowl.
5. One at a time, dip each shrimp first in the flour mixture, then the egg white, and then in the coconut mixture, patting on the coconut with your fingers to make sure it sticks.
6. Place the shrimp in the basket of the air fryer.
7. Cook for 10 minutes, turning once halfway through.

Nutrition: Calories 350.3, Total Fat 12.3 g, Saturated Fat 9.4 g, Total Carbohydrate 31.9 g, Dietary Fiber 2.9 g, Sugars 1.1 g, Protein 28.1 g

282. Prosciutto Wrapped Shrimp
Preparation Time: 1o minutes
Cooking Time: 10 minutes
Servings: 4
Ingredients:
- 1-pound shrimp, cleaned and deveined
- 2 teaspoons lemon juice
- ½ teaspoon salt
- 1 teaspoon black pepper
- ½ teaspoon garlic powder
- ½ pound prosciutto, or enough to wrap each shrimp with one piece

Directions:
1. Set the air fryer to 350°F.
2. Season the shrimp with the lemon juice, salt, black pepper, and garlic powder.
3. Take one piece of prosciutto and wrap it completely around one piece of shrimp.
4. Repeat until all the shrimp is wrapped, and place it in the basket of the air fryer.
5. Cook for 10 minutes, or until the shrimp is cooked all the way through.

Nutrition: Calories 260.1, Total Fat 12.0 g Saturated Fat 4.4 g Total Carbohydrate 3.0 g Dietary Fiber 0.0 g Sugars 0.0 g Protein 34.0 g

283. Shrimp Spring Rolls
Preparation Time: 10 minutes
Cooking Time: 15 minutes
Servings: 4
Ingredients:
- 1 tablespoon peanut oil
- 1 teaspoon sesame oil
- 2 cloves garlic, crushed and minced
- 1 teaspoon fresh ginger, grated
- ¼ cup water chestnuts, cut into small strips
- ½ cup carrots, shredded
- ½ cup cabbage, shredded
- ¼ cup scallions, sliced
- 1 tablespoon soy sauce
- 1 teaspoon five spice powder
- 1 teaspoon salt
- 1 teaspoon pepper
- ¼ pound shrimp, cleaned, deveined and sliced
- ½ cup bean sprouts
- 12-14 spring roll wrappers
- 1 egg, lightly beaten

Directions:
1. Heat the peanut oil and sesame oil in a large skillet over medium heat.
2. Add the garlic, ginger, chestnuts, carrots, cabbage, scallions, and soy sauce.
3. Season the mixture with five spice powder, salt, and pepper. Sauté the mixture for 3-5 minutes.
4. Add the shrimp and bean sprouts. Cook just until the shrimp is pink, and then remove the skillet from the heat.
5. Lay the spring roll wrappers out on the counter or other flat surface.
6. Brush the ends with the beaten egg mixture.
7. Place a generous spoonful of the mixture onto each spring roll wrapper.
8. Roll each one up, fold in the ends, and press the edge to seal.
9. Lightly brush the spring roll with the egg mixture again, if desired.
10. Set the air fryer to 390°F.
11. Place the spring rolls in the basket of the air fryer and cook for 5 minutes.
12. Serve with your favorite dipping sauce, if desired.

Nutrition: Calories 172.9, Total Fat 5.1 g Saturated Fat 0.8 g Total Carbohydrate 24.5 g Dietary Fiber 1.3 g Sugars 20.8 g Protein 6.7 g

284. Flakey Fried Whitefish
Preparation Time: 15 minutes
Cooking Time: 15 minutes
Servings: 4
Ingredients:
- 1-pound whitefish fillets, cut into 3-4-inch pieces
- 2 teaspoons fresh lemon juice
- 1 teaspoon salt
- 1 teaspoon black pepper

- ½ cup flour
- 2 eggs, lightly beaten
- 1 cup panko bread crumbs
- 1 tablespoon fresh tarragon, chopped
- 1 tablespoon fresh parsley chopped
- 1 tablespoon olive oil

Directions:
1. Set the air fryer to 390°F.
2. Sprinkle the whitefish fillets with lemon juice and season them with salt and black pepper.
3. Place the flour in one bowl and the eggs in a second bowl.
4. In a third bowl, combine the panko bread crumbs, tarragon, parsley, and olive oil. Mix until the olive oil is worked through the crumbs.
5. Dust a piece of whitefish with the flour, and then dip it into the egg mixture.
6. Next, place it into the panko mixture and use your hands to pat the crumbs onto the fish. Repeat until all the pieces are coated.
7. Place the whitefish pieces in the basket of the air fryer.
8. Cook for 12-15 minutes, or until the fish is cooked through.

Nutrition: Calories 372.8 Total Fat 14.8 g Saturated Fat 2.6 g Total Carbohydrate 24.1 g Dietary Fiber 0.9 g Sugars 1.1 g Protein 34.0 g

285. Cod with Simple Olive Caper Sauce

Preparation Time: 10 minutes
Cooking Time: 15 minutes
Servings: 4

Ingredients:
- 1-pound cod pieces
- 1 tablespoon plus 1 teaspoon olive oil
- 1 teaspoon lemon juice
- 1 teaspoon salt
- 1 teaspoon black pepper
- 1 cup cherry tomatoes, halved
- 2 cloves garlic, crushed and minced
- ¼ cup Kalamata olives, diced
- 1 tablespoon capers
- ¼ cup fresh basil, chopped

Directions:
1. Set the air fryer to 355°F.
2. Lightly brush the cod with 1 teaspoon of the olive oil.
3. Sprinkle the cod with lemon juice and season it with salt and black pepper.
4. Place the cod in the basket of the air fryer.
5. Cook for 12 minutes, or until the cod is flakey and tender.
6. While the cod is cooking, heat the remaining olive oil in a large skillet over medium.
7. Add the tomatoes and cook for 2-3 minutes, or until they begin to break down and release their juices.
8. Next, add the garlic, olives, capers, and basil to the skillet. Cook, stirring frequently, for 4-5 minutes.
9. Remove the cod from the air fryer and transfer it to serving plates.
10. Top the cod with the olive caper sauce before serving.

Nutrition: Calories 164.7 Total Fat 5.2 g Saturated Fat 0.8 g Total Carbohydrate 2.2 g Dietary Fiber 0.8 g Sugars 1.0 g Protein 25.7 g

286. Sesame Soy Striped Bass

Preparation Time: 15 minutes
Cooking Time: 10 minutes
Servings: 4
Ingredients:
- 1-pound striped bass steaks
- 1 cup soy sauce
- ½ cup mirin
- 2 tablespoons sesame oil
- 2 tablespoons brown sugar
- 1 tablespoon lime juice
- 1 tablespoon garlic chili paste
- ¼ cup apple juice

Directions:
1. Place the bass steaks in a shallow baking dish.
2. In a bowl, combine the soy sauce, mirin, sesame oil, brown sugar, lime juice, garlic chili paste, and apple juice. Use a whisk to blend.
3. Cover the steaks with the sesame soy sauce, cover, and refrigerate for one hour.
4. Set the air fryer to 390°F.
5. Remove the bass from the marinade and blot up any extra.
6. Place the steaks in the air fryer and cook for approximately 10 minutes, or until the fish is cooked through and flakey.
7. Remove the bass from the air fryer and let it rest several minutes before serving.

Nutrition: Calories 311.0 Total Fat 10.2 g Saturated Fat 1.7 g Total Carbohydrate 23.1 g Dietary Fiber 0.5 g Sugars 18.3 g Protein 29.8 g

287. Crab And Herb Croquettes

Preparation Time: 15 minutes
Cooking Time: 15 minutes
Servings: 4

Ingredients:
- 1 tablespoon olive oil
- ½ cup red onion, diced
- ¼ cup celery, diced
- ¼ cup red bell pepper, diced
- 3 cloves garlic, crushed and minced
- 1 teaspoon salt
- 1 teaspoon black pepper
- 1 tablespoon fresh tarragon, chopped
- 1 tablespoon fresh parsley, chopped
- 1-pound lump crab meat, shredded
- ¼ cup sour cream
- 2 eggs
- ½ cup flour
- 1 cup panko bread crumbs
- 1 teaspoon fresh lemon zest
- 1-2 teaspoon crushed red pepper flakes

Directions:
1. Place the olive oil in a skillet over medium heat.
2. Add the red onion, celery, red bell pepper, and garlic. Cook, stirring frequently, for approximately 5 minutes, or until the vegetables begin to become tender.
3. Season the mixture with salt, black pepper, tarragon, and parsley. Remove the skillet from the heat and allow it to cool enough so the mixture can be handled.
4. Next, transfer the vegetables to a bowl and add the lump crab meat, sour cream, and 1 egg. Mix well.
5. Set the air fryer to 390°F.
6. Place the flour in a bowl. In a second bowl, lightly beat the remaining egg.
7. In a blender or food processor, combine the panko bread crumbs, lemon zest, and crushed red pepper flakes. Transfer the contents to a third bowl.
8. Take the large spoonfuls of the lump crab mixture and form them into golf ball sized fritters.

9. Dip each one first into the flour, then the egg, and finally the panko mixture.
10. Place them in the air fryer and cook for 10 minutes.
11. Serve with your favorite seafood dipping sauce.

Nutrition: Calories 339.4 Total Fat 10.3 g Saturated Fat 3.1 g Total Carbohydrate 28.3 g Dietary Fiber 1.5 g Sugars 1.4 g Protein 32.3 g

288. Garlic Tarragon Buttered Salmon

Preparation Time: 30 minutes
Cooking Time: 20 minutes
Servings: 4
Ingredients:
- ¼ cup butter
- 1 tablespoon shallot, diced
- 1 tablespoon fresh tarragon, chopped
- 1 teaspoon fresh lemon zest
- 1-pound salmon fillets
- 1 teaspoon salt
- 1 teaspoon black pepper
- Fresh lemon slices for garnish

Directions:
1. Set the air fryer to 350°F.
2. Melt the butter in a saucepan over medium heat.
3. Once the butter has melted, add the shallot, tarragon, and lemon zest. Cook, stirring frequently, for 2-3 minutes. Remove it from the heat and set it aside.
4. Season the salmon fillets with salt and black pepper.
5. Liberally brush both sides of each piece of salmon with the garlic tarragon butter.
6. Place the salmon pieces in the air fryer and cook for 15 minutes, turning once halfway through.
7. Remove the salmon from the air fryer and garnish with any remaining butter sauce and fresh lemon slices.

Nutrition: Calories 272.6 Total Fat 16.5 g Saturated Fat 8.1 g Total Carbohydrate 0.4 g Dietary Fiber 0.0 g Sugars 0.0 g Protein 29.1 g

289. Crab-Stuffed Mushrooms

Preparation Time: 10 minutes
Cooking Time: 20 minutes
Servings: 6
Ingredients:
- 2 ounces cream cheese, at room temperature
- ½ cup lump crabmeat, shells discarded
- 1 teaspoon prepared horseradish
- 1 teaspoon lemon juice
- ½ teaspoon salt
- ½ teaspoon freshly ground black pepper
- 16 ounces baby bella (cremini) mushrooms, stems removed
- 2 tablespoons panko bread crumbs
- 2 tablespoons butter, melted
- ¼ cup chopped fresh parsley

Directions:
1. 2 ounces cream cheese, at room temperature
2. ½ cup lump crabmeat, shells discarded
3. 1 teaspoon prepared horseradish
4. 1 teaspoon lemon juice
5. ½ teaspoon salt
6. ½ teaspoon freshly ground black pepper
7. 16 ounces baby bella (cremini) mushrooms, stems removed
8. 2 tablespoons panko bread crumbs
9. 2 tablespoons butter, melted
10. ¼ cup chopped fresh parsley

Nutrition: Calories: 99 Protein: 5g Fiber: 1g Net carbohydrates: 4g Fat: 7g Sodium: 274mg Carbohydrates: 5g Sugar: 2g

290. Oysters Rockefeller

Preparation Time: 10 minutes
Cooking Time: 16 minutes
Servings: 2
Ingredients:
- 2 tablespoons butter
- 1 medium shallot, peeled and minced
- 1 clove garlic, peeled and minced
- 1 cup chopped fresh baby spinach
- 4 teaspoons grated Parmesan cheese
- ⅛ teaspoon Tabasco original hot sauce
- ½ teaspoon fresh lemon juice
- ¼ cup crushed garlic pork rinds
- 12 oysters, on the half shell, rinsed and patted dry

Directions:
1. In a small skillet, heat butter over medium heat 30 seconds. Add shallot, garlic, and spinach. Stir-fry 3 minutes until shallot is translucent.
2. Add Parmesan cheese, Tabasco sauce, lemon juice, and pork rinds to skillet. Distribute mixture to tops of oysters.
3. Preheat air fryer at 400°F for 3 minutes.
4. Place half of oysters in ungreased air fryer basket. Cook 6 minutes.
5. Transfer cooked oysters to a large serving plate and repeat cooking with remaining oysters. Serve warm.

Nutrition: Calories: 198 Protein: 9g Fiber: 1g Net carbohydrates: 5g Fat: 15g Sodium: 213mg Carbohydrates: 6g Sugar: 2g

291. Steamer Clams

Preparation Time: 20 minutes
Cooking Time: 7 minutes
Servings: 2
Ingredients:
- 25 littleneck clams, scrubbed
- 2 tablespoons water
- 2 tablespoons butter, melted
- 2 lemon wedges

Directions:
1. Place clams in a large bowl filled with water. Let stand 10 minutes. Drain. Refill bowl with water and let stand an additional 10 minutes. Drain.
2. Preheat air fryer at 350°F for 3 minutes.
3. Pour 2 tablespoons water into bottom of air fryer. Add clams to ungreased air fryer basket. Cook 7 minutes. Discard any clams that don't open.
4. Remove clams from shells and add to a large serving dish with melted butter. Squeeze lemon on top and serve.

Nutrition: Calories: 279 Protein: 30g Fiber: 0g Net carbohydrates: 7g Fat: 14g Sodium: 1,429mg Carbohydrates: 7g Sugar: 0g

292. Bay Scallops

Preparation Time: 5 minutes
Cooking Time: 5 minutes
Servings: 4
Ingredients:
- 2 tablespoons butter, melted
- Juice from 1 medium lime
- ¼ teaspoon salt
- 1-pound bay scallops

Directions:
1. Preheat air fryer at 350°F for 3 minutes.
2. In a medium bowl, whisk together butter, lime juice, and salt. Add scallops and toss.

SEAFOOD RECIPES

3. Place scallops in ungreased air fryer basket. Cook 2 minutes. Toss scallops. Cook an additional 3 minutes.
4. Transfer scallops to a serving dish. Serve warm.

Nutrition: Calories: 132 Protein: 14g Fiber: 0g Net carbohydrates: 4g Fat: 6g Sodium: 591mg Carbohydrates: 4g Sugar: 0g

293. Smoky Fried Calamari

Preparation Time: 15 minutes
Cooking Time: 8 minutes
Servings: 4

Ingredients:
- 2 tablespoons no-sugar-added tomato paste
- 1 tablespoon gochujang
- 1 tablespoon fresh lime juice
- 1 teaspoon smoked paprika
- ½ teaspoon salt
- 1 cup crushed pork rinds
- ⅓ pound (about 6) calamari tubes, cut into ¼" rings

Directions:
1. Preheat air fryer at 400°F for 3 minutes.
2. In a medium bowl, whisk together tomato paste, gochujang, lime juice, paprika, and salt. Add pork rinds to a separate shallow dish.
3. Dredge a calamari ring in tomato mixture. Shake off excess. Roll through pork rind crumbs. Repeat with remaining rings.
4. Place half of calamari rings in air fryer basket lightly greased with olive oil. Cook 2 minutes. Gently flip and cook an additional 2 minutes.
5. Transfer cooked calamari to a large serving dish and repeat cooking with remaining calamari. Serve warm.

Nutrition: Calories: 99 Protein: 11g Fiber: 1g Net carbohydrates: 5g Fat: 3g Sodium: 545mg Carbohydrates: 6g Sugar: 2g

294. Breaded Fish Sticks with Tartar Sauce

Preparation Time: 10 minutes
Cooking Time: 20 minutes
Servings: 4

Ingredients:
- For Tartar Sauce
- ½ cup mayonnaise
- 1 tablespoon Dijon mustard
- ½ cup small-diced dill pickles
- ⅛ teaspoon salt
- ¼ teaspoon freshly ground black pepper
- For Fish Sticks
- 1 large egg, beaten
- ¼ cup arrowroot flour
- ¼ cup almond flour
- ½ teaspoon salt
- ¼ teaspoon freshly ground black pepper
- 1-pound cod, cut into 1" sticks

Directions:
1. To make Tartar Sauce: Combine all ingredients in a small bowl and refrigerate covered until ready to use.
2. To make Fish Sticks: Preheat air fryer at 350°F for 3 minutes.
3. Place egg in a small bowl. Combine arrowroot flour, almond flour, salt, and pepper in a separate shallow dish.
4. Dip a fish stick in egg. Shake off excess egg. Roll in flour mixture. Transfer to a large plate. Repeat with remaining fish sticks.
5. Place half of fish sticks in air fryer basket lightly greased with olive oil. Cook 5 minutes. Carefully flip fish sticks. Cook an additional 5 minutes.
6. Transfer cooked fish sticks to a large serving plate and repeat cooking with remaining fish sticks. Serve warm with tartar sauce on the side.

Nutrition: Calories: 363 Protein: 21g Fiber: 1g Net carbohydrates: 8g Fat: 26g Sodium: 855mg Carbohydrates: 9g Sugar: 1g

295. Crab Cakes With Arugula And Blackberry Salad

Preparation Time: 15 minutes
Cooking Time: 10 minutes
Servings: 2

Ingredients:
For Crab Cakes
- 8 ounces lump crabmeat, shells discarded
- 2 tablespoons mayonnaise
- ½ teaspoon Dijon mustard
- ½ teaspoon lemon juice
- 2 teaspoons peeled and minced yellow onion
- ¼ teaspoon prepared horseradish
- ¼ cup almond meal
- 1 large egg white, beaten
- ½ teaspoon Old Bay Seasoning

For Salad
- 1 tablespoon olive oil
- 2 teaspoons lemon juice
- ⅛ teaspoon salt
- ⅛ teaspoon freshly ground black pepper
- 4 ounces fresh arugula
- ½ cup fresh blackberries
- ¼ cup walnut pieces
- 2 lemon wedges

Directions:
1. To make Crab Cakes: Preheat air fryer at 400°F for 3 minutes.
2. In a medium bowl, combine all ingredients. Form into four patties.
3. Place patties into air fryer basket lightly greased with olive oil. Cook 5 minutes. Flip patties. Cook an additional 5 minutes.
4. Transfer crab cakes to a large plate. Set aside.
5. To make Salad: In a large bowl, whisk together olive oil, lemon juice, salt, and pepper. Add arugula and toss. Distribute into two medium bowls.
6. Add two crab cakes to each bowl. Garnish with blackberries, walnuts, and lemon wedges. Serve.

Nutrition: Calories: 406 Protein: 29g Fiber: 4g Net carbohydrates: 6g Fat: 29g Sodium: 790mg Carbohydrates: 10g Sugar: 4g

296. Bacon-Wrapped Stuffed Shrimp

Preparation Time: 10 minutes
Cooking Time: 18 minutes
Servings: 4

Ingredients:
- 1-pound (about 20) large raw shrimp, deveined and shelled
- 3 tablespoons crumbled goat cheese
- 2 tablespoons panko bread crumbs
- ¼ teaspoon Worcestershire sauce
- ½ teaspoon prepared horseradish
- ¼ teaspoon garlic powder

- 2 teaspoons mayonnaise
- ¼ teaspoon freshly ground black pepper
- 2 tablespoons water
- 5 slices bacon, quartered
- ¼ cup chopped fresh parsley

Directions:
1. Butterfly shrimp by cutting down the spine of each shrimp without going all the way through.
2. In a medium bowl, combine goat cheese, bread crumbs, Worcestershire sauce, horseradish, garlic powder, mayonnaise, and pepper.
3. Preheat air fryer at 400°F for 3 minutes. Pour 2 tablespoons water into bottom of air fryer.
4. Evenly press goat cheese mixture into shrimp. Wrap a piece of bacon around each piece of shrimp to hold in cheese mixture.
5. Place half of shrimp in fryer basket. Cook 5 minutes. Flip shrimp. Cook an additional 4 minutes. Transfer to serving plate. Repeat with remaining shrimp.
6. Garnish with chopped parsley. Serve warm.

Nutrition: Calories: 174 Protein: 20g Fiber: 0g Net carbohydrates: 3g Fat: 8g Sodium: 833mg Carbohydrates: 4g Sugar: 0g

297. Simply Shrimp

Preparation Time: 5 minutes
Cooking Time: 6 minutes
Servings: 2

Ingredients:
- 1-pound medium raw shrimp, tail on, deveined, and thawed or fresh
- 2 tablespoons butter, melted
- 1 tablespoon fresh lemon juice (about ½ medium lemon)

Directions:
1. Preheat air fryer at 350°F for 3 minutes.
2. In a large bowl, toss shrimp in butter.
3. Place shrimp in air fryer basket lightly greased with olive oil. Cook 4 minutes. Gently flip shrimp. Cook an additional 2 minutes.
4. Transfer shrimp to a large serving plate. Squeeze lemon juice over shrimp and serve.

Nutrition: Calories: 265 Protein: 31g Fiber: 0g Net carbohydrates: 3g Fat: 14g Sodium: 1,285mg Carbohydrates: 3g Sugar: 0g

298. Chili Lime–Crusted Halibut

Preparation Time: 10 minutes
Cooking Time: 10 minutes
Servings: 2

Ingredients:
- 2 tablespoons butter, melted
- ½ cup crushed chili lime–flavored pork rinds
- 2 (6-ounce) halibut fillets

Directions:
1. Preheat air fryer at 350°F for 3 minutes.
2. Combine butter and pork rinds in a small bowl. Press mixture onto tops of halibut fillets.
3. Place fish in air fryer basket lightly greased with olive oil. Cook 10 minutes until fish is opaque and flakes easily with a fork.
4. Transfer fish to two medium plates and serve warm.

Nutrition: Calories: 269 Protein: 32g Fiber: 0g Net carbohydrates: 0g Fat: 15g Sodium: 239mg Carbohydrates: 0g Sugar: 0g

299. Tuna Croquettes

Preparation Time: 15 minutes
Cooking Time: 24 minutes
Servings: 4

Ingredients:
- 1 (12-ounce) can tuna in water, drained
- ⅓ cup mayonnaise
- 1 tablespoon minced fresh celery
- 2 teaspoons dried dill, divided
- 1 teaspoon fresh lime juice
- 1 cup crushed pork rinds, divided
- 1 large egg
- 1 teaspoon prepared horseradish

Directions:
1. Preheat air fryer at 375°F for 3 minutes.
2. In a medium bowl, combine tuna, mayonnaise, celery, 1 teaspoon dill, lime juice, ¼ cup pork rinds, egg, and horseradish.
3. Form mixture into twelve rectangular mound shapes (about 2 tablespoons each). Roll each croquette in a shallow dish with remaining crushed pork rinds.
4. Place six croquettes in air fryer basket lightly greased with olive oil. Cook 4 minutes. Gently turn one third. Cook an additional 4 minutes. Gently turn another third. Cook an additional 4 minutes.
5. Transfer cooked croquettes to a large serving dish. Repeat cooking with remaining croquettes and garnish with remaining dill. Serve warm.

Nutrition: Calories: 241 Protein: 19g Fiber: 0g Net carbohydrates: 0g Fat: 18g Sodium: 440mg Carbohydrates: 0g Sugar: 0g

300. Tuna Melts On Tomatoes

Preparation Time: 10 minutes
Cooking Time: 4 minutes
Servings: 2

Ingredients:
- 1 (6-ounce) can tuna in water, drained
- ¼ cup mayonnaise
- 2 teaspoons yellow mustard
- 1 tablespoon minced dill pickle
- 1 tablespoon minced celery
- 1 tablespoon peeled and minced yellow onion
- ⅛ teaspoon salt
- ⅛ teaspoon freshly ground black pepper
- 4 thick slices large beefsteak tomato
- 1 small avocado, peeled, pitted, and cut into 8 slices
- ½ cup grated mild Cheddar cheese

Directions:
1. Combine tuna, mayonnaise, mustard, pickles, celery, onion, salt, and pepper in a medium bowl.
2. Preheat air fryer at 350°F for 3 minutes.
3. Cut a piece of parchment paper to fit the bottom of the air fryer basket. Place tomato slices on paper in single layer. Place two avocado slices on each tomato slice. Distribute tuna salad over avocado slices. Top evenly with cheese.
4. Place stacks in ungreased air fryer basket and cook 4 minutes until cheese starts to brown. Serve warm.

Nutrition: Calories: 532 Protein: 22g Fiber: 8g Net carbohydrates: 5g Fat: 46g Sodium: 762mg Carbohydrates: 13g Sugar: 3g

301. Classic Lobster Salad

Preparation Time: 10 minutes
Cooking Time: 8 minutes
Servings: 2

Ingredients:
- 2 (6-ounce) uncooked lobster tails, thawed
- ¼ cup mayonnaise
- 2 teaspoons fresh lemon juice
- 1 small stalk celery, sliced

- 2 teaspoons chopped fresh chives
- 2 teaspoons chopped fresh tarragon
- ¼ teaspoon salt
- ⅛ teaspoon freshly ground black pepper
- 2 thick slices large beefsteak tomato
- 1 small avocado, peeled, pitted, and diced

Directions:
1. Preheat air fryer at 400°F for 3 minutes.
2. Using kitchen shears, cut down the middle of each lobster tail on the softer side. Carefully run your finger between the lobster meat and the shell to loosen meat.
3. Place lobster tails, cut sides up, in ungreased air fryer basket. Cook 8 minutes.
4. Transfer tails to a large plate and let cool about 3 minutes until easy to handle, then pull lobster meat from shell. Roughly chop meat and add to a medium bowl.
5. Add mayonnaise, lemon juice, celery, chives, tarragon, salt, and pepper to bowl. Combine.
6. Divide lobster salad between two medium plates, top with tomato slices, and garnish with avocado. Serve.

Nutrition: Calories: 463 Protein: 24g Fiber: 7g Net carbohydrates: 5g Fat: 36g Sodium: 1,343mg Carbohydrates: 12g Sugar: 3g

302. Baked Avocados with Smoked Salmon
Preparation Time: 10 minutes
Cooking Time: 8 minutes
Servings: 2
Ingredients:
- ¼ cup apple cider vinegar
- 1 teaspoon granular erythritol
- ¼ cup peeled and sliced red onion
- 2 ounces cream cheese, room temperature
- 1 tablespoon capers, drained
- 2 large avocados, peeled, halved, and pitted
- 4 ounces smoked salmon
- 2 medium cherry tomatoes, halved

Directions:
1. In a small saucepan, heat apple cider vinegar and erythritol over high heat 4 minutes until boiling. Add onion and remove saucepan from heat. Let set while preparing remaining ingredients. Drain when ready to use onions.
2. Combine cream cheese and capers in a small bowl. Cover and refrigerate until ready to use.
3. Preheat air fryer at 350°F for 3 minutes.
4. Place avocado halves, cut sides up, in ungreased air fryer basket and cook 4 minutes.
5. Transfer avocados to two medium plates and garnish with cream cheese mixture, smoked salmon, pickled onions, and tomato halves. Serve.

Nutrition: Calories: 501 Protein: 16g Fiber: 14g Net carbohydrates: 6g Fat: 42g Sodium: 590mg Carbohydrates: 22g Sugar: 3g

303. Breaded Cod Sticks
Preparation Time: 10 minutes
Cooking Time: 12 minutes
Servings: 5
Ingredients:
- 2 Large eggs
- 3 tbsp. Milk
- 2 cups Breadcrumbs
- 1 cup Almond flour
- 1 lb. Cod

Directions:
1. Heat the Air Fryer at 350° Fahrenheit.
2. Prepare three bowls; one with the milk and eggs, one with the breadcrumbs (salt and pepper if desired), and another with almond flour.
3. Dip the sticks in the flour, egg mixture, and breadcrumbs.
4. Place in the basket and set the timer for 12 minutes. Toss the basket halfway through the cooking process.
5. Serve with your favorite sauce.

Nutrition: Calories: 107 kcal Protein: 16.56 g Fat: 3.69 g Carbohydrates: 0.74 g

304. Cod Fish Nuggets
Preparation Time: 10 minutes
Cooking Time: 20 minutes
Servings: 4
Ingredients:
- 1 lb. Cod fillet
- 3 Eggs
- 4 tbsp. Olive oil
- 1 cup Almond flour
- 1 cup Gluten-free breadcrumbs

Directions:
1. Warm the Air Fryer at 390° Fahrenheit.
2. Slice the cod into nuggets.
3. Prepare three bowls. Whisk the eggs in one. Combine the salt, oil, and breadcrumbs in another. Sift the almond flour into the third one.
4. Cover each of the nuggets with the flour, dip in the eggs, and the breadcrumbs.
5. Arrange the nuggets in the basket and set the timer for 20 minutes.
6. Serve the fish with your favorite dips or sides.

Nutrition: Calories: 595 kcal Protein: 35.06 g Fat: 42.98 g Carbohydrates: 17.21 g

305. Easy Crab Sticks
Preparation Time: 10 minutes
Cooking Time: 20 minutes
Servings: 2-3
Ingredients:
- 1 pkg. Crab sticks
- Cooking oil spray (as needed)

Directions:
1. Take each of the sticks out of the package and unroll it until the stick is flat. Tear the sheets into thirds.
2. Arrange them on a baking tray and lightly spritz using cooking spray. Set the timer for 10 minutes.

Note: If you shred the crab meat, you can cut the time in half, but they will also easily fall through the holes in the basket.

Nutrition: Calories: 34 kcal Protein: 3.4 g Fat: 2.17 g Carbohydrates: 0.02 g

306. Caspian Cod
Preparation Time: 10 minutes
Cooking Time: 12 minutes
Servings: 5
Ingredients:
- 2 Large eggs
- 3 tbsp. Milk
- 2 cups Breadcrumbs
- 1 cup Almond flour
- 1 lb. Cod

Directions:
1. Heat the Air Fryer at 350° Fahrenheit.
2. Prepare three bowls; one with the milk and eggs, one with the breadcrumbs (salt and pepper if desired), and another with almond flour.

3. Dip the sticks in the flour, egg mixture, and breadcrumbs.
4. Place in the basket and set the timer for 12 minutes. Toss the basket halfway through the cooking process.
5. Serve with your favorite sauce.

Nutrition: Calories: 107 kcal Protein: 16.56 g Fat: 3.69 g Carbohydrates: 0.74 g

307. Sesame Seeds Fish Fillet

Preparation Time: 10 minutes
Cooking Time: 30 minutes
Servings: 3-5

Ingredients:
- 5 frozen fish fillets (if it's not frozen, just cut the cooking time by roughly 3 minutes)
- 3 tbsp. plain flour
- 1 egg, beaten
- Coating:
- Handful of sesame seeds
- 3 tbsp. oil Pinch of ground black pepper
- Pinch of sea salt
- 5-6 soda biscuit crumbs (or any plain biscuits you have or breadcrumbs)
- Pinch of rosemary herbs, optional

Directions:
1. Coating Without adding oil to the pan, fry the sesame seed in it for 2 minutes while stirring consis-tently. Once they become brown, remove them from pan.
2. Get a large plate and make a mixture of all the coating ingredients.
3. Ensure that your Air Fryer is preheated to 3 60 F and lined with aluminum foil.
4. Proceed to arrange your ingredients to en-sure efficiency following the order below.
5. Dip the fish in the flour, then the egg, and finally in the coating mixture.
6. Place the coated fish inside the air fryer.
7. Cook for 10 minutes if it's frozen fillet, flip the fish and cook for extra 4 minutes.
8. If the fillet is not frozen, cook the first side for 8 minutes and for 2 minutes
9. Serve!

Nutrition: Calories: 200 kcal Protein: 6.48 g Fat: 7.49 g Carbohydrates: 27.07 g

308. Chili Tuna Puff

Preparation Time: 10 minutes
Cooking Time: 10 minutes
Servings: 2

Ingredients:
- ½ cup chili tuna
- 1 sheet puff pastry (thawed)

Directions:
1. Ensure that your Air Fryer is preheated to 375 F.
2. Make four equal squares out of the pastry.
3. Spread the Chili Tuna on each square pas-try, right at the center.
4. Fold the square pastry into a triangle or a rectangle, and press the edges with a fork to seal them off.
5. Transfer the pastry in the baking tray and allow to air bake for 10-12 minutes, or until you have the golden brown color.

Nutrition: Calories: 131 kcal Protein: 7.51 g Fat: 7.6 g Carbohydrates: 15.9 g

309. Shrimp Spring Rolls with Sweet Chili Sauce

Preparation Time: 20 minutes
Cooking Time: 20 minutes
Servings: 4

Ingredients:
- 2 ½ tbsp. sesame oil, divided
- 1 cup julienne-cut red bell pepper
- 1 cup matchstick carrots
- 2 cups pre-shredded cabbage
- ¼ cup chopped fresh cilantro
- 2 tsp fish sauce
- ¼ tsp crushed red pepper
- 1 tbsp. fresh lime juice
- 3/4 cup julienne-cut snow peas
- 4 oz. peeled, deveined raw shrimp, chopped
- 8 (8-inch-square) spring roll wrappers
- ½ cup sweet chili sauce

Directions:
1. Get a large skillet, pour in 1.5 teaspoons of the oil and let it heat over high heat until it smokes slightly. Now toss in the bell pepper, carrots, and cabbage. Allow it to cook while continually stirring until the mixture is lightly wilted (this takes 1 or 1.5 minutes). Spread on a rimmed baking sheet and allow to cool for 5 minutes.
2. Get a large bowl and combine cilantro, fish sauce, crushed red pepper, lime juice, snow peas, shrimps, and the cabbage mixture. Stir slightly.
3. Place the spring roll wrappers on the work surface such that one corner is facing you. Using your spoon, transfer ¼ cup filling into the center of each spring roll wrapper, while spreading it from left to right and into a 3-inch long strip.
4. Fold the bottom corner of each wrapper over the filling, while tucking the tip of the corner under the filling. Fold right and left corners over filling. Brush the re-maining corner lightly using water, and roll the filled end of the wrapper towards the remaining corner. Finally, press gently to seal. Brush the spring rolls with the un-used two teaspoons oil.
5. Transfer the first four spring rolls in the air fryer basket and allow them to cook for about 7 minutes at 390 F. After the first five minutes, turn the spring rolls. Do the same for the other spring rolls.
6. Serve the cooked spring rolls alongside sweet chili sauce.

Nutrition: Calories: 1712 kcal Protein: 61.22 g Fat: 21.1 g Carbohydrates: 310.7 g

310. Gambas with Sweet Potato

Preparation Time: 10 minutes
Cooking Time: 25 minutes
Servings: 3-4

Ingredients:
- 12 King prawns
- 4 garlic cloves
- 1 red chili pepper, de-seeded
- 1 shallot
- 4 tbsp. olive oil
- Smoked paprika powder
- 5 large sweet potatoes
- 2 tbsp. olive oil
- 1 tbsp. honey
- 2 tbsp. fresh rosemary, finely chopped
- 4 stalks lemongrass
- 2 limes

Directions:
1. Clean and gut the prawns.

2. Gut the garlic and red chili pepper finely, and chop the shallots.
3. Combine the red chili pepper, garlic, and olive oil alongside the paprika to form a marinade. Let the prawns marinate for about 2 hours in the marinade.
4. Make fine slices by cutting the sweet potato. Mix the potato slices with 2 table-spoons of olive oil, honey, and the chopped rosemary. Bake the potatoes in the air fryer at 360 F for 15 minutes.
5. While baking the potatoes, thread the prawns on the lemongrass stalks. Increase the temperature to 390 F and include the prawn skewers.
6. Allow the combination to cook for 5 min-utes.
7. Serve alongside lime wedges.

Nutrition: Calories: 465 kcal Protein: 10.07 g Fat: 22.6 g Carbohydrates: 60.98 g

311. Wasabi Crab Cakes
Preparation Time: 20 minutes
Cooking Time: 15 minutes
Servings: 2
Ingredients:
- 2 large egg whites
- 1 celery rib, finely chopped
- 1 medium sweet red pepper, finely chopped
- 3 green onions, finely chopped
- ¼ tsp prepared wasabi
- 3 tbsp. reduced-fat mayonnaise
- ¼ tsp salt 1/3 cup plus
- ½ cup dry bread crumbs, divided
- 1-½ cups lump crabmeat, drained
- Cooking spray
- Sauce:
- ½ tsp prepared wasabi
- 1 green onion, chopped
- 1 celery rib, chopped
- 1 tbsp. sweet pickle relish
- ¼ tsp celery salt
- 1/3 cup reduced-fat mayonnaise

Directions:
1. Ensure that your Air Fryer is preheated to 375 F, and the air fryer basket spritzed with cooking spray.
2. Get a mixing bowl and make a mixture of the first seven ingredients, alongside 1/3 cup breadcrumbs. Fold gently in crab.
3. Get a shallow bowl and transfer the re-maining bread crumbs in it. Then add heaping tablespoonful of crab mixture into the bowl. Coat and shape the crumbs into patties of ¾-inches thick.
4. You may work in batches if required - each batch of crab cakes should be arranged in the air fryer basket to form a single layer.
5. Only cook after spritzing the crab cakes with cooking spray.
6. The cooking should last for 8 to 12 min-utes, or until the cakes turn golden brown. Halfway through cooking, turn the cakes, and spritz again with extra cooking spray.
7. Once cooked, withdraw and keep warm.
8. Do the same for the other batches.
9. While cooking the cakes, place the sauce ingredients in your food processor and blend to the preferred consistency.
10. Serve cooked crabs while hot, along-side the dipping sauce.

Nutrition: Calories: 482 kcal Protein: 18.17 g Fat: 25.4 g Carbohydrates: 46.72 g

312. Crab Legs
Preparation Time: 10 minutes
Cooking Time: 10 minutes
Servings: 3
Ingredients:
- 3 lb. crab legs
- ¼ cup salted butter, melted and divided
- ½ lemon, juiced
- ¼ tsp. garlic powder

Directions:
1. In a bowl, toss the crab legs and two tablespoons of the melted butter together. Place the crab legs in the basket of the fryer.
2. Cook at 400°F for fifteen minutes, giving the basket a good shake halfway through.
3. Combine the remaining butter with the lemon juice and garlic powder.
4. Crack open the cooked crab legs and remove the meat. Serve with the butter dip on the side and enjoy!

Nutrition: Calories: 515 kcal Protein: 84.23 g Fat: 17.16 g Carbohydrates: 0.93 g

313. Avocado Shrimp
Preparation Time: 10 minutes
Cooking Time: 10 minutes
Servings: 2
Ingredients:
- ½ cup onion, chopped
- 2 lb. shrimp
- 1 tbsp. seasoned salt
- 1 avocado
- ½ cup pecans, chopped

Directions:
1. Pre-heat the fryer at 400°F.
2. Put the chopped onion in the basket of the fryer and spritz with some cooking spray. Leave to cook for five minutes.
3. Add the shrimp and set the timer for a further five minutes. Sprinkle with some seasoned salt, then allow to cook for an additional five minutes.
4. During these last five minutes, halve your avocado and remove the pit. Cube each half, then scoop out the flesh.
5. Take care when removing the shrimp from the fryer. Place it on a dish and top with the avocado and the chopped pecans.

Nutrition: Calories: 770 kcal Protein: 98.97 g Fat: 37.92 g Carbohydrates: 14.69 g

314. Cheesy Lemon Halibut
Preparation Time: 10 minutes
Cooking Time: 12 minutes
Servings: 2
Ingredients:
- 1 lb. halibut fillet
- ½ cup butter
- 2 ½ tbsp. mayonnaise
- 2 ½ tbsp. lemon juice
- ¾ cup parmesan cheese, grated

Directions:
1. Pre-heat your fryer at 375°F.
2. Spritz the halibut fillets with cooking spray and season as desired.
3. Put the halibut in the fryer and cook for twelve minutes.

4. In the meantime, combine the butter, mayonnaise, and lemon juice in a bowl with a hand mixer. Ensure a creamy texture is achieved.
5. Stir in the grated parmesan.
6. When the halibut is ready, open the drawer and spread the butter over the fish with a butter knife. Allow to cook for a further two minutes, then serve hot.

Nutrition: Calories: 1328 kcal Protein: 67.69 g Fat: 106.33 g Carbohydrates: 27.55 g

315. Spicy Mackerel
Preparation Time: 15 minutes
Cooking Time: 5 minutes
Servings: 2
Ingredients:
- 2 mackerel fillets
- 2 tbsp. red chili flakes
- 2 tsp. garlic, minced
- 1 tsp. lemon juice

Directions:
1. Season the mackerel fillets with the red pepper flakes, minced garlic, and a drizzle of lemon juice. Allow to sit for five minutes.
2. Preheat your fryer at 350°F.
3. Cook the mackerel for five minutes, before opening the drawer, flipping the fillets, and allowing to cook on the other side for another five minutes.
4. Plate the fillets, making sure to spoon any remaining juice over them before serving.

Nutrition: Calories: 464 kcal Protein: 83.8 g Fat: 10.98 g Carbohydrates: 1.65 g

316. Thyme Scallops
Preparation Time: 5 minutes
Cooking Time: 7 minutes
Servings: 1
Ingredients:
- 1 lb. scallops
- Salt and pepper
- ½ tbsp. butter
- ½ cup thyme, chopped

Directions:
1. Wash the scallops and dry them completely. Season with pepper and salt, then set aside while you prepare the pan.
2. Grease a foil pan in several spots with the butter and cover the bottom with the thyme. Place the scallops on top.
3. Pre-heat the fryer at 400°F and set the rack inside.
4. Place the foil pan on the rack and allow to cook for seven minutes.
5. Take care when removing the pan from the fryer and transfer the scallops to a serving dish. Spoon any remaining butter in the pan over the fish and enjoy.

Nutrition: Calories: 484 kcal Protein: 62.9 g Fat: 14.51 g Carbohydrates: 23.58 g

317. Whitefish Cakes
Preparation Time: 5 minutes + 1 hour marinate
Cooking Time: 15 minutes
Servings: 4
Ingredients:
- 1 ½ cups whitefish fillets, minced
- 1 ½ cups green beans, finely chopped
- ½ cup scallions, chopped
- 1 chili pepper, deveined and minced
- 1 tbsp. red curry paste
- 1 tsp. sugar
- 1 tbsp. fish sauce
- 2 tbsp. apple cider vinegar
- 1 tsp. water
- Sea salt flakes, to taste
- ½ tsp. cracked black peppercorns
- 1 ½ teaspoons butter, at room temperature
- 1 lemon

Directions:
1. Place all of the ingredients a bowl, following the order in which they are listed.
2. Combine well with a spatula or your hands.
3. Mold the mixture into several small cakes and refrigerate for 1 hour.
4. Put a piece of aluminum foil in the cooking basket and lay the cakes on top.
5. Cook at 390°F for 10 minutes. Turn each fish cake over before air-frying for another 5 minutes.
6. Serve the fish cakes with a side of cucumber relish.

Nutrition: Calories: 162 kcal Protein: 17.16 g Fat: 7.65 g Carbohydrates: 6.19 g

318. Marinated Sardines
Preparation Time: 5 minutes + 30 minutes marinate
Cooking Time: 45 minutes
Servings: 4
Ingredients:
- ¾ lb. sardines, cleaned and rinsed
- Salt and ground black pepper, to taste
- 1 tsp. smoked cayenne pepper
- 1 tbsp. lemon juice
- 1 tbsp. soy sauce
- 2 tbsp. olive oil
- For the Potatoes:
- 8 medium Russet potatoes, peeled and quartered
- ½ stick melted butter
- Salt and pepper, to taste
- 1 tsp. granulated garlic

Directions:
1. Dry the sardines with a paper towel.
2. Cover the sardines in the salt, black pepper, cayenne pepper, lemon juice, soy sauce, and olive oil, and leave to marinate for half an hour.
3. Air-fry the sardines at 350°F for roughly 5 minutes.
4. Raise the heat to 385°F and cook for an additional 7 - 8 minutes. Remove the sardines and plate up.
5. Wipe the cooking basket clean and pour in the potatoes, butter, salt, pepper, and garlic.
6. Roast at 390°F for 30 minutes. Serve the vegetables and the sardines together.

Nutrition: Calories: 935 kcal Protein: 40.98 g Fat: 19.55 g Carbohydrates: 153.39 g

319. Halibut Steaks
Preparation Time: 10 minutes
Cooking Time: 15 minutes
Servings: 4
Ingredients:
- 1 lb. halibut steaks
- Salt and pepper to taste
- 1 tsp. dried basil
- 2 tbsp. honey
- ¼ cup vegetable oil
- 2 ½ tbsp. Worcester sauce
- 1 tbsp. freshly squeezed lemon juice
- 2 tbsp. vermouth

- 1 tbsp. fresh parsley leaves, coarsely chopped

Directions:
1. Put all of the ingredients in a large bowl. Combine and cover the fish completely with the seasoning.
2. Transfer to your Air Fryer and cook at 390°F for 5 minutes.
3. Turn the fish over and allow to cook for a further 5 minutes.
4. Ensure the fish is cooked through, leaving it in the fryer for a few more minutes if necessary.
5. Serve with a side of potato salad.

Nutrition: Calories: 402 kcal Protein: 18.42 g Fat: 30.9 g Carbohydrates: 11.89 g

320. Fish Taco

Preparation Time: 10 minutes
Cooking Time: 13 minutes
Servings: 4

Ingredients:
- 12 oz. cod filet
- 1 cup friendly bread crumbs
- 4 – 6 friendly flour tortillas
- 1 cup tempura butter
- ½ cup salsa
- ½ cup guacamole
- 2 tbsp. freshly chopped cilantro
- ½ tsp. salt
- ¼ tsp. black pepper
- Lemon wedges for garnish

Directions:
1. Slice the cod filets lengthwise and sprinkle salt and pepper on all sides.
2. Put the tempura butter in a bowl and coat each cod piece in it. Dip the fillets into the bread crumbs.
3. Pre-heat the Air Fryer to 340°F.
4. Fry the cod sticks for about 10 – 13 minutes in the fryer. Flip each one once while cooking.
5. In the meantime, coat one side of each tortilla with an even spreading of guacamole.
6. Put a cod stick in each tortilla and add the chopped cilantro and salsa on top. Lightly drizzle over the lemon juice. Fold into tacos.

Nutrition: Calories: 705 kcal Protein: 20.71 g Fat: 55.2 g Carbohydrates: 34.02 g

321. Seafood Fritters

Preparation Time: 20 minutes
Cooking Time: 30 minutes
Servings: 2-4

Ingredients:
- 2 cups clam meat
- 1 cup shredded carrot
- ½ cup shredded zucchini
- 1 cup flour, combined with 3/4 cup water to make a batter
- 2 tbsp. olive oil
- ¼ tsp. pepper

Directions:
1. Pre-heat your Air Fryer to 390°F.
2. Combine the clam meat with the olive oil, shredded carrot, pepper and zucchini.
3. Using your hands, shape equal portions of the mixture into balls and roll each ball in the chickpea mixture.
4. Put the balls in the fryer and cook for 30 minutes, ensuring they turn nice and crispy before serving.

Nutrition: Calories: 265 kcal Protein: 5.9 g Fat: 8.89 g Carbohydrates: 40.02 g

POULTRY RECIPES

322. Pretzel Crusted Chicken with Spicy Mustard Sauce

Preparation Time: 15 minutes
Cooking Time: 20 minutes
Servings: 6
Ingredients:
- 2 eggs
- 1 ½ pound chicken breasts, boneless, skinless, cut into bite-sized chunks
- 1/2 cup crushed pretzels
- 1 teaspoon shallot powder
- 1 teaspoon paprika
- Sea salt and ground black pepper, to taste
- 1/2 cup vegetable broth
- 1 tablespoon cornstarch
- 3 tablespoons Worcestershire sauce
- 3 tablespoons tomato paste
- 1 tablespoon apple cider vinegar
- 2 tablespoons olive oil
- 2 garlic cloves, chopped
- 1 jalapeno pepper, minced
- 1 teaspoon yellow mustard

Directions:
1. Start by preheating your Air Fryer to 390 degrees F.
2. In a mixing dish, whisk the eggs until frothy; toss the chicken chunks into the whisked eggs and coat well.
3. In another dish, combine the crushed pretzels with shallot powder, paprika, salt and pepper. Then, lay the chicken chunks in the pretzel mixture; turn it over until well coated.
4. Place the chicken pieces in the air fryer basket. Cook the chicken for 12 minutes, shaking the basket halfway through.
5. Meanwhile, whisk the vegetable broth with cornstarch, Worcestershire sauce, tomato paste, and apple cider vinegar.
6. Preheat a cast-iron skillet over medium flame. Heat the olive oil and sauté the garlic with jalapeno pepper for 30 to 40 seconds, stirring frequently.
7. Add the cornstarch mixture and let it simmer until the sauce has thickened a little. Now, add the air-fried chicken and mustard; let it simmer for 2 minutes more or until heated through.
8. Serve immediately and enjoy!

Nutrition: 357 Calories 17.6g Fat 20.3g Carbs 28.1g Protein 2.8g Sugars

323. Chinese-Style Sticky Turkey Thighs

Preparation Time: 20 minutes
Cooking Time: 35 minutes
Servings: 6
Ingredients:
- 1 tablespoon sesame oil
- 2 pounds turkey thighs
- 1 teaspoon Chinese Five-spice powder
- 1 teaspoon pink Himalayan salt
- 1/4 teaspoon Sichuan pepper
- 6 tablespoons honey
- 1 tablespoon Chinese rice vinegar
- 2 tablespoons soy sauce
- 1 tablespoon sweet chili sauce
- 1 tablespoon mustard

Directions:
1. Preheat your Air Fryer to 360 degrees F.
2. Brush the sesame oil all over the turkey thighs. Season them with spices.
3. Cook for 23 minutes, turning over once or twice. Make sure to work in batches to ensure even cooking
4. In the meantime, combine the remaining ingredients in a wok (or similar type pan) that is preheated over medium-high heat. Cook and stir until the sauce reduces by about a third.
5. Add the fried turkey thighs to the wok; gently stir to coat with the sauce.
6. Let the turkey rest for 10 minutes before slicing and serving. Enjoy!

Nutrition: 279 Calories 10.1g Fat 19g Carbs 27.7g Protein 17.9g Sugars

324. Easy Hot Chicken Drumsticks

Preparation Time: 40 minutes
Cooking Time: 30 minutes
Servings: 6
Ingredients:
- 6 chicken drumsticks
- Sauce:
- 6 ounces hot sauce
- 3 tablespoons olive oil
- 3 tablespoons tamari sauce
- 1 teaspoon dried thyme
- 1/2 teaspoon dried oregano

Directions:
1. Spritz the sides and bottom of the cooking basket with a nonstick cooking spray.
2. Cook the chicken drumsticks at 380 degrees F for 35 minutes, flipping them over halfway through.
3. Meanwhile, heat the hot sauce, olive oil, tamari sauce, thyme, and oregano in a pan over medium-low heat; reserve.
4. Drizzle the sauce over the prepared chicken drumsticks; toss to coat well and serve. Bon appétit!

Nutrition: 280 Calories 18.7g Fat 2.6g Carbs 24.1g Protein 1.4g Sugars

325. Crunchy Munchy Chicken Tenders With Peanuts

Preparation Time: 25 minutes
Cooking Time: 20 minutes
Servings: 4
Ingredients:
- 1 ½ pounds chicken tenderloins
- 2 tablespoons peanut oil
- 1/2 cup tortilla chips, crushed
- Sea salt and ground black pepper, to taste
- 1/2 teaspoon garlic powder
- 1 teaspoon red pepper flakes
- 2 tablespoons peanuts, roasted and roughly chopped

Directions:
1. Start by preheating your Air Fryer to 360 degrees F.
2. Brush the chicken tenderloins with peanut oil on all sides.

POULTRY RECIPES

3. In a mixing bowl, thoroughly combine the crushed chips, salt, black pepper, garlic powder, and red pepper flakes. Dredge the chicken in the breading, shaking off any residual coating.
4. Lay the chicken tenderloins into the cooking basket. Cook for 12 to 13 minutes or until it is no longer pink in the center. Work in batches; an instant-read thermometer should read at least 165 degrees F.
5. Serve garnished with roasted peanuts. Bon appétit!

Nutrition: 343 Calories 16.4g Fat 10.6g Carbs 36.8g Protein 1g Sugar

326. Tarragon Turkey Tenderloins with Baby Potatoes

Preparation Time: 50 minutes
Cooking Time: 50 minutes
Servings: 6

Ingredients:
- 2 pounds turkey tenderloins
- 2 teaspoons olive oil
- Salt and ground black pepper, to taste
- 1 teaspoon smoked paprika
- 2 tablespoons dry white wine
- 1 tablespoon fresh tarragon leaves, chopped
- 1-pound baby potatoes, rubbed

Directions:
1. Brush the turkey tenderloins with olive oil. Season with salt, black pepper, and paprika.
2. Afterwards, add the white wine and tarragon.
3. Cook the turkey tenderloins at 350 degrees F for 30 minutes, flipping them over halfway through. Let them rest for 5 to 9 minutes before slicing and serving.
4. After that, spritz the sides and bottom of the cooking basket with the remaining 1 teaspoon of olive oil.
5. Then, preheat your Air Fryer to 400 degrees F; cook the baby potatoes for 15 minutes. Serve with the turkey and enjoy!

Nutrition: 317 Calories 7.4g Fat 14.2g Carbs 45.7g Protein 1.1g Sugars

327. Mediterranean Chicken Breasts with Roasted Tomatoes

Preparation Time: 1 hour
Cooking Time: 30 minutes
Servings: 8

Ingredients:
- 2 teaspoons olive oil, melted
- 3 pounds chicken breasts, bone-in
- 1/2 teaspoon black pepper, freshly ground
- 1/2 teaspoon salt
- 1 teaspoon cayenne pepper
- 2 tablespoons fresh parsley, minced
- 1 teaspoon fresh basil, minced
- 1 teaspoon fresh rosemary, minced
- 4 medium-sized Roma tomatoes, halved

Directions:
1. Start by preheating your Air Fryer to 370 degrees F. Brush the cooking basket with 1 teaspoon of olive oil.
2. Sprinkle the chicken breasts with all seasonings listed above.
3. Cook for 25 minutes or until chicken breasts are slightly browned. Work in batches.
4. Arrange the tomatoes in the cooking basket and brush them with the remaining teaspoon of olive oil. Season with sea salt.
5. Cook the tomatoes at 350 degrees F for 10 minutes, shaking halfway through the cooking time. Serve with chicken breasts. Bon appétit!

Nutrition: 315 Calories 17.1g Fat 2.7g Carbs 36g Protein 1.7g Sugars

328. Thai Red Duck with Candy Onion

Preparation Time: 25 minutes
Cooking Time: 25 minutes
Servings: 4

Ingredients:
- 1 ½ pounds duck breasts, skin removed
- 1 teaspoon kosher salt
- 1/2 teaspoon cayenne pepper
- 1/3 teaspoon black pepper
- 1/2 teaspoon smoked paprika
- 1 tablespoon Thai red curry paste
- 1 cup candy onions, halved
- 1/4 small pack coriander, chopped

Directions:
1. Place the duck breasts between 2 sheets of foil; then, use a rolling pin to bash the duck until they are 1-inch thick.
2. Preheat your Air Fryer to 395 degrees F.
3. Rub the duck breasts with salt, cayenne pepper, black pepper, paprika, and red curry paste. Place the duck breast in the cooking basket.
4. Cook for 11 to 12 minutes. Top with candy onions and cook for another 10 to 11 minutes.
5. Serve garnished with coriander and enjoy!

Nutrition: 362 Calories 18.7g Fat 4g Carbs 42.3g Protein 1.3g Sugars

329. Rustic Chicken Legs With Turnip Chips

Preparation Time: 30 minutes
Cooking Time: 20 minutes
Servings: 3

Ingredients:
- 1-pound chicken legs
- 1 teaspoon Himalayan salt
- 1 teaspoon paprika
- 1/2 teaspoon ground black pepper
- 1 teaspoon butter, melted
- 1 turnip, trimmed and sliced

Directions:
1. Spritz the sides and bottom of the cooking basket with a nonstick cooking spray.
2. Season the chicken legs with salt, paprika, and ground black pepper.
3. Cook at 370 degrees F for 10 minutes. Increase the temperature to 380 degrees F.
4. Drizzle turnip slices with melted butter and transfer them to the cooking basket with the chicken. Cook the turnips and chicken for 15 minutes more, flipping them halfway through the cooking time.
5. As for the chicken, an instant-read thermometer should read at least 165 degrees F.
6. Serve and enjoy!

Nutrition: 207 Calories 7.8g Fat 3.4g Carbs 29.5g Protein 1.6g Sugars

330. Old-Fashioned Chicken Drumettes

Preparation Time: 30 minutes
Cooking Time: 22 minutes

Servings: 3

Ingredients:
- 1/3 cup all-purpose flour
- 1/2 teaspoon ground white pepper
- 1 teaspoon seasoning salt
- 1 teaspoon garlic paste
- 1 teaspoon rosemary
- 1 whole egg + 1 egg white
- 6 chicken drumettes
- 1 heaping tablespoon fresh chives, chopped

Directions:
1. Start by preheating your Air Fryer to 390 degrees.
2. Mix the flour with white pepper, salt, garlic paste, and rosemary in a small-sized bowl.
3. In another bowl, beat the eggs until frothy.
4. Dip the chicken into the flour mixture, then into the beaten eggs; coat with the flour mixture one more time.
5. Cook the chicken drumettes for 22 minutes. Serve warm, garnished with chives.

Nutrition: 347 Calories 9.1g Fat 11.3g Carbs 41g Protein 0.1g Sugars

331. Easy Ritzy Chicken Nuggets

Preparation Time: 20 minutes
Cooking Time: 8 minutes
Servings: 4

Ingredients:
- 1 ½ pounds chicken tenderloins, cut into small pieces
- 1/2 teaspoon garlic salt
- 1/2 teaspoon cayenne pepper
- 1/4 teaspoon black pepper, freshly cracked
- 4 tablespoons olive oil
- 1/3 cup saltines (e.g. Ritz crackers), crushed
- 4 tablespoons Parmesan cheese, freshly grated

Directions:
1. Start by preheating your Air Fryer to 390 degrees F.
2. Season each piece of the chicken with garlic salt, cayenne pepper, and black pepper.
3. In a mixing bowl, thoroughly combine the olive oil with crushed saltines. Dip each piece of chicken in the cracker mixture.
4. Finally, roll the chicken pieces over the Parmesan cheese. Cook for 8 minutes, working in batches.
5. Later, if you want to warm the chicken nuggets, add them to the basket and cook for 1 minute more. Serve with French fries, if desired.

Nutrition: 355 Calories; 20.1g Fat; 5.3g Carbs; 36.6g Protein; 0.2g Sugars

332. Asian Chicken Filets With Cheese

Preparation Time: 50 minutes
Cooking Time: 20 minutes
Servings: 2

Ingredients:
- 4 rashers smoked bacon
- 2 chicken filets
- 1/2 teaspoon coarse sea salt
- 1/4 teaspoon black pepper, preferably freshly ground
- 1 teaspoon garlic, minced
- 1 (2-inch) piece ginger, peeled and minced
- 1 teaspoon black mustard seeds
- 1 teaspoon mild curry powder
- 1/2 cup coconut milk
- 1/3 cup tortilla chips, crushed
- 1/2 cup Pecorino Romano cheese, freshly grated

Directions:
1. Start by preheating your Air Fryer to 400 degrees F. Add the smoked bacon and cook in the preheated Air Fryer for 5 to 7 minutes. Reserve.
2. In a mixing bowl, place the chicken fillets, salt, black pepper, garlic, ginger, mustard seeds, curry powder, and milk. Let it marinate in your refrigerator about 30 minutes.
3. In another bowl, mix the crushed chips and grated Pecorino Romano cheese.
4. Dredge the chicken fillets through the chips mixture and transfer them to the cooking basket. Reduce the temperature to 380 degrees F and cook the chicken for 6 minutes.
5. Turn them over and cook for a further 6 minutes. Repeat the process until you have run out of ingredients.
6. Serve with reserved bacon. Enjoy!

Nutrition: 376 Calories 19.6g Fat 12.1g Carbs 36.2g Protein 3.4g Sugars

333. Paprika Chicken Legs With Brussels Sprouts

Preparation Time: 30 minutes
Cooking Time: 20 minutes
Servings: 2

Ingredients:
- 2 chicken legs
- 1/2 teaspoon paprika
- 1/2 teaspoon kosher salt
- 1/2 teaspoon black pepper
- 1-pound Brussels sprouts
- 1 teaspoon dill, fresh or dried

Directions:
1. Start by preheating your Air Fryer to 370 degrees F.
2. Now, season your chicken with paprika, salt, and pepper. Transfer the chicken legs to the cooking basket. Cook for 10 minutes.
3. Flip the chicken legs and cook an additional 10 minutes. Reserve.
4. Add the Brussels sprouts to the cooking basket; sprinkle with dill. Cook at 380 degrees F for 15 minutes, shaking the basket halfway through.
5. Serve with the reserved chicken legs. Bon appétit!

Nutrition: 355 Calories 20.1g Fat 5.3g Carbs 36.6g Protein 0.2g Sugars

334. Chinese Duck

Preparation Time: 30 minutes
Cooking Time: 20 minutes
Servings: 6

Ingredients:
- 2 pounds duck breast, boneless
- 2 green onions, chopped
- 1 tablespoon light soy sauce
- 1 teaspoon Chinese 5-spice powder
- 1 teaspoon Szechuan peppercorns
- 3 tablespoons Shaoxing rice wine
- 1 teaspoon coarse salt
- 1/2 teaspoon ground black pepper
- Glaze:
- 1/4 cup molasses
- 3 tablespoons orange juice
- 1 tablespoon soy sauce

Directions:

POULTRY RECIPES

1. In a ceramic bowl, place the duck breasts, green onions, light soy sauce, Chinese 5-spice powder, Szechuan peppercorns, and Shaoxing rice wine. Let it marinate for 1 hour in your refrigerator.
2. Preheat your Air Fryer to 400 degrees F for 5 minutes.
3. Now, discard the marinade and season the duck breasts with salt and pepper. Cook the duck breasts for 12 to 15 minutes or until they are golden brown. Repeat with the other ingredients.
4. In the meantime, add the reserved marinade to the saucepan that is preheated over medium-high heat. Add the molasses, orange juice, and 1 tablespoon of soy sauce.
5. Bring to a simmer and then, whisk constantly until it gets syrupy. Brush the surface of duck breasts with glaze so they are completely covered.
6. Place duck breasts back in the Air Fryer basket; cook an additional 5 minutes. Enjoy!

Nutrition: 403 Calories 25.3g Fat 16.4g Carbs 27.5g Protein 13.2g Sugars

335. Turkey Bacon with Scrambled Eggs

Preparation Time: 25 minutes
Cooking Time: 20 minutes
Servings: 4
Ingredients:
- 1/2-pound turkey bacon
- 4 eggs
- 1/3 cup milk
- 2 tablespoons yogurt
- 1/2 teaspoon sea salt
- 1 bell pepper, finely chopped
- 2 green onions, finely chopped
- 1/2 cup Colby cheese, shredded

Directions:
1. Place the turkey bacon in the cooking basket.
2. Cook at 360 degrees F for 9 to 11 minutes. Work in batches. Reserve the fried bacon.
3. In a mixing bowl, thoroughly whisk the eggs with milk and yogurt. Add salt, bell pepper, and green onions.
4. Brush the sides and bottom of the baking pan with the reserved 1 teaspoon of bacon grease.
5. Pour the egg mixture into the baking pan. Cook at 355 degrees F about 5 minutes. Top with shredded Colby cheese and cook for 5 to 6 minutes more.
6. Serve the scrambled eggs with the reserved bacon and enjoy!

Nutrition: 456 Calories 38.3g Fat 6.3g Carbs 1.4g Protein 4.5g Sugars

336. Italian Chicken And Cheese Frittata

Preparation Time: 25 minutes ago
Cooking Time: 20 minutes
Servings: 4
Ingredients:
- 1 (1-pound) fillet chicken breast
- Sea salt and ground black pepper, to taste
- 1 tablespoon olive oil
- 4 eggs
- 1/2 teaspoon cayenne pepper
- 1/2 cup Mascarpone cream
- 1/4 cup Asiago cheese, freshly grated

Directions:
1. Flatten the chicken breast with a meat mallet. Season with salt and pepper.
2. Heat the olive oil in a frying pan over medium flame. Cook the chicken for 10 to 12 minutes; slice into small strips, and reserve.
3. Then, in a mixing bowl, thoroughly combine the eggs, and cayenne pepper; season with salt to taste. Add the cheese and stir to combine.
4. Add the reserved chicken. Then, pour the mixture into a lightly greased pan; put the pan into the cooking basket.
5. Cook in the preheated Air Fryer at 355 degrees F for 10 minutes, flipping over halfway through.

Nutrition: 329 Calories 25.3g Fat 3.4g Carbs 21.1g Protein 2.3g Sugars

337. Parmigiana Chicken

Preparation Time: 3 minutes
Cooking Time: 12 minutes
Servings: 4
Ingredients:
- 2 eggs
- ½ cup Parmesan cheese, grated
- 1 cup seasoned bread crumbs
- 1-pound (454 g) chicken breast halves
- 2 sprigs rosemary, chopped
- From the cupboard:
- Salt and ground black pepper, to taste

Directions:
1. Preheat the air fryer to 380°F (193°C). Spritz the air fryer basket with cooking spray.
2. Beat the egg in a first bowl and sprinkle with salt and black pepper. Combine the Parmesan and bread crumbs in the second bowl.
3. Dredge the chicken in the first bowl to coat well, then in the second bowl. Shake the excess off.
4. Cook the chicken in the preheated air fryer for 12 minutes or until the internal temperature reaches at least 165°F (74°C). Flip the chicken halfway through the cooking time.
5. Transfer the chicken to a plate and serve with rosemary on top.

Nutrition: Calories: 430 Fat: 25.0g Carbs: 21.5g Protein: 48.0g

338. Easy Paprika Chicken

Preparation Time: 7 minutes
Cooking Time: 18 minutes
Servings: 4
Ingredients:
- 4 chicken breasts
- 1 tablespoon paprika
- ¼ teaspoon garlic powder
- 2 tablespoons fresh thyme, chopped
- From the cupboard:
- Salt and ground black pepper, to taste
- 2 tablespoons butter, melted

Directions:
1. Preheat the air fryer to 360°F (182°C). Spritz the air fryer basket with cooking spray.
2. On a clean work surface, rub the chicken breasts with paprika, garlic powder, salt, and black pepper, then brush with butter.
3. Cook the chicken in the preheated air fryer for 18 minutes or until the internal temperature reaches at least 165°F (74°C). Flip the chicken with tongs halfway through the cooking time.

4. Serve the cooked chicken on a plate immediately with thyme on top.

Nutrition: Calories: 368 Fat: 14.1g Carbs: 2.3g Protein: 57.9g

339. Spinach and Cheese Stuffed Chicken Breasts

Preparation Time: 3 minutes
Cooking Time: 12 minutes
Servings: 4

Ingredients:
- 1 cup spinach, chopped
- 4 tablespoons cottage cheese
- 2 chicken breasts
- 2 tablespoons Italian seasoning
- Juice of ½ lime
- Special Equipment:
- 2 or 4 toothpicks, soaked for at least 30 minutes

Directions:
1. Preheat the air fryer to 390°F (199°C). Spritz the air fryer basket with cooking spray.
2. Combine the chopped spinach and cheese in a large bowl. Set aside.
3. Butterfly the chicken breasts and flatten with a rolling pin. Sprinkle with Italian seasoning, then wrap the spinach and cheese mixture in the butterflied chicken breasts. Secure with toothpicks.
4. Place the chicken in the air fryer basket and spritz with cooking spray.
5. Cook for 12 minutes or until the internal temperature reaches at least 165°F (74°C). Flip the chicken halfway through the cooking time.
6. Remove the chicken from the air fryer basket. Discard the toothpicks and serve drizzled with lemon juice.

Nutrition: Calories: 248 Fat: 11.0g Carbs: 4.1g Protein: 31.0g

340. Texas Thighs

Preparation Time: 10 minutes
Cooking Time: 20 minutes
Servings: 8

Ingredients:
- 8 chicken thighs
- 2 teaspoons Texas BBQ Jerky seasoning
- 2 tablespoons cilantro, chopped
- From the Cupboard:
- 1 tablespoon olive oil
- Salt and ground black pepper, to taste

Directions:
1. Preheat air fryer to 380°F (193°C). Spritz the air fryer basket with cooking spray.
2. Arrange the chicken thighs in the air fryer basket, then brush with olive oil on all sides. Sprinkle with BBQ seasoning, salt, and black pepper.
3. Cook for 20 minutes or until the internal temperature of the thighs reaches at least 165°F (74°C). Flip the thighs three times during the cooking time.
4. Remove the chicken thighs from the air fryer basket and serve with cilantro on top.

Nutrition: Calories: 444 Fat: 33.8g Carbs: 1.0g Protein: 31.9g

341. Chicken Wings with Sweet Chili Sauce

Preparation Time: 6 minutes
Cooking Time: 14 minutes
Servings: 4

Ingredients:
- 1-pound (454 g) chicken wings
- 1 teaspoon garlic powder
- 1 tablespoon tamarind powder
- ¼ cup sweet chili sauce
- From the Cupboard:
- Salt and ground black pepper, to taste

Directions:
1. Preheat the air fryer to 390°F (199°C). Spritz the air fryer with cooking spray.
2. On a clean work surface, rub the chicken wings with garlic powder, tamarind powder, salt, and black pepper.
3. Place the wings in the basket and cook for 6 minutes, then spread the chili sauce on top and cook for an additional 8 minutes or until the internal temperature of the wings reaches at least 165°F (74°C).
4. Remove the wings from the air fryer. Allow to cool for a few minutes and serve.

Nutrition: Calories: 165 Fat: 4.1g Carbs: 4.5g Protein: 25.5g

342. Crunchy Golden Nuggets

Preparation Time: 5 minutes
Cooking Time: 10 minutes
Servings: 4

Ingredients:
- 2 chicken breasts, cut into nuggets
- 4 tablespoons sour cream
- ½ cup bread crumbs
- ½ tablespoon garlic powder
- From the Cupboard:
- ½ teaspoon cayenne pepper
- Salt and ground black pepper, to taste

Directions:
1. Preheat the air fryer to 360°F (182°C). Spritz the air fryer basket with cooking spray.
2. Put the sour cream in a large bowl. Combine the bread crumbs, cayenne pepper, garlic powder, salt, and black pepper on a large plate.
3. Dredge the chicken nuggets in the bowl of sour cream, shake the excess off, then roll the nuggets through the bread crumbs mixture to coat well.
4. Place the nuggets in the air fryer basket and cook for 10 minutes or until the chicken nuggets are golden brown and crispy. Flip the nuggets halfway through the cooking time.
5. Remove the nuggets from the basket and serve warm.

Nutrition: Calories: 324 Fat: 15.5g Carbs: 11.7g Protein: 32.7g

343. Roasted Whole Chicken

Preparation Time: 10 minutes
Cooking Time: 40 minutes
Servings: 4

Ingredients:
- 1 (3-pound / 1.4-kg) chicken, rinsed and patted dry
- 1 garlic bulb
- 1 sprig fresh tarragon
- 1 lemon, cut into wedges
- From the Cupboard:
- 2 tablespoons butter, melted
- Salt and ground black pepper, to taste

Directions:
1. Preheat the air fryer to 380°F (193°C). Spritz the air fryer basket with cooking spray.
2. On a clean work surface, brush the chicken with butter and rub with salt and black pepper. Stuff the chicken with garlic, tarragon, and lemon wedges.
3. Arrange the chicken in the air fryer basket and roast for 40 minutes or until an instant-read thermometer inserted

in the thickest part of the chicken registers at least 165°F (74°C).
4. Remove the chicken from the basket and put on a large platter. Carve the chicken and slice to serve.

Nutrition: Calories: 440 Fat: 15.0g Carbs: 2.6g Protein: 69.7g

344. Cheesy Chicken Thighs With Marinara Sauce

Preparation Time: 10 minutes
Cooking Time: 10 minutes
Servings: 4
Ingredients:
- 2 tablespoons grated Parmesan cheese
- ½ cup Italian bread crumbs
- 4 chicken thighs
- ½ cup shredded Monterrey Jack cheese
- ½ cup marinara sauce
- From the Cupboard:
- 1 tablespoon butter, melted

Directions:
1. Preheat the air fryer to 380°F (193°C). Spritz the air fryer basket with cooking spray.
2. Combine the Parmesan and bread crumbs in a bowl.
3. On a clean work surface, brush the chicken thighs with butter, then dredge the thighs in the Parmesan mixture to coat.
4. Place the chicken thighs in the preheated air fryer and cook for 5 minutes, then spread the Monterrey Jack cheese over and pour the marinara sauce on the thighs, and then cook for 4 more minutes until the thighs are golden brown and the cheese melts.
5. Transfer the thighs onto a plate and serve warm.

Nutrition: Calories: 617 Fat: 42.1g Carbs: 17.7g Protein: 39.6g

345. Chicken In Bacon Wrap

Preparation Time: 5 minutes
Cooking Time: 15 minutes
Servings: 4
Ingredients:
- 2 chicken breasts
- 8 ounces (227 g) onion and chive cream cheese
- 6 slices turkey bacon
- 1 tablespoon fresh parsley, chopped
- Juice from ½ lemon
- From the Cupboard:
- 1 tablespoon butter
- Salt, to taste
- Special Equipment:
- 2 or 4 toothpicks, soaked for at least 30 minutes

Directions:
1. Preheat the air fryer to 390°F (199°C). Spritz the air fryer basket with cooking spray.
2. On a clean work surface, brush the chicken breasts with cream cheese and butter on both sides. Sprinkle with salt.
3. Wrap each chicken breast with 3 slices of bacon and secure with 1 or 2 toothpicks.
4. Arrange the bacon-wrapped chicken in the preheated air fryer and cook for 14 minutes or until the bacon is well browned and a meat thermometer inserted in the chicken reads at least 165°F (74°C). Flip them halfway through the cooking time.
5. Remove them from the air fryer basket and serve with parsley and lemon juice on top.

Nutrition: Calories: 437 Fat: 28.6g Carbs: 5.2g Protein: 39.8g

346. Chicken Thighs With Honey-Dijon Sauce

Preparation Time: 5 minutes
Cooking Time: 35 minutes
Servings: 4
Ingredients:
- 8 bone-in and skinless chicken thighs
- Chicken seasoning or rub, to taste
- ½ cup honey
- ¼ cup Dijon mustard
- 2 garlic cloves, minced
- From the Cupboard:
- Salt and ground black pepper, to taste

Directions:
1. Preheat the air fryer to 400°F (205°C). Spritz the air fryer basket with cooking spray.
2. On a clean work surface, rub the chicken thighs with chicken seasoning, salt, and black pepper.
3. Cook the chicken thighs in the preheated air fryer for 15 minutes or until the internal temperature of the chicken thighs reaches at least 165°F (74°C). Flip the thighs halfway through the cooking time. You may need to work in batches to avoid overcrowding.
4. Meanwhile, combine the honey, Dijon mustard, and garlic in a saucepan, and cook over medium-high heat for 3 to 4 minutes until the sauce reduced by one third. Keep stirring during the cooking.
5. Remove the chicken thighs from the air fryer basket and put on a dish. Baste the thighs with the cooked sauce and serve warm.

Nutrition: Calories: 382 Fat: 18.0g Carbs: 36.0g Protein: 21.0g

347. Lemon and Honey Glazed Game Hen

Preparation Time: 10 minutes
Cooking Time: 20 minutes
Servings: 2
Ingredients:
- 1 (2-pound / 907-g) Cornish game hen, split in half
- ¼ teaspoon dried thyme
- Juice and zest of 1 lemon
- ¼ cup honey
- 1½ teaspoons chopped fresh thyme leaves
- From the Cupboard:
- 1 tablespoon olive oil
- Salt and ground black pepper, to taste
- ½ teaspoon soy sauce

Directions:
1. Preheat the air fryer to 390°F (199°C). Spritz the air fryer basket with cooking spray.
2. On a clean work surface, brush the game hen halves with olive oil, then sprinkle with dried thyme, salt, and black pepper to season.
3. Cook the hen in the preheated air fryer for 15 minutes or until the hen is lightly browned. Flip the hen halfway through.
4. Meanwhile, mix the lemon juice and zest, honey, thyme leaves, soy sauce, and black pepper in a bowl.
5. Baste the game hen with the honey glaze, then cook for an additional 4 minutes or until the hen is well glazed and a meat thermometer inserted in the hen reads at least 165°F (74°C).
6. Remove the game hen from the air fryer basket. Allow to cool for a few minutes and slice to serve.

Nutrition: Calories: 724 Fat: 22.0g Carbs: 37.5g Protein: 91.3g

348. Cheesy Spinach Stuffed Chicken Breasts

Preparation Time: 20 minutes
Cooking Time: 25 minutes
Servings: 4

Ingredients:
- 1 (10-ounce / 284-g) package frozen spinach, thawed and drained well
- 1 cup feta cheese, crumbled
- 4 boneless chicken breasts
- From the Cupboard:
- Salt and ground black pepper, to taste
- Special Equipment:
- 4 or 8 toothpicks, soaked for at least 30 minutes

Directions:
1. Preheat the air fryer to 380°F (193°C). Spritz the air fryer basket with cooking spray.
2. Make the filling: Chop the spinach and put in a large bowl, then add the feta cheese and ½ teaspoon of ground black pepper. Stir to mix well.
3. On a clean work surface, using a knife, cut a 1-inch incision into the thicker side of each chicken breast horizontally. Make a 3-inch long pocket from the incision and keep the sides and bottom intact.
4. Stuff the chicken pockets with the filling and secure with 1 or 2 toothpicks.
5. Arrange the stuffed chicken breasts in the preheated air fryer. Sprinkle with salt and black pepper and spritz with cooking spray. You may need to work in batches to avoid overcrowding.
6. Cook for 12 minutes or until the internal temperature of the chicken reads at least 165°F (74°C). Flip the chicken halfway through the cooking time.
7. Remove the chicken from the air fryer basket. Discard the toothpicks and allow to cool for 10 minutes before slicing to serve.

Nutrition: Calories: 648 Fat: 38.7g Carbs: 4.5g Protein: 68.2g

349. Turkey And Pepper Sandwich

Preparation Time: 5 minutes
Cooking Time: 5 minutes
Servings: 1

Ingredients:
- 2 slices whole grain bread
- 2 teaspoons Dijon mustard
- 2 ounces (57 g) cooked turkey breast, thinly sliced
- 2 slices low-fat Swiss cheese
- 3 strips roasted red bell pepper
- From the Cupboard:
- Salt and ground black pepper, to taste

Directions:
1. Preheat the air fryer to 330°F (166°C). Spritz the air fryer basket with cooking spray.
2. Assemble the sandwich: On a dish, place a slice of bread, then top the bread with 1 teaspoon of Dijon mustard, use a knife to smear the mustard evenly.
3. Layer the turkey slices, Swiss cheese slices, and red pepper strips on the bread according to your favorite order. Top them with remaining teaspoon of Dijon mustard and remaining bread slice.
4. Place the sandwich in the preheated air fryer and spritz with cooking spray. Sprinkle with salt and black pepper.
5. Cook for 5 minutes until the cheese melts and the bread is lightly browned. Flip the sandwich halfway through the cooking time.
6. Serve the sandwich immediately.

Nutrition: Calories: 328 Fat: 5.0g Carbs: 38.0g Protein: 29.0g

350. Spicy Turkey Breast

Preparation Time: 5 minutes
Cooking Time: 40 minutes
Servings: 4

Ingredients:
- 2-pound (907 g) turkey breast
- 2 teaspoons taco seasonings
- 1 teaspoon ground cumin
- 1 teaspoon red pepper flakes
- From the Cupboard:
- Salt and ground black pepper, to taste

Directions:
1. Preheat the air fryer to 350°F (180°C). Spritz the air fryer basket with cooking spray.
2. On a clean work surface, rub the turkey breast with taco seasoning, ground cumin, red pepper flakes, salt, and black pepper.
3. Arrange the turkey in the preheated air fryer and cook for 40 minutes or until the internal temperature of the turkey reads at least 165°F (74°C). Flip the turkey breast halfway through the cooking time.
4. Remove the turkey from the basket. Allow to cool for 15 minutes before slicing to serve.

Nutrition: Calories: 235 Fat: 5.6g Carbs: 6.6g Protein: 37.3g

351. Chicken, Mushroom, And Pepper Kabobs

Preparation Time: 1 hour 5 minutes
Cooking Time: 15-20 minutes
Servings: 4

Ingredients:
- ⅓ cup raw honey
- 2 tablespoons sesame seeds
- 2 boneless chicken breasts, cut into cubes
- 6 white mushrooms, cut in halves
- 3 green or red bell peppers, diced
- From the Cupboard:
- ⅓ cup soy sauce
- Salt and ground black pepper, to taste
- Special Equipment:
- 4 wooden skewers, soaked for at least 30 minutes

Directions:
1. Combine the honey, soy sauce, sesame seeds, salt, and black pepper in a large bowl. Stir to mix well.
2. Dunk the chicken cubes in this bowl, then wrap the bowl in plastic and refrigerate to marinate for at least an hour.
3. Preheat the air fryer to 390°F (199°C). Spritz the air fryer basket with cooking spray.
4. Remove the chicken cubes from the marinade, then run the skewers through the chicken cubes, mushrooms, and bell peppers alternatively.
5. Baste the chicken, mushrooms, and bell peppers with the marinade, then arrange them in the preheated air fryer.
6. Spritz them with cooking spray and cook for 15 to 20 minutes or until the mushrooms and bell peppers are tender and the chicken cubes are well browned. Flip them halfway through the cooking time.
7. Transfer the skewers to a large plate and serve hot.

Nutrition: Calories: 380 Fat: 16.0g Carbs: 26.1g Protein: 34.0g

352. Chicken & Zucchini

Preparation Time: 30 minutes
Cooking Time: 20 minutes
Servings: 6

Ingredients:
- 1/4 cup olive oil
- 1 tablespoon lemon juice
- 2 tablespoons red wine vinegar
- 1 teaspoon oregano
- 1 tablespoon garlic, chopped
- 2 chicken breast fillet, sliced into cubes
- 1 zucchini, sliced
- 1 red onion, sliced
- 1 cup cherry tomatoes, sliced
- Salt and pepper to taste

Directions:
1. In a bowl, mix the olive oil, lemon juice, vinegar, oregano and garlic.
2. Pour half of mixture into another bowl.
3. Toss chicken in half of the mixture.
4. Cover and marinate for 15 minutes.
5. Toss the veggies in the remaining mixture.
6. Season both chicken and veggies with salt and pepper.
7. Add chicken to the air fryer basket.
8. Spread veggies on top.
9. Select air fry function. Seal and cook at 380 degrees f for 15 to 20 minutes.

Nutrition: Calories: 282 kcal Protein: 21.87 g Fat: 19.04 g Carbohydrates: 5.31 g

353. Chicken Quesadilla

Preparation Time: 20 minutes
Cooking Time: 30 minutes
Servings: 8

Ingredients:
- 4 tortillas
- Cooking spray
- 1/2 cup sour cream
- 1/2 cup salsa
- Hot sauce
- 12 oz. chicken breast fillet, chopped and grilled
- 3 jalapeño peppers, diced
- 2 cups cheddar cheese, shredded
- Chopped scallions

Directions:
1. Add grill grate to the Ninja Foodi Grill.
2. Close the hood.
3. Choose grill setting.
4. Preheat for 5 minutes.
5. While waiting, spray tortillas with oil.
6. In a bowl, mix sour cream, salsa and hot sauce. Set aside.
7. Add tortilla to the grate.
8. Grill for 1 minute.
9. Repeat with the other tortillas.
10. Spread the toasted tortilla with the salsa mixture, chicken, jalapeño peppers, cheese and scallions.
11. Place a tortilla on top. Press.
12. Repeat these steps with the remaining 2 tortillas.
13. Take the grill out of the pot.
14. Choose roast setting.
15. Cook the Quesadillas at 350F for 25 minutes.

Nutrition: Calories: 184 kcal Protein: 12.66 g Fat: 7.66 g Carbohydrates: 15.87 g

354. Buffalo Chicken Wings

Preparation Time: 15 minutes
Cooking Time: 30 minutes
Servings: 4

Ingredients:
- 2 lb. chicken wings
- 2 tablespoons oil
- 1/2 cup Buffalo sauce

Directions:
1. Coat the chicken wings with oil.
2. Add these to an air fryer basket.
3. Choose air fry function.
4. Cook at 390 degrees F for 15 minutes.
5. Shake and then cook for another 15 minutes.
6. Dip in Buffalo sauce before serving.

Nutrition: Calories: 376 kcal Protein: 51.93 g Fat: 16.4 g Carbohydrates: 2.18 g

355. Mustard Chicken

Preparation Time: 20 minutes
Cooking Time: 50 minutes
Servings: 4

Ingredients:
- 1/4 cup Dijon mustard
- 1/4 cup cooking oil
- Salt and pepper to taste
- 2 tablespoons honey
- 1 tablespoon dry oregano
- 2 teaspoons dry Italian seasoning
- 1 tablespoon lemon juice
- 6 chicken pieces

Directions:
1. Combine all the ingredients except chicken in a bowl.
2. Mix well.
3. Toss the chicken in the mixture.
4. Add roasting rack to your Ninja Foodi Grill.
5. Choose roast function.
6. Set it to 350 degrees F.
7. Cook for 30 minutes.
8. Flip and cook for another 15 to 20 minutes.

Nutrition: Calories: 1781 kcal Protein: 293.44 g Fat: 54.33 g Carbohydrates: 11.71 g

356. Honey & Rosemary Chicken

Preparation Time: 15 minutes
Cooking Time: 35 minutes
Servings: 6

Ingredients:
- 1 teaspoon paprika
- Salt to taste
- 1/2 teaspoon baking powder
- 2 lb. chicken wings
- 1/4 cup honey
- 1 tablespoon lemon juice
- 1 tablespoon garlic, minced
- 1 tablespoon rosemary, chopped

Directions:
1. Choose air fry setting in your Ninja Foodi Grill.
2. Set it to 390 degrees F.
3. Set the time to 30 minutes.
4. Press start to preheat.
5. While waiting, mix the paprika, salt and baking powder in a bowl.
6. Add the wings to the crisper basket.
7. Close and cook for 15 minutes.
8. Flip and cook for another 15 minutes.
9. In a bowl, mix the remaining ingredients.

POULTRY RECIPES

10. Coat the wings with the sauce and cook for another 5 minutes.

Nutrition: Calories: 251 kcal Protein: 34.49 g Fat: 6.44 g Carbohydrates: 12.56 g

357. Grilled Chicken with Veggies

Preparation Time: 20 minutes
Cooking Time: 25 minutes
Servings: 2
Ingredients:
- 2 chicken thighs and legs
- 2 tablespoons oil, divided
- Salt and pepper to taste
- 1 onion, diced
- 1/4 cup mushrooms, sliced
- 1 cup potatoes, diced
- 1 tablespoon lemon juice
- 1 tablespoon honey
- 4 sprigs fresh thyme, chopped
- 2 cloves garlic, crushed and minced

Directions:
1. Add the grill grate to your Ninja Foodi Grill.
2. Put the veggie tray on top of the grill grate.
3. Close the hood.
4. Choose grill function and set it to high.
5. Press start to preheat.
6. Brush the chicken with half of oil.
7. Season with salt and pepper.
8. Toss the onion, mushrooms and potatoes in the remaining oil.
9. Sprinkle with salt and pepper.
10. Add chicken to the grill grate.
11. Add the potato mixture to the veggie tray.
12. Close the hood and cook for 10 to 15 minutes.
13. Flip chicken and toss potatoes.
14. Cook for another 10 minutes.

Nutrition: 715 kcal Protein: 37.93 g Fat: 48.89 g Carbohydrates: 31.05 g

358. Grilled Garlic Chicken

Preparation Time: 10 minutes
Cooking Time: 20 minutes
Servings: 8
Ingredients:
- 3 lb. chicken thigh fillets
- Garlic salt to taste

Directions:
1. Add grill plate to the Ninja Foodi Grill.
2. Preheat to medium heat.
3. Sprinkle chicken with garlic salt on both sides.
4. Cook for 8 to 10 minutes.
5. Flip and cook for another 7 minutes.

Nutrition: Calories: 386 kcal Protein: 28.9 g Fat: 29.01 g Carbohydrates: 0.43 g

359. Grilled Balsamic Chicken Breast

Preparation Time: 45 minutes
Cooking Time: 45 minutes
Servings: 4
Ingredients:
- 1/4 cup olive oil
- 2 tablespoons balsamic vinegar
- 3 teaspoon garlic, minced
- 3 tablespoons soy sauce
- 1 tablespoon Worcestershire sauce
- 1/4 cup brown sugar
- Salt and pepper to taste
- 4 chicken breast fillets

Directions:
1. In a bowl, mix all ingredients except chicken.
2. Reserve 1/4 cup of the mixture for later.
3. Marinate the chicken breast in the remaining mixture for 30 minutes.
4. Add grill grate to the Ninja Foodi Grill.
5. Set it to grill and for 25 minutes.
6. Add the chicken breast and close the hood.
7. Cook for 10 minutes.
8. Flip and cook for another 5 minutes.
9. Baste with remaining sauce. Cook for 5 more minutes.
10. Serve with remaining sauce if any.

Nutrition: Calories: 716 kcal Protein: 63.31 g Fat: 44.04 g Carbohydrates: 13.16

360. Barbecue Chicken Breast

Preparation Time: 15 minutes
Cooking Time: 50 minutes
Servings: 4
Ingredients:
- 4 chicken breast fillets
- 2 tablespoons vegetable oil
- Salt and pepper to taste
- 1 cup barbecue sauce

Directions:
1. Add grill grate to the Ninja Foodi Grill.
2. Close the hood.
3. Choose grill setting.
4. Preheat to medium for 25 minutes.
5. Press start.
6. Brush chicken breast with oil.
7. Sprinkle both sides with salt and pepper.
8. Add chicken and cook for 10 minutes.
9. Flip and cook for another 10 minutes.
10. Brush chicken with barbecue sauce.
11. Cook for 5 minutes.
12. Brush the other side and cook for another 5 minutes.

Nutrition: Calories: 707 kcal Protein: 62.88 g Fat: 35.61 g Carbohydrates: 30.21 g

361. Chicken, Potatoes & Cabbage

Preparation Time: 30 minutes
Cooking Time: 40 minutes
Servings: 8
Ingredients:
- 1 cup apple cider vinegar
- 2 lb. chicken thigh fillets
- 6 oz. barbecue sauce
- 2 lb. cabbage, sliced into wedges and steamed
- 1 lb. potatoes, roasted
- Salt and pepper to taste

Directions:
1. Pour apple cider vinegar to the inner pot.
2. Add grill grate to the Ninja Foodi Grill.
3. Place the chicken on top of the grill.
4. Sprinkle both sides with salt and pepper.
5. Grill the chicken for 15 to 20 minutes per side at 350 degrees F.
6. Baste the chicken with the barbecue sauce.
7. Serve chicken with potatoes and cabbage.

Nutrition: Calories: 385 kcal Protein: 22.59 g Fat: 19.97 g Carbohydrates: 28.03 g

362. Roasted Chicken

POULTRY RECIPES

Preparation Time: 30 minutes
Cooking Time: 1 hour and 10 minutes
Servings: 6
Ingredients:
- 1 whole chicken
- 1/2 teaspoon onion powder
- 1 teaspoon garlic powder
- 1 teaspoon paprika
- Salt and pepper to taste
- 2 drops liquid smoke
- 1 cup water
- 2 tablespoons butter
- 1/4 cup flour
- 2 cups chicken broth
- Basting Butter
- 2 tablespoons butter
- Dash garlic powder

Directions:
1. Season chicken with a mixture of onion powder, garlic powder, paprika, salt and pepper.
2. Add the chicken to the air frying basket.
3. Combine liquid smoke and butter.
4. Pour into the pot of your Ninja Foodi grill.
5. Seal the unit and cook at 350 degrees F for 45 minutes.
6. Drain the pot.
7. Sprinkle chicken with butter and flour.
8. Air fry at 400 degrees F for 15 minutes.
9. Baste with a mixture of the basting butter ingredients.
10. Cook for another 10 minutes.

Nutrition: Calories: 410 kcal Protein: 51.61 g Fat: 18.64 g Carbohydrates: 6.05 g

363. Sugar Glazed Chicken

Preparation Time: 15 minutes
Cooking Time: 45 minutes
Servings: 8
Ingredients:
- 1 tablespoon olive oil
- 1/2 tablespoon apple cider vinegar
- 3 teaspoon garlic, minced
- 1 tablespoon honey
- 1/4 cup light brown sugar
- 1/3 cup soy sauce
- 8 chicken thigh fillets

Directions:
1. Combine all the ingredients except chicken.
2. Reserve 1/4 cup of this mixture for later.
3. Marinate the chicken with the remaining mixture for 30 minutes.
4. Add grill grate to your Ninja Foodi Grill.
5. Select grill button.
6. Set it to 25 minutes.
7. Add chicken to the grill.
8. Close the hood.
9. Cook for 10 minutes.
10. Flip and cook for 5 minutes.
11. Brush with the remaining mixture.
12. Cook for another 5 minutes.

Nutrition: Calories: 518 kcal Protein: 33.52 g Fat: 36.41 g Carbohydrates: 12.36 g

364. Lemon Garlic Chicken

Preparation Time: 15 minutes
Cooking Time: 40 minutes
Servings: 4
Ingredients:
- 4 chicken breast fillets
- 1 tablespoon lemon juice
- 1 tablespoon melted butter
- 1 teaspoon garlic powder
- Salt and pepper to taste

Directions:
1. Mix lemon juice and melted butter in a bowl.
2. Brush both sides of chicken with this mixture.
3. Season with garlic powder, salt and pepper.
4. Insert grill grate to your Ninja Foodi Grill.
5. Place chicken on top of the grill.
6. Close the hood.
7. Grill at 350 degrees F for 15 to 20 minutes per side.

Nutrition: Calories: 553 kcal Protein: 62.46 g Fat: 31.26 g Carbohydrates: 1.89 g

365. Grilled Ranch Chicken

Preparation Time: 30 minutes
Cooking Time: 30 minutes
Servings: 6
Ingredients:
- 6 chicken thigh fillets
- 3 tablespoons ranch dressing
- Garlic salt and pepper

Directions:
1. Spread both sides of chicken with ranch dressing.
2. Sprinkle with garlic salt and pepper.
3. Set your Ninja Foodi Grill to grill.
4. Preheat it to medium.
5. Add chicken to the grill grate.
6. Cook for 15 minutes per side.

Nutrition: Calories: 475 kcal Protein: 33.16 g Fat: 36.43 g Carbohydrates: 1.66 g

366. Chicken Breast Pita Sandwiches

Preparation Time: 20 minutes
Cooking Time: 10 minutes
Servings: 4
Ingredients:
- 2 boneless, skinless chicken breasts, cut into 1-inch cubes
- 4 pita pockets, split in half
- 1 red bell pepper, sliced
- 1 small red onion, sliced
- ⅓ cup Italian salad dressing
- ½ teaspoon dried thyme
- 1 cup cherry tomatoes, chopped
- 2 cups butter lettuce, tear into slices
- Cooking spray

Directions:
1. Place the chicken, bell pepper and onion in the air fryer basket. Sprinkle with 1 tablespoon Italian salad dressing and thyme. Spritz with cooking spray.
2. Put the air fryer lid on and bake in the preheated instant pot at 375°F for 9 to 11 minutes. Shake the basket once when it shows 'TURN FOOD' on the air fryer lid screen halfway through cooking time, or until the chicken is cooked through.
3. Transfer the chicken to a bowl and pour in the remaining salad dressing. Combine well.
4. To assemble the sandwiches, start with the pita halves, then add the butter lettuce slices, and cherry tomatoes. Serve immediately.

Nutrition: Calories: 1493 Total Fat: 146.77g Saturated Fat: 75.456g Total Carbs: 36.38g Fiber: 3.7g Protein: 46.36g Sugar: 9.78g Sodium: 1611mg

367. Asian Style Turkey Meatballs

Preparation Time: 24 minutes
Cooking Time: 13 minutes
Servings: 4

Ingredients:
- 1-pound ground turkey
- 1 small onion, minced
- 2 tablespoons peanut oil
- ¼ cup water chestnuts, finely chopped
- 2 tablespoons low-sodium soy sauce
- ½ teaspoon ground ginger
- ¼ cup panko bread crumbs
- 1 egg, beaten

Directions:
1. In a 6×6×2 inch baking pan, add the onion and peanut oil. Stir well.
2. Place the pan in the instant pot and put the air fryer lid on. Cook in the preheated instant pot at 375°F for 1 to 2 minutes, or until the onion is soft and translucent. Transfer the cooked onion into a large bowl.
3. Add the water chestnuts, soy sauce, ground ginger, and bread crumbs into the onion. Stir in the beaten egg and whisk well, then add in the turkey. Toss until well combined.
4. On your cutting board, scoop out the mixture and shape into 1-inch meatballs.
5. Arrange the meatballs in the pan and drizzle with the oil.
6. Place the pan in the instant pot and put the air fryer lid on. Bake in batches at 400°F for 10 to 12 minutes, or until the meatballs are cooked through.
7. Remove the meatballs from the pan to a plate. Let cool for 3 minutes before serving.

Nutrition: Calories: 683 Total Fat: 33.29g Saturated Fat: 15.591g Total Carbs: 3.23g Fiber: 0.6g Protein: 24.77g Sugar: 1.17g Sodium: 342mg Cholesterol: 271mg

368. Sweet and Spicy Chicken Stir-Fry

Preparation Time: 15 minutes
Cooking Time: 15 minutes
Servings: 4

Ingredients:
- ¾ pound boneless, skinless chicken thighs, cut into 1-inch pieces
- 1 small red onion, sliced
- 1 yellow bell pepper, cut into 1½-inch pieces
- ¼ cup chicken stock
- 1 tablespoon olive oil
- 2 to 3 teaspoons curry powder
- 2 tablespoons honey
- ¼ cup orange juice
- 1 tablespoon cornstarch

Directions:
1. Place the red onion, chicken thighs, and pepper in the air fryer basket and drizzle with olive oil.
2. Put the air fryer lid on and cook in the preheated instant pot at 375°F for 12 to 14 minutes. Flip the chicken thighs when it shows 'TURN FOOD' on the lid screen halfway through cooking time, or until the chicken reaches 165°F.
3. Transfer the chicken and vegetables to a 6-inch metal bowl. Add the chicken stock, curry powder, honey, orange juice, and cornstarch into the bowl. Combine well.
4. Place the metal bowl inside the basket and put the air fryer lid on. Cook for 3 minutes more.
5. Remove the bowl from the basket. Let cool for 3 minutes before serving.

Nutrition: Calories: 746 Total Fat: 22.98g Saturated Fat: 16.852g Total Carbs: 25.2g Fiber: 2.1g Protein: 12.61g Sugar: 14.48g Sodium: 471mg

369. Crispy Chicken Parmigiana

Preparation Time: 15 minutes
Cooking Time: 15 minutes
Servings: 4

Ingredients:
- 2 (4-ounce) boneless, skinless chicken breasts
- ½ cup grated Parmesan cheese
- 1 cup Italian bread crumbs
- 2 teaspoons Italian seasoning
- Salt and pepper to taste
- 2 egg whites
- ¾ cup marinara sauce
- ½ cup shredded mozzarella cheese
- Cooking spray

Directions:
1. On a flat work surface, pound the chicken into ¼-inch pieces.
2. In a large bowl, mix together the bread crumbs, Parmesan cheese, Italian seasoning, salt and pepper. Stir until well combined. In another bowl, pour in the egg whites. Set aside.
3. Spritz the air fryer basket with cooking spray.
4. Dredge the chicken cutlets in the egg whites, and then in the bread crumbs mixture to coat.
5. Arrange the breaded cutlets in the air fryer basket and mist with cooking spray.
6. Put the air fryer lid on and cook in the preheated instant pot at 375°F for 7 minutes.
7. Transfer the fried chicken cutlets to a serving plate.
8. Drizzle with the marinara sauce and sprinkle mozzarella cheese on top. Cook for an additional 3 minutes until the cheese is bubbly.
9. Let cool for 3 minutes and serve.

Nutrition: Calories: 944 Total fat: 70g Saturated fat: 3g Cholesterol: 46mg Sodium: 593mg Carbohydrates: 220g Fiber: 1g, Protein: 105g

370. Chicken Fajitas With Avocados

Preparation Time: 15 minutes
Cooking Time: 10 minutes
Servings: 4

Ingredients:
- 4 boneless, skinless chicken breasts, sliced
- 2 avocados, peeled and chopped
- 1 small red onion, sliced
- 2 red bell peppers, sliced
- ½ cup spicy ranch salad dressing
- ½ teaspoon dried oregano
- 8 corn tortillas
- 2 cups torn butter lettuce

Directions:
1. Put the onion, chicken and pepper in the air fryer basket. Drizzle with 1 tablespoon of salad dressing and sprinkle with the oregano.
2. Put the air fryer lid on and grill in the preheated instant pot at 375°F for 10 to 14 minutes. Flip the chicken when it shows 'TURN FOOD' on the lid screen halfway through cooking time, or until the chicken is browned and slightly charred.

3. Remove the vegetables and chicken from the basket to a serving dish. Drizzle over the remaining salad dressing.
4. Serve warm.

Nutrition: Calories: 887, Total Fat: 34.25g Saturated Fat: 22.931g Total Carbs: 14.29g Fiber: 7.3g Protein: 22.2g Sugar: 4.2g Sodium: 2841mg

371. Fried Chicken with Buttermilk

Preparation Time: 15 minutes
Cooking Time: 15 minutes
Servings: 4

Ingredients:
- 6 chicken pieces: drumsticks, breasts, and thighs
- ⅓ cup buttermilk
- 1 cup flour
- 2 teaspoons paprika
- 2 eggs, beaten
- 1½ cups bread crumbs
- 2 tablespoons olive oil
- Freshly ground black pepper and salt to taste

Directions:
1. On your cutting board, thoroughly dry the chicken with paper towels. In a shallow bowl, mix the flour, paprika, salt and pepper.
2. In another bowl, whisk the eggs and buttermilk until well combined.
3. In a third bowl, combine the bread crumbs with olive oil.
4. Dredge the chicken in the flour mixture, then dip into the eggs, and finally dunk into the bread crumbs. Gently but firmly press the crumbs onto the skin of chicken pieces to fully coat.
5. Place the breaded chicken into the air fryer basket. Put the air fryer lid on and cook in the preheated instant pot at 375ºF for 15 minutes. Flip the chicken when it shows 'TURN FOOD' on the lid screen halfway through cooking time.
6. Transfer the chicken to a serving dish. Let cool for 5 minutes before serving.

Nutrition: Calories: 651 Total Fat: 22.34g Saturated Fat: 13.684g Total Carbs: 27.54g Fiber: 2.2g Protein: 14.38g Sugar: 6.14g Sodium: 1257mg

372. Panko-Crusted Chicken Nuggets

Preparation Time: 15 minutes
Cooking Time: 15 minutes
Servings: 4

Ingredients:
- 1-pound boneless, skinless chicken breasts
- Chicken seasoning or rub
- Salt and pepper to taste
- 2 eggs
- 6 tablespoons bread crumbs
- 2 tablespoons panko bread crumbs
- Cooking spray

Directions:
1. On your cutting board, slice the chicken breast into 1-inch cutlets.
2. In a large bowl, mix together the chicken cutlets, chicken seasoning, salt and pepper. Toss to fully coat. Set aside.
3. In another bowl, whisk the eggs. In a third bowl, combine the bread crumbs with panko.
4. Dredge the chicken cutlets in the whisked eggs, and then into the bread crumbs to coat well.
5. Arrange the breaded chicken cutlets in the air fryer basket and spray them with cooking spray.
6. Put the air fryer lid on and cook in batches in the preheated instant pot at 400ºF for 4 minutes. Shake the air fryer basket when the lid screen indicates 'TURN FOOD' during cooking time, and cook for an additional 4 minutes.
7. Transfer the cooked chicken cutlets to a serving bowl. Let cool for 3 minutes and serve.

Nutrition: Calories: 508 Total Fat: 24g Saturated Fat: 1g Cholesterol: 147mg Sodium: 267mg Carbohydrates: 67g Fiber: 1g Protein: 24g

373. Crusted Chicken Tenders

Preparation Time: 27 minutes
Cooking Time: 12 minutes
Servings: 4

Ingredients:
- 8 chicken tenders
- ½ cup all-purpose flour
- 1 egg
- ½ cup dry bread crumbs
- 2 tablespoons vegetable oil

Directions:
1. Put the flour in a bowl. Set aside.
2. In a second bowl, whisk the egg. Set aside.
3. In a third bowl, mix the bread crumbs and oil together. Set aside.
4. Dredge the chicken tenders in the flour, then in the whisked egg, and finally in the crumb mixture to coat well.
5. Lay the tenders in the air fryer basket. Put the air fry lid on and cook in the preheated instant pot at 350ºF for about 12 minutes or until lightly browned.
6. Remove the chicken tenders from the basket and serve on a platter.

Nutrition: Calories: 253 Total Fat: 11.4g Carbohydrates: 9.8g Protein: 26.2g Cholesterol: 109mg Sodium: 171mg

374. Chicken With Greek Yogurt Buffalo Sauce

Preparation Time: 36 minutes
Cooking Time: 15 minutes
Servings: 4

Ingredients:
- 1-pound skinless, boneless chicken breasts, cut into 1-inch strips
- ½ cup plain fat-free Greek yogurt
- 1 cup panko bread crumbs
- 1 tablespoon sweet paprika
- 1 tablespoon cayenne pepper
- 1 tablespoon garlic pepper
- ¼ cup egg substitute
- 1 tablespoon hot sauce
- 1 teaspoon hot sauce

Directions:
1. In a bowl, mix the bread crumbs, sweet paprika, cayenne pepper, and garlic pepper. Set aside.
2. In a second bowl, whisk together the Greek yogurt, egg substitute, and 1 tablespoon plus 1 teaspoon hot sauce.
3. Dunk the chicken strips into the buffalo sauce, then coat with bread crumb mixture.
4. Arrange the well-coated chicken strips in the air fryer basket. Put the air fry lid on and cook in the preheated instant pot at 400ºF for 15 minutes or until well browned. Flip the strips when the lid screen indicates 'TURN FOOD' halfway through.
5. Remove the chicken from the basket and serve on a plate.

Nutrition: Calories: 234, Fat: 4.6g, Carbohydrates: 22.1g Protein: 31.2g Cholesterol: 65mg Sodium: 696mg

375. Baked Chicken Fajita Roll-Ups

Preparation Time: 35 minutes
Cooking Time: 12 minutes
Servings: 4
Ingredients:
- 2 (4-ounce) boneless, skinless chicken breasts
- Juice of ½ lime
- 2 tablespoons fajita seasoning
- ½ red bell pepper, cut into strips
- ½ green bell pepper, cut into strips
- ¼ onion, sliced
- Cooking spray
- 4 toothpicks, soaked for at least 30 minutes

Directions:
1. On a flat work surface, carefully butterfly or pound the chicken into ¼-inch cutlets.
2. Sprinkle the lemon juice over cutlets and season with fajita seasoning to taste. Toss well.
3. To make the chicken roll-ups, evenly spread the bell pepper strips and onion slices on each chicken cutlet. Roll each cutlet into a tight cylinder and secure with a toothpick through the center.
4. Arrange 4 chicken roll-ups in the air fryer basket. Spray them with cooking spray.
5. Put the air fryer lid on and cook in the preheated instant pot at 400°F for 12 minutes.
6. Transfer to a serving dish and cool for 5 minutes before serving.

Nutrition: Calories: 770 Total Fat: 65g Saturated Fat: 0g Cholesterol: 32mg Sodium: 302mg Carbohydrates: 212g Fiber: 0g Protein: 94g

376. Garlicky Chicken and Potatoes

Preparation Time: 15 minutes
Cooking Time: 15 minutes
Servings: 4
Ingredients:
- 1 broiler-fryer whole chicken (2½ to 3 pounds)
- 12 to 16 creamer potatoes, scrubbed
- 8 cloves garlic, peeled
- 2 tablespoons olive oil
- ½ teaspoon garlic salt
- 1 slice of lemon
- ½ teaspoon dried thyme
- ½ teaspoon dried marjoram

Directions:
1. Rinse the chicken and pat it dry using paper towels.
2. In a small bowl, combine 1 tablespoon of the olive oil and salt. Rub half of the olive mixture evenly on all sides of the chicken. Stuff the lemon slice and garlic cloves inside the chicken. Sprinkle the thyme and marjoram on top.
3. Arrange the chicken in the air fryer basket and spread out the scrubbed potatoes. Drizzle the remaining olive oil mixture on top.
4. Put the air fryer lid on and roast in the preheated instant pot at 375°F for 25 minutes, or until the chicken registers 165°F on a meat thermometer (inserted into the center of the chicken's thickest part). If not fully cooked through, return the chicken to the basket and roast for another 5 minutes.
5. Transfer the chicken and potatoes to a plate. Let rest for 5 minutes before serving.

Nutrition: Calories: 1523 Total Fat: 22.77g Saturated Fat: 14.11g Total Carbs: 24.16g Fiber: 1.5g Protein: 13.35g Sugar: 0.24g Sodium: 1013mg

377. Chicken Thighs with Lemon Garlic

Preparation Time: 15 minutes
Cooking Time: 20 minutes
Servings: 4
Ingredients:
- 4 skin-on, bone-in chicken thighs
- 4 lemon wedges
- ¼ cup lemon juice
- 2 cloves garlic, minced
- 2 tablespoons olive oil
- 1 teaspoon Dijon mustard
- ¼ teaspoon salt
- ⅛ teaspoon ground black pepper

Directions:
1. Mix the lemon juice, Dijon mustard, olive oil, garlic, salt, and pepper together in a bowl. Refrigerate to marinate for an hour.
2. Put the chicken thighs into a zip lock bag and pour the marinade all over the chicken and zip the bag. Refrigerate for at least 2 hours.
3. Take the chicken out from the bag. Pat dry with paper towels. Arrange them in the air fryer basket.
4. Put the air fry lid on and cook in batches in the preheated instant pot at 350°F for 15 to 18 minutes or until cooked through.
5. Transfer the chicken thighs to a platter. Squeeze the lemon wedges over before serving.

Nutrition: Calories: 258, Total Fat: 18.6g, Cholesterol: 71mg, Carbohydrates: 3.6g, Sodium: 242mg, Protein: 19.4g

378. Lemony Chicken with Barbecue Sauce

Preparation Time: 10 minutes
Cooking Time: 12 minutes
Servings: 4
Ingredients:
- 6 boneless, skinless chicken thighs
- 2 tablespoons lemon juice
- ¼ cup barbecue sauce, gluten-free
- 2 cloves garlic, minced

Directions:
1. In a medium bowl, mix together the chicken, cloves, barbecue sauce and lemon juice. Set aside for 10 minutes to marinate.
2. Transfer the marinated chicken thighs into the air fryer basket, shaking off excess sauce. You may need to work in batches to avoid overcrowding.
3. Put the air fryer lid on and grill in the preheated instant pot at 375°F for 12 minutes. Flip the chicken thighs when it shows 'TURN FOOD' on the lid screen halfway through cooking time, or until the chicken registers at least 165°F using a meat thermometer inserted into the center of the chicken.
4. Transfer to a platter and repeat with remaining chicken thighs. Serve warm.

Nutrition: Calories: 113 Total Fat: 12.31g Saturated Fat: 8.531g Total Carbs: 27g Fiber: 0.2g Protein: 6.61g Sugar: 2.874g Sodium: 803mg

379. Chicken Popcorn

Preparation time: 10 minutes
Cooking time: 10 minutes
Servings: 6
Ingredients:
- 4 eggs
- 1 1/2 lb. Chicken breasts, cut into small chunks
- 1 tsp paprika
- 1/2 tsp garlic powder
- 1 tsp onion powder
- 2 1/2 cups pork rind, crushed
- 1/4 cup coconut flour
- Pepper
- Salt

Directions:
1. In a small bowl, mix together coconut flour, pepper, and salt.
2. In another bowl, whisk eggs until combined.
3. Take one more bowl and mix together pork panko, paprika, garlic powder, and onion powder.
4. Add chicken pieces in a large mixing bowl. Sprinkle coconut flour mixture over chicken and toss well.
5. Dip chicken pieces in the egg mixture and coat with pork panko mixture and place on a plate.
6. Spray air fryer basket with cooking spray.
7. Preheat the air fryer to 400 f.
8. Add half prepared chicken in air fryer basket and cook for 10-12 minutes. Shake basket halfway through.
9. Cook remaining half using the same method.
10. Serve and enjoy.

Nutrition: Calories 265 Fat 11 g Carbohydrates 3 g Sugar 0.5 g Protein 35 g Cholesterol 195 mg

380. Quick & Easy Meatballs

Preparation time: 10 minutes
Cooking time: 10 minutes
Servings: 4
Ingredients:
- 1 lb. Ground chicken
- 1 egg, lightly beaten
- 1/2 cup mozzarella cheese, shredded
- 1 1/2 tbsp taco seasoning
- 3 garlic cloves, minced
- 3 tbsp fresh parsley, chopped
- 1 small onion, minced
- Pepper
- Salt

Directions:
1. Add all ingredients into the large mixing bowl and mix until well combined.
2. Make small balls from mixture and place in the air fryer basket.
3. Cook meatballs for 10 minutes at 400 f.
4. Serve and enjoy.

Nutrition: Calories 253 Fat 10 g Carbohydrates 2 g Sugar 0.9 g Protein 35 g Cholesterol 144 mg

381. Lemon Pepper Chicken Wings

Preparation time: 10 minutes
Cooking time: 16 minutes
Servings: 4
Ingredients:
- 1 lb. Chicken wings
- 1 tsp lemon pepper
- 1 tbsp. olive oil
- 1 tsp salt

Directions:
1. Add chicken wings into the large mixing bowl.
2. Add remaining ingredients over chicken and toss well to coat.
3. Place chicken wings in the air fryer basket.
4. Cook chicken wings for 8 minutes at 400 f.
5. Turn chicken wings to another side and cook for 8 minutes more.
6. Serve and enjoy.

Nutrition: Calories 247 Fat 11 g Carbohydrates 0.3 g Sugar 0 g Protein 32 g Cholesterol 101 mg

382. Bbq Chicken Wings

Preparation time: 10 minutes
Cooking time: 20 minutes
Servings: 4
Ingredients:
- 1 1/2 lbs. Chicken wings
- 2 tbsp unsweetened bbq sauce
- 1 tsp paprika
- 1 tbsp. olive oil
- 1 tsp garlic powder
- Pepper
- Salt

Directions:
1. In a large bowl, toss chicken wings with garlic powder, oil, paprika, pepper, and salt.
2. Preheat the air fryer to 360 f.
3. Add chicken wings in air fryer basket and cook for 12 minutes.
4. Turn chicken wings to another side and cook for 5 minutes more.
5. Remove chicken wings from air fryer and toss with bbq sauce.
6. Return chicken wings in air fryer basket and cook for 2 minutes more.
7. Serve and enjoy.

Nutrition: Calories 372 Fat 16.2 g Carbohydrates 4.3g Sugar 3.7 g Protein 49.4 g Cholesterol 151 mg

383. Yummy Chicken Nuggets

Preparation time: 10 minutes
Cooking time: 12 minutes
Servings: 4
Ingredients:
- 1 lb. Chicken breast, skinless, boneless and cut into chunks
- 6 tbsp sesame seeds, toasted
- 4 egg whites
- 1/2 tsp ground ginger
- 1/4 cup coconut flour
- 1 tsp sesame oil
- Pinch of salt

Directions:
1. Preheat the air fryer to 400 f.
2. Toss chicken with oil and salt in a bowl until well coated.
3. Add coconut flour and ginger in a zip-lock bag and shake to mix. Add chicken to the bag and shake well to coat.
4. In a large bowl, add egg whites. Add chicken in egg whites and toss until well coated.
5. Add sesame seeds in a large zip-lock bag.
6. Shake excess egg off from chicken and add chicken in sesame seed bag. Shake bag until chicken well coated with sesame seeds.
7. Spray air fryer basket with cooking spray.

8. Place chicken in air fryer basket and cook for 6 minutes.
9. Turn chicken to another side and cook for 6 minutes more.
10. Serve and enjoy.

Nutrition: Calories 265 Fat 11.5 g Carbohydrates 8.6 g Sugar 0.3 g Protein 31.1 g Cholesterol 73 mg

384. Italian Seasoned Chicken Tenders

Preparation time: 10 minutes
Cooking time: 10 minutes
Servings: 2

Ingredients:
- 2 eggs, lightly beaten
- 1 1/2 lbs. Chicken tenders
- 1/2 tsp onion powder
- 1/2 tsp garlic powder
- 1 tsp paprika
- 1 tsp italian seasoning
- 2 tbsp ground flax seed
- 1 cup almond flour
- 1/2 tsp pepper
- 1 tsp sea salt

Directions:
1. Preheat the air fryer to 400 f.
2. Season chicken with pepper and salt.
3. In a medium bowl, whisk eggs to combine.
4. In a shallow dish, mix together almond flour, all seasonings, and flaxseed.
5. Dip chicken into the egg then coats with almond flour mixture and place on a plate.
6. Spray air fryer basket with cooking spray.
7. Place half chicken tenders in air fryer basket and cook for 10 minutes. Turn halfway through.
8. Cook remaining chicken tenders using same steps.
9. Serve and enjoy.

Nutrition: Calories 315 Fat 21 g Carbohydrates 12 g Sugar 0.6 g Protein 17 g Cholesterol 184 mg

385. Classic Chicken Wings

Preparation time: 10 minutes
Cooking time: 40 minutes
Servings: 4

Ingredients:
- 2 lbs. Chicken wings
- For sauce:
- 1/4 tsp tabasco
- 1/4 tsp worcestershire sauce
- 6 tbsp. butter, melted
- 12 oz. hot sauce

Directions:
1. Spray air fryer basket with cooking spray.
2. Add chicken wings in air fryer basket and cook for 25 minutes at 380 f. Shake basket after every 5 minutes.
3. After 25 minutes turn temperature to 400 f and cook for 10-15 minutes more.
4. Meanwhile, in a large bowl, mix together all sauce ingredients.
5. Add cooked chicken wings in a sauce bowl and toss well to coat.
6. Serve and enjoy.

Nutrition: Calories 593 Fat 34.4 g Carbohydrates 1.6 g Sugar 1.1 g Protein 66.2 g Cholesterol 248 mg

386. Simple Spice Chicken Wings

Preparation time: 10 minutes
Cooking time: 30 minutes
Servings: 3

Ingredients:
- 1 1/2 lbs. Chicken wings
- 1 tbsp. baking powder, gluten-free
- 1/2 tsp onion powder
- 1/2 tsp garlic powder
- 1/2 tsp smoked paprika
- 1 tbsp. olive oil
- 1/2 tsp pepper
- 1/4 tsp sea salt

Directions:
1. Add chicken wings and oil in a large mixing bowl and toss well.
2. Mix together remaining ingredients and sprinkle over chicken wings and toss to coat.
3. Spray air fryer basket with cooking spray.
4. Add chicken wings in air fryer basket and cook at 400 f for 15 minutes. Toss well.
5. Turn chicken wings to another side and cook for 15 minutes more.
6. Serve and enjoy.

Nutrition: Calories 280 Fat 19 g Carbohydrates 2 g Sugar 0 g Protein 22 g Cholesterol 94 mg

387. Herb Seasoned Turkey Breast

Preparation time: 10 minutes
Cooking time: 35 minutes
Servings: 4

Ingredients:
- 2 lbs. Turkey breast
- 1 tsp fresh sage, chopped
- 1 tsp fresh rosemary, chopped
- 1 tsp fresh thyme, chopped
- Pepper
- Salt

Directions:
1. Spray air fryer basket with cooking spray.
2. In a small bowl, mix together sage, rosemary, and thyme.
3. Season turkey breast with pepper and salt and rub with herb mixture.
4. Place turkey breast in air fryer basket and cook at 390 f for 30-35 minutes.
5. Slice and serve.

Nutrition: Calories 238 Fat 3.9 g Carbohydrates 10 g Sugar 8 g Protein 38.8 g Cholesterol 98 mg

388. Tasty Rotisserie Chicken

Preparation time: 10 minutes
Cooking time: 20 minutes
Servings: 6

Ingredients:
- 3 lbs. Chicken, cut into eight pieces
- 1/4 tsp cayenne
- 1 tsp paprika
- 2 tsp onion powder
- 1 1/2 tsp garlic powder
- 1 1/2 tsp dried oregano
- 1/2 tbsp dried thyme
- Pepper
- Salt

Directions:
1. Season chicken with pepper and salt.
2. In a bowl, mix together spices and herbs and rub spice mixture over chicken pieces.

POULTRY RECIPES

3. Spray air fryer basket with cooking spray.
4. Place chicken in air fryer basket and cook at 350 f for 10 minutes.
5. Turn chicken to another side and cook for 10 minutes more or until the internal temperature of chicken reaches at 165 f.
6. Serve and enjoy.

Nutrition: Calories 350 Fat 7 g Carbohydrates 1.8 g Sugar 0.5 g Protein 66 g Cholesterol 175 mg

389. Spicy Asian Chicken Thighs

Preparation time: 10 minutes
Cooking time: 20 minutes
Servings: 4

Ingredients:
- 4 chicken thighs, skin-on, and bone-in
- 2 tsp ginger, grated
- 1 lime juice
- 2 tbsp. chili garlic sauce
- 1/4 cup olive oil
- 1/3 cup soy sauce

Directions:
1. In a large bowl, whisk together ginger, lime juice, chili garlic sauce, oil, and soy sauce.
2. Add chicken in bowl and coat well with marinade and place in the refrigerator for 30 minutes.
3. Place marinated chicken in air fryer basket and cook at 400 f for 15-20 minutes or until the internal temperature of chicken reaches at 165 f. Turn chicken halfway through.
4. Serve and enjoy.

Nutrition: Calories 403 Fat 23.5 g Carbohydrates 3.2 g Sugar 0.6 g Protein 43.7 g Cholesterol 130 mg

390. Tomato, Eggplant 'n Chicken Skewers

Preparation time: 10 minutes
Cooking time: 30 minutes
Servings: 4

Ingredients:
- ¼ teaspoon cayenne pepper
- ¼ teaspoon ground cardamom
- 1 ½ teaspoon ground turmeric
- 1 can coconut milk
- 1 cup cherry tomatoes
- 1 medium eggplant, cut into cubes
- 1 onion, cut into wedges
- 1-inch ginger, grated
- 2 pounds boneless chicken breasts, cut into cubes
- 2 tablespoons fresh lime juice
- 2 tablespoons tomato paste
- 3 teaspoons lime zest
- 4 cloves of garlic, minced
- Salt and pepper to taste

Directions:
1. Place in a bowl the garlic, ginger, coconut milk, lime zest, lime juice, tomato paste, salt, pepper, turmeric, cayenne pepper, cardamom, and chicken breasts. Allow to marinate in the fridge for at least for 2 hours.
2. Preheat the air fryer to 390oF.
3. Place the grill pan accessory in the air fryer.
4. Skewer the chicken cubes with eggplant, onion, and cherry tomatoes on bamboo skewers.
5. Place on the grill pan and cook for 25 minutes making sure to flip the chicken every 5 minutes for even cooking.

Nutrition: Calories:485 Carbs:19.7 g Protein: 55.2g Fat: 20.6g

391. Teriyaki Glazed Chicken Bake

Preparation time: 10 minutes
Cooking time: 30 minutes
Servings: 2

Ingredients:
- 2 tablespoons cider vinegar
- 4 skinless chicken thighs
- 1-1/2 teaspoons cornstarch
- 1-1/2 teaspoons cold water
- 1/2 clove garlic, minced
- 1/4 cup white sugar
- 1/4 cup soy sauce
- 1/4 teaspoon ground ginger
- 1/8 teaspoon ground black pepper

Directions:
1. Lightly grease baking pan of air fryer with cooking spray. Add all Ingredients and toss well to coat. Spread chicken in a single layer on bottom of pan.
2. For 15 minutes, cook on 390oF.
3. Turnover chicken while brushing and covering well with the sauce.
4. Cook for 15 minutes at 330oF.
5. Serve and enjoy.

Nutrition: Calories:267 Carbs: 19.9g Protein: 24.7g Fat: 9.8g

392. Sriracha-Ginger Chicken

Preparation time: 10 minutes
Cooking time: 35 minutes
Servings: 3

Ingredients:
- ¼ cup fish sauce
- ¼ cup sriracha
- ½ cup light brown sugar
- ½ cup rice vinegar
- 1 ½ pounds chicken breasts, pounded
- 1/3 cup hot chili paste
- 2 teaspoons grated and peeled ginger

Directions:
1. Place all Ingredients in a Ziploc bag and allow to marinate for at least 2 hours in the fridge.
2. Preheat the air fryer to 390oF.
3. Place the grill pan accessory in the air fryer.
4. Grill the chicken for 25 minutes.
5. Flip the chicken every 10 minutes for even grilling.
6. Meanwhile, pour the marinade in a saucepan and heat over medium flame until the sauce thickens.
7. Before serving the chicken, brush with the sriracha glaze.

Nutrition: Calories: 415 Carbs: 5.4g Protein: 49.3g Fat: 21.8g

393. Naked Cheese, Chicken Stuffing 'n Green Beans

Preparation time: 10 minutes
Cooking time: 20 minutes
Servings: 3

Ingredients:
- 1 cup cooked, cubed chicken breast meat
- 1/2 (10.75 ounce) can condensed cream of chicken soup
- 1/2 (14.5 ounce) can green beans, drained
- 1/2 cup shredded Cheddar cheese
- 6-ounce unseasoned dry bread stuffing mix
- salt and pepper to taste

Directions:

1. Mix well pepper, salt, soup, and chicken in a medium bowl.
2. Make the stuffing according to package Directions for Cooking.
3. Lightly grease baking pan of air fryer with cooking spray. Evenly spread chicken mixture on bottom of pan. Top evenly with stuffing. Sprinkle cheese on top.
4. Cover pan with foil.
5. For 15 minutes, cook on 390oF.
6. Remove foil and cook for 5 minutes at 390oF until tops are lightly browned.
7. Serve and enjoy.

Nutrition: Calories: 418 Carbs: 48.8g Protein: 27.1g Fat: 12.7g

394. Grilled Chicken Pesto

Preparation time: 10 minutes
Cooking time: 30 minutes
Servings: 8
Ingredients:
- 1 ¾ cup commercial pesto
- 8 chicken thighs
- Salt and pepper to taste

Directions:
1. Place all Ingredients in the Ziploc bag and allow to marinate in the fridge for at least 2 hours.
2. Preheat the air fryer to 3900F.
3. Place the grill pan accessory in the air fryer.
4. Grill the chicken for at least 30 minutes.
5. Make sure to flip the chicken every 10 minutes for even grilling.

Nutrition: Calories: 477 Carbs: 3.8g Protein: 32.6g Fat: 36.8g

395. Healthy Turkey Shepherd's Pie

Preparation time: 10 minutes
Cooking time: 50 minutes
Servings: 2
Ingredients:
- 1 tablespoon butter, room temperature
- 1/2 clove garlic, minced
- 1/2 large carrot, shredded
- 1/2 onion, chopped
- 1/2 teaspoon chicken bouillon powder
- 1/2-pound ground turkey
- 1/8 teaspoon dried thyme
- 1-1/2 large potatoes, peeled
- 1-1/2 teaspoons all-purpose flour
- 1-1/2 teaspoons chopped fresh parsley
- 1-1/2 teaspoons olive oil
- 2 tablespoons warm milk
- 4.5-ounce can sliced mushrooms
- ground black pepper to taste
- salt to taste

Directions:
1. Until tender, boil potatoes. Drain and transfer to a bowl. Mash with milk and butter until creamy. Set aside.
2. Lightly grease baking pan of air fryer with olive oil. Add onion and for 5 minutes, cook on 360oF. Add chicken bouillon, garlic, thyme, parsley, mushrooms, carrot, and ground turkey. Cook for 10 minutes while stirring and crumbling halfway through cooking time.
3. Season with pepper and salt. Stir in flour and mix well. Cook for 2 minutes.
4. Evenly spread turkey mixture. Top with mashed potatoes, evenly.
5. Cook for 20 minutes or until potatoes are lightly browned.
6. Serve and enjoy.

Nutrition: Calories: 342 Carbs: 38.0g Protein: 18.3g Fat: 12.9g

396. Chicken Fillet Strips

Preparation time: 10 minutes
Cooking time: 11 minutes
Servings: 4
Ingredients:
- 1 lb. Chicken fillets
- 1 tsp. Paprika
- 1 tbsp. Heavy cream
- .5 tsp. Black pepper
- Butter (as needed)

Directions:
1. Heat the Air Fryer at 365° Fahrenheit.
2. Slice the fillets into strips and dust with salt and pepper.
3. Add a light coating of butter to the basket.
4. Arrange the strips in the basket and air-fry for six minutes.
5. Flip the strips and continue frying for another five minutes.
6. When done, garnish with the cream and paprika. Serve warm.

Nutrition: Calories: 162 kcal Protein: 24.85 g Fat: 6.05 g Carbohydrates: 0.65 g

397. Chicken Chili Verde

Preparation time: 10 minutes
Cooking time: 25 minutes
Servings: 6
Ingredients:
- 2 pounds of chicken breasts or thighs
- ½ of a teaspoon of cumin, ground
- ¼ of a teaspoon of garlic powder
- 16 ounces of salsa verde
- Salt and pepper, to taste

Directions:
1. Place the chicken meat inside the cooker. Sprinkle with seasonings and pour the salsa on top.
2. Set the pressure to high and cook for 25 minutes.
3. After that time, release the pressure quickly. Using two forks, shred the meat inside the pot and mix with the juices and salsa. Taste for seasoning and adjust as necessary.

Nutrition: Cal.: 206 Total fat: 4.8 g Total Carbs: 3.9 g Proteins: 33 g

398. Lemon Curry Chicken

Preparation time: 5 minutes
Cooking time: 35 minutes
Servings: 6
Ingredients:
- 1 can of coconut milk
- ¼ of a cup of cup freshly squeezed lemon juice
- 1 tablespoon of curry powder
- 1 teaspoon of turmeric
- 4 pounds chicken thighs and/or breasts

Directions:
1. In a measuring cup (or a bowl – but the cup makes it easier later) combine the coconut milk, spices and lemon juice.
2. First, pour a little of the coconut milk mix into the pot. Place the meat over it, and cover it with the rest of the milk. Don't worry about little lumps in the cream. Close the lid and seal the valve.

3. Choose the poultry setting and set the pressure to high and the timer for 15 minutes. Add 10 extra minutes if you're using frozen chicken meat.
4. Once it finishes cooking, quickly release the pressure. Check the chicken by cutting through the thickest part – you should not see any pink. If it looks pinkish, close the lid back, again select high pressure and cook for 10-15 more minutes.
5. When the chicken is cooked through, shred it with two forks without removing it from the pot. Mix it well with the sauce. If you find it hard to manoeuvre inside the pot, take the meat to the plate and add it shredded to the sauce. Taste for seasoning and adjust as necessary with salt and pepper.
6. This chicken goes great served with your favourite vegetables – roasted or steamed!

Nutrition: Cal.: 615 Fat: 25.2 g Carbs: 3.3 g Protein: 89.6 g

399. Turkey Joint

Preparation time: 10 minutes
Cooking time: 11 minutes
Servings: 6

Ingredients:
- 2 lb. Turkey breast
- 4 tbsp. Melted butter
- 3 cloves Garlic
- 1 tsp. Thyme
- 1 tsp. Rosemary

Directions:
1. Warm the Air Fryer to reach 375° Fahrenheit.
2. Pat the turkey breast dry. Mince the garlic and chop the rosemary and thyme.
3. Melt the butter and mix with the garlic, thyme, and rosemary in a small mixing bowl. Brush the butter over turkey breast.
4. Place in the Air Fryer basket, skin side up, and cook for 40 minutes or until internal temperature reaches 160° Fahrenheit, flipping halfway through.
5. Wait for five minutes before slicing.

Nutrition: Calories: 321 kcal Protein: 34.35 g Fat: 19.32 g Carbohydrates: 0.56 g

400. Cilantro Drumsticks

Preparation time: 12 minutes
Cooking time: 18 minutes
Servings: 4

Ingredients:
- 8 chicken drumsticks
- ½ cup chimichurri sauce
- ¼ cup lemon juice

Directions:
1. Coat the chicken drumsticks with chimichurri sauce and refrigerate in an airtight container for no less than an hour, ideally overnight.
2. When it's time to cook, pre-heat your fryer to 400°F.
3. Remove the chicken from refrigerator and allow return to room temperature for roughly twenty minutes.
4. Cook for eighteen minutes in the fryer. Drizzle with lemon juice to taste and enjoy.

Nutrition: Calories: 452 kcal Protein: 49.16 g Fat: 25.53 g Carbohydrates: 3.52 g

401. Mozzarella Turkey Rolls

Preparation time: 10 minutes
Cooking time: 10 minutes
Servings: 4

Ingredients:
- 4 slices turkey breast
- 1 cup sliced fresh mozzarella
- 1 tomato, sliced
- ½ cup fresh basil
- 4 chive shoots

Directions:
1. Pre-heat your Air Fryer to 390°F.
2. Lay the slices of mozzarella, tomato and basil on top of each turkey slice.
3. Roll the turkey up, enclosing the filling well, and secure by tying a chive shoot around each one.
4. Put in the Air Fryer and cook for 10 minutes. Serve with a salad if desired.

Nutrition: Calories: 3616 kcal Protein: 506.27 g Fat: 160.48 g Carbohydrates: 1.21 g

402. Sage & Onion Turkey Balls

Preparation time: 25 minutes
Cooking time: 15 minutes
Servings: 2

Ingredients:
- 3.5 oz. turkey mince
- ½ small onion, diced
- 1 medium egg
- 1 tsp. sage
- ½ tsp. garlic, pureed
- 3 tbsp. friendly bread crumbs
- Salt to taste
- Pepper to taste

Directions:
1. Put all of the ingredients in a bowl and mix together well.
2. Take equal portions of the mixture and mold each one into a small ball. Transfer to the Air Fryer and cook for 15 minutes at 350°F.
3. Serve with tartar sauce and mashed potatoes.

Nutrition: Calories: 516 kcal Protein: 22.1 g Fat: 30.22 g Carbohydrates: 37.75 g

403. Turkey Loaf

Preparation time: 10 minutes
Cooking time: 40 minutes
Servings: 4

Ingredients:
- 2/3 cup of finely chopped walnuts
- 1 egg
- 1 tbsp. organic tomato paste
- 1 ½ lb. turkey breast, diced
- 1 tbsp. Dijon mustard
- ½ tsp. dried savory or dill
- 1 tbsp. onion flakes
- ½ tsp. ground allspice
- 1 small garlic clove, minced
- ½ tsp. sea salt
- ¼ tsp. black pepper
- 1 tbsp. liquid aminos
- 2 tbsp. grated parmesan cheese

Directions:
1. Pre-heat Air Fryer to 375°F.
2. Coat the inside of a baking dish with a little oil.
3. Mix together the egg, dill, tomato paste, liquid aminos, mustard, salt, dill, garlic, pepper and allspice using a whisk. Stir in the diced turkey, followed by the walnuts, cheese and onion flakes.
4. Transfer the mixture to the greased baking dish and bake in the Air Fryer for 40 minutes.
5. Serve hot.

Nutrition: Calories: 432 kcal Protein: 44.43 g Fat: 25.61 g Carbohydrates: 5.18 g

404. Moroccan Chicken

Preparation time: 15 minutes
Cooking time: 15 minutes
Servings: 2
Ingredients:
- ½ lb. shredded chicken
- 1 cup broth
- 1 carrot
- 1 broccoli, chopped
- Pinch of cinnamon
- Pinch of cumin
- Pinch of red pepper
- Pinch of sea salt

Directions:
1. In a bowl, cover the shredded chicken with cumin, red pepper, sea salt and cinnamon.
2. Chop up the carrots into small pieces. Put the carrot and broccoli into the bowl with the chicken.
3. Add the broth and stir everything well. Set aside for about 30 minutes.
4. Transfer to the Air Fryer. Cook for about 15 minutes at 390°F. Serve hot.

Nutrition: Calories: 212 kcal Protein: 30.03 g Fat: 7.1 g Carbohydrates: 5.96 g

MEAT RECIPES

405. Pork And Mixed Greens Salad
Preparation Time: 10 minutes
Cooking Time: 15 minutes
Servings: 4
Ingredients:
- 2 pounds pork tenderloin, cut into 1-inch slices (see Tip)
- 1 teaspoon olive oil
- 1 teaspoon dried marjoram
- ⅛ teaspoon freshly ground black pepper
- 6 cups mixed salad greens
- 1 red bell pepper, sliced (see Tip)
- 1 (8-ounce) package button mushrooms, sliced (see Tip)
- ⅓ cup low-sodium low-fat vinaigrette dressing

Directions:
1. In a medium bowl, mix the pork slices and olive oil. Toss to coat.
2. Sprinkle with the marjoram and pepper and rub these into the pork.
3. Grill the pork in the air fryer, in batches, for about 4 to 6 minutes, or until the pork reaches at least 145°F on a meat thermometer.
4. Meanwhile, in a serving bowl, mix the salad greens, red bell pepper, and mushrooms. Toss gently.
5. When the pork is cooked, add the slices to the salad. -Drizzle with the vinaigrette and toss gently. Serve immediately.

Nutrition: Calories: 172 Fat: 5 g Saturated Fat: 1g Protein: 27g Carbohydrates: 28g Sodium: 124mg Fiber: 2g Sugar: 3g

406. Pork Satay
Preparation Time: 15 minutes
Cooking Time: 9-14 minutes
Servings: 4
Ingredients:
- 1 (1-pound) pork tenderloin, cut into 1½-inch cubes
- ¼ cup minced onion
- 2 garlic cloves, minced
- 1 jalapeño pepper, minced
- 2 tablespoons freshly squeezed lime juice
- 2 tablespoons coconut milk
- 2 tablespoons unsalted peanut butter
- 2 teaspoons curry powder

Directions:
1. In a medium bowl, mix the pork, onion, garlic, jalapeño, lime juice, coconut milk, peanut butter, and curry powder until well combined. Let stand for 10 minutes at room temperature.
2. With a slotted spoon, remove the pork from the marinade. Reserve the marinade.
3. Thread the pork onto about 8 bamboo (see Tip, here) or metal skewers. Grill for 9 to 14 minutes, brushing once with the reserved marinade, until the pork reaches at least 145°F on a meat thermometer. Discard any remaining marinade. Serve immediately.

Nutrition: Calories: 194 Fat: 7g Saturated Fat: 3g Protein: 25g Carbohydrates: 7g Sodium: 65mg Fiber: 1g Sugar: 3g

407. Pork Burgers With Red Cabbage Salad
Preparation Time: 20 minutes
Cooking Time: 7-9 minutes
Servings: 4
Ingredients:
- ½ cup Greek yogurt
- 2 tablespoons low-sodium mustard, divided
- 1 tablespoon lemon juice
- ¼ cup sliced red cabbage
- ¼ cup grated carrots
- 1-pound lean ground pork
- ½ teaspoon paprika
- 1 cup mixed baby lettuce greens
- 2 small tomatoes, sliced
- 8 small low-sodium whole-wheat sandwich buns, cut in half

Directions:
1. In a small bowl, combine the yogurt, 1 tablespoon mustard, lemon juice, cabbage, and carrots; mix and refrigerate.
2. In a medium bowl, combine the pork, remaining 1 tablespoon mustard, and paprika. Form into 8 small patties.
3. Put the sliders into the air fryer basket. Grill for 7 to 9 minutes, or until the sliders register 165°F as tested with a meat thermometer.
4. Assemble the burgers by placing some of the lettuce greens on a bun bottom. Top with a tomato slice, the -burgers, and the cabbage mixture. Add the bun top and serve immediately.

Nutrition: Calories: 472 Fat 15g Saturated Fat: 0g Protein: 35g Carbohydrates: 51g Sodium 138mg Sugar 8g Fiber 8g

408. Crispy Mustard Pork Tenderloin
Preparation Time: 10 minutes
Cooking Time: 12-16 minutes
Servings: 4
Ingredients:
- 3 tablespoons low-sodium grainy mustard
- 2 teaspoons olive oil
- ¼ teaspoon dry mustard powder
- 1 (1-pound) pork tenderloin, silverskin and excess fat trimmed and discarded (see Tip, here)
- 2 slices low-sodium whole-wheat bread, crumbled
- ¼ cup ground walnuts (see Tip)
- 2 tablespoons cornstarch

Directions:
1. In a small bowl, stir together the mustard, olive oil, and mustard powder. Spread this mixture over the pork.
2. On a plate, mix the bread crumbs, walnuts, and cornstarch. Dip the mustard-coated pork into the crumb -mixture to coat.
3. Air-fry the pork for 12 to 16 minutes, or until it registers at least 145°F on a meat thermometer. Slice to serve.

Nutrition: Calories: 239 Fat: 9g Saturated Fat: 2g Protein: 26g Carbohydrates: 15g Sodium: 118m Fiber: 2g Sugar: 3g

409. Apple Pork Tenderloin
Preparation Time: 10 minutes
Cooking Time: 14-19 minutes
Servings: 4
Ingredients:
- 1 (1-pound) pork tenderloin, cut into 4 pieces (see Tip)
- 1 tablespoon apple butter
- 2 teaspoons olive oil

MEAT RECIPES

- 2 Granny Smith apples or Jonagold apples, sliced
- 3 celery stalks, sliced
- 1 onion, sliced
- ½ teaspoon dried marjoram
- ⅓ cup apple juice

Directions:
1. Rub each piece of pork with the apple butter and olive oil.
2. In a medium metal bowl, mix the pork, apples, celery, onion, marjoram, and apple juice.
3. Place the bowl into the air fryer and roast for 14 to 19 minutes, or until the pork reaches at least 145°F on a meat thermometer and the apples and vegetables are tender. Stir once during cooking. Serve immediately.

Nutrition: Calories: 213 Fat: 5g Saturated Fat: 1g Protein: 24g Carbohydrates: 20g Sodium: 88mg Fiber: 3g Sugar: 15g

410. Espresso-Grilled Pork Tenderloin

Preparation Time: 15 minutes
Cooking Time: 9-11 minutes
Servings: 4
Ingredients:
- 1 tablespoon packed brown sugar
- 2 teaspoons espresso powder
- 1 teaspoon ground paprika
- ½ teaspoon dried marjoram
- 1 tablespoon honey
- 1 tablespoon freshly squeezed lemon juice
- 2 teaspoons olive oil
- 1 (1-pound) pork tenderloin

Directions:
1. In a small bowl, mix the brown sugar, espresso powder, paprika, and marjoram.
2. Stir in the honey, lemon juice, and olive oil until well mixed.
3. Spread the honey mixture over the pork and let stand for 10 minutes at room temperature.
4. Roast the tenderloin in the air fryer basket for 9 to 11 minutes, or until the pork registers at least 145°F on a meat thermometer. Slice the meat to serve.

Nutrition: Calories: 177 Fat: 5g Saturated Fat: 1g Protein: 23g Carbohydrates: 10g Sodium: 61mg Fiber: 1g Sugar: 8g

411. Pork And Potatoes

Preparation Time: 5 minutes
Cooking Time: 25 minutes
Servings: 4
Ingredients:
- 2 cups creamer potatoes, rinsed and dried
- 2 teaspoons olive oil (see Tip)
- 1 (1-pound) pork tenderloin, cut into 1-inch cubes
- 1 onion, chopped
- 1 red bell pepper, chopped
- 2 garlic cloves, minced
- ½ teaspoon dried oregano
- 2 tablespoons low-sodium chicken broth

Directions:
1. In a medium bowl, toss the potatoes and olive oil to coat.
2. Transfer the potatoes to the air fryer basket. Roast for 15 minutes.
3. In a medium metal bowl, mix the potatoes, pork, onion, red bell pepper, garlic, and oregano.
4. Drizzle with the chicken broth. Put the bowl in the air fryer basket. Roast for about 10 minutes more, shaking the basket once during cooking, until the pork reaches at least 145°F on a meat thermometer and the potatoes are tender. Serve immediately.

Nutrition: Calories: 235 Fat: 5g Saturated Fat: 1g Protein: 26g Carbohydrates: 22g Sodium: 66mg Fiber: 3g Sugar: 4g

412. Pork And Fruit Kebabs

Preparation Time: 15 minutes
Cooking Time: 9-12 minutes
Servings: 4
Ingredients:
- ⅓ cup apricot jam
- 2 tablespoons freshly squeezed lemon juice
- 2 teaspoons olive oil
- ½ teaspoon dried tarragon
- 1 (1-pound) pork tenderloin, cut into 1-inch cubes
- 4 plums, pitted and quartered (see Tip)
- 4 small apricots, pitted and halved (see Tip)

Directions:
1. In a large bowl, mix the jam, lemon juice, olive oil, and tarragon.
2. Add the pork and stir to coat. Let stand for 10 minutes at room temperature.
3. Alternating the items, thread the pork, plums, and apricots onto 4 metal skewers that fit into the air fryer. Brush with any remaining jam mixture. Discard any remaining marinade.
4. Grill the kebabs in the air fryer for 9 to 12 minutes, or until the pork reaches 145°F on a meat thermometer and the fruit is tender. Serve immediately.

Nutrition: Calories: 256 Fat; 5g Saturated Fat; 1g Protein: 24g Carbohydrates: 30g Sodium: 60mg Fiber: 2g Sugar: 22g

413. Steak And Vegetable Kebabs

Preparation Time: 15 minutes
Cooking Time: 5 to 7 minutes
Servings: 4
Ingredients:
- 2 tablespoons balsamic vinegar
- 2 teaspoons olive oil
- ½ teaspoon dried marjoram
- ⅛ teaspoon freshly ground black pepper
- ¾ pound round steak, cut into 1-inch pieces
- 1 red bell pepper, sliced
- 16 button mushrooms
- 1 cup cherry tomatoes (

Directions:
1. In a medium bowl, stir together the balsamic vinegar, olive oil, marjoram, and black pepper.
2. Add the steak and stir to coat. Let stand for 10 minutes at room temperature.
3. Alternating items, thread the beef, red bell pepper, mushrooms, and tomatoes onto 8 bamboo (see Tip, here) or metal skewers that fit in the air fryer.
4. Grill in the air fryer for 5 to 7 minutes, or until the beef is browned and reaches at least 145°F on a meat thermo-meter. Serve immediately.

Nutrition: Calories: 194 Fat: 6g Saturated Fat: 2g Protein: 31g Carbohydrates: 7g Sodium: 53mg Fiber: 2g Sugar: 2g

414. Spicy Grilled Steak

Preparation Time: 7 minutes
Cooking Time: 6 to 9 minutes
Servings: 4
Ingredients:
- 2 tablespoons low-sodium salsa
- 1 tablespoon minced chipotle pepper

- 1 tablespoon apple cider vinegar
- 1 teaspoon ground cumin
- ⅛ teaspoon freshly ground black pepper
- ⅛ teaspoon red pepper flakes
- ¾ pound sirloin tip steak, cut into 4 pieces and gently pounded to about ⅓ inch thick

Directions:
1. In a small bowl, thoroughly mix the salsa, chipotle pepper, cider vinegar, cumin, black pepper, and red pepper flakes. Rub this mixture into both sides of each steak piece. Let stand for 15 minutes at room temperature.
2. Grill the steaks in the air fryer, two at a time, for 6 to 9 minutes, or until they reach at least 145°F on a meat thermometer.
3. Remove the steaks to a clean plate and cover with aluminum foil to keep warm. Repeat with the remaining steaks.
4. Slice the steaks thinly against the grain and serve.

Nutrition: Calories: 160 Fat: 6g Saturated Fat: 3g Protein: 24g Carbohydrates: 1g Sodium: 87mg Fiber: 0g Sugar: 0g

415. Greek Vegetable Skillet

Preparation Time: 10 minutes
Cooking Time: 9 to 19 minutes
Servings: 4

Ingredients:
- ½ pound 96 percent lean ground beef
- 2 medium tomatoes, chopped
- 1 onion, chopped
- 2 garlic cloves, minced
- 2 cups fresh baby spinach (see Tip)
- 2 tablespoons freshly squeezed lemon juice
- ⅓ cup low-sodium beef broth
- 2 tablespoons crumbled low-sodium feta cheese

Directions:
1. In a 6-by-2-inch metal pan, crumble the beef. Cook in the air fryer for 3 to 7 minutes, stirring once during cooking, until browned. Drain off any fat or liquid.
2. Add the tomatoes, onion, and garlic to the pan. Air-fry for 4 to 8 minutes more, or until the onion is tender.
3. Add the spinach, lemon juice, and beef broth. Air-fry for 2 to 4 minutes more, or until the spinach is wilted.
4. Sprinkle with the feta cheese and serve immediately

Nutrition: Calories: 97 Fat: 1g Saturated Fat: 1g Protein: 15g Carbohydrates: 5g Sodium: 123mg Fiber: 1g Sugar: 2g

416. Light Herbed Meatballs

Preparation Time: 10 minutes
Cooking Time: 12 to 17 minutes
Servings: 24

Ingredients:
- 1 medium onion, minced
- 2 garlic cloves, minced
- 1 teaspoon olive oil
- 1 slice low-sodium whole-wheat bread, crumbled
- 3 tablespoons 1 percent milk
- 1 teaspoon dried marjoram
- 1 teaspoon dried basil
- 1-pound 96 percent lean ground beef

Directions:
1. In a 6-by-2-inch pan, combine the onion, garlic, and olive oil. Air-fry for 2 to 4 minutes, or until the vegetables are crisp-tender.
2. Transfer the vegetables to a medium bowl, and add the bread crumbs, milk, marjoram, and basil. Mix well.
3. Add the ground beef. With your hands, work the mixture gently but thoroughly until combined. Form the meat mixture into about 24 (1-inch) meatballs.
4. Bake the meatballs, in batches, in the air fryer basket for 12 to 17 minutes, or until they reach 160°F on a meat thermometer. Serve immediately.

Nutrition: Calories: 190 Fat: 6g Saturated Fat: 2g Protein: 25g Carbohydrates: 8g Sodium: 120mg Fiber: 1g; Sugar: 2g 1% DV vitamin A 3% DV vitamin C

417. Brown Rice And Beef-Stuffed Bell Peppers

Preparation Time: 10 minutes
Cooking Time: 11 to 16 minutes
Servings: 4

Ingredients:
- 4 medium bell peppers, any colors, rinsed, tops removed
- 1 medium onion, chopped
- ½ cup grated carrot
- 2 teaspoons olive oil
- 2 medium beefsteak tomatoes, chopped
- 1 cup cooked brown rice
- 1 cup chopped cooked low-sodium roast beef (see Tip)
- 1 teaspoon dried marjoram

Directions:
1. Remove the stems from the bell pepper tops and chop the tops.
2. In a 6-by-2-inch pan, combine the chopped bell pepper tops, onion, carrot, and olive oil. Cook for 2 to 4 minutes, or until the vegetables are crisp-tender.
3. Transfer the vegetables to a medium bowl. Add the -tomatoes, brown rice, roast beef, and marjoram. Stir to mix.
4. Stuff the vegetable mixture into the bell peppers. Place the bell peppers in the air fryer basket. Bake for 11 to 16 minutes, or until the peppers are tender and the filling is hot. Serve immediately.

Nutrition: Calories: 206 Fat: 6g Saturated Fat: 1g Protein: 18g Carbohydrates: 20g Sodium: 105mg Fiber: 3g Sugar: 5g

418. Beef And Broccoli

Preparation Time: 10 minutes
Cooking Time: 14 to 18 minutes
Servings: 4

Ingredients:
- 2 tablespoons cornstarch
- ½ cup low-sodium beef broth
- 1 teaspoon low-sodium soy sauce
- 12 ounces sirloin strip steak, cut into 1-inch cubes
- 2½ cups broccoli florets
- 1 onion, chopped
- 1 cup sliced cremini mushrooms (see Tip)
- 1 tablespoon grated fresh ginger
- Brown rice, cooked (optional)

Directions:
1. In a medium bowl, stir together the cornstarch, beef broth, and soy sauce.
2. Add the beef and toss to coat. Let stand for 5 minutes at room temperature.
3. With a slotted spoon, transfer the beef from the broth mixture into a medium metal bowl. Reserve the broth.
4. Add the broccoli, onion, mushrooms, and ginger to the beef. Place the bowl into the air fryer and cook for 12 to

15 minutes, or until the beef reaches at least 145°F on a meat thermometer and the vegetables are tender.
5. Add the reserved broth and cook for 2 to 3 minutes more, or until the sauce boils.
6. Serve immediately over hot cooked brown rice, if desired.

Nutrition: Calories: 240 Fat: 6g Saturated Fat: 2g Protein: 19g Carbohydrates: 11g Sodium: 107mg Fiber: 2g Sugar: 3g

419. Beef And Fruit Stir-Fry

Preparation Time: 15 minutes
Cooking Time: 6 to 11 minutes
Servings: 4
Ingredients:
- 12 ounces sirloin tip steak, thinly sliced
- 1 tablespoon freshly squeezed lime juice
- 1 cup canned mandarin orange segments, drained, juice reserved (see Tip)
- 1 cup canned pineapple chunks, drained, juice reserved (see Tip)
- 1 teaspoon low-sodium soy sauce
- 1 tablespoon cornstarch
- 1 teaspoon olive oil
- 2 scallions, white and green parts, sliced
- Brown rice, cooked (optional)

Directions:
1. In a medium bowl, mix the steak with the lime juice. Set aside.
2. In a small bowl, thoroughly mix 3 tablespoons of reserved mandarin orange juice, 3 tablespoons of reserved pineapple juice, the soy sauce, and cornstarch.
3. Drain the beef and transfer it to a medium metal bowl, reserving the juice. Stir the reserved juice into the mandarin-pineapple juice mixture. Set aside.
4. Add the olive oil and scallions to the steak. Place the metal bowl in the air fryer and cook for 3 to 4 minutes, or until the steak is almost cooked, shaking the basket once during cooking.
5. Stir in the mandarin oranges, pineapple, and juice -mixture. Cook for 3 to 7 minutes more, or until the sauce is bubbling and the beef is tender and reaches at least 145°F on a meat thermometer.
6. Stir and serve over hot cooked brown rice, if desired.

Nutrition: Calories: 212 Fat: 4g Saturated Fat: 1g Protein: 19g Carbohydrates: 28g Sodium: 105mg Fiber: 2g Sugar: 22g

420. Simple Beef Sirloin Roast

Preparation Time: 10 minutes
Cooking Time: 50 minutes
Servings: 8
Ingredients:
- 2½ pounds sirloin roast
- Salt and ground black pepper, as required

Directions:
1. Rub the roast with salt and black pepper generously.
2. Insert the rotisserie rod through the roast.
3. Insert the rotisserie forks, one on each side of the rod to secure the rod to the chicken.
4. Arrange the drip pan in the bottom of Instant Vortex Plus Air Fryer Oven cooking chamber.
5. Select "Roast" and then adjust the temperature to 350 degrees F.
6. Set the timer for 50 minutes and press the "Start".
7. When the display shows "Add Food" press the red lever down and load the left side of the rod into the Vortex.
8. Now, slide the rod's left side into the groove along the metal bar so it doesn't move.
9. Then, close the door and touch "Rotate".
10. When cooking time is complete, press the red lever to release the rod.
11. Remove from the Vortex and place the roast onto a platter for about 10 minutes before slicing.
12. With a sharp knife, cut the roast into desired sized slices and serve.

Nutrition: Calories 201 Total Fat 8.8 g Saturated Fat 3.1 g Cholesterol 94 mg Sodium 88 mg Total Carbs 0 g Fiber 0 g Sugar 0 g Protein 28.9 g

421. Seasoned Beef Roast

Preparation Time: 10 minutes
Cooking Time: 45 minutes
Servings: 10
Ingredients:
- 3 pounds beef top roast
- 1 tablespoon olive oil
- 2 tablespoons Montreal steak seasoning

Directions:
1. Coat the roast with oil and then rub with the seasoning generously.
2. With kitchen twines, tie the roast to keep it compact.
3. Arrange the roast onto the cooking tray.
4. Arrange the drip pan in the bottom of Instant Vortex Plus Air Fryer Oven cooking chamber.
5. Select "Air Fry" and then adjust the temperature to 360 degrees F.
6. Set the timer for 45 minutes and press the "Start".
7. When the display shows "Add Food" insert the cooking tray in the center position.
8. When the display shows "Turn Food" do nothing.
9. When cooking time is complete, remove the tray from Vortex and place the roast onto a platter for about 10 minutes before slicing.
10. With a sharp knife, cut the roast into desired sized slices and serve.

Nutrition: Calories 269 Total Fat 9.9 g Saturated Fat 3.4 g Cholesterol 122 mg Sodium 538 mg

422. Bacon Wrapped Filet Mignon

Preparation Time: 10 minutes
Cooking Time: 15 minutes
Servings: 2
Ingredients:
- 2 bacon slices
- 2 (4-ounce) filet mignon
- Salt and ground black pepper, as required
- Olive oil cooking spray

Directions:
1. Wrap 1 bacon slice around each filet mignon and secure with toothpicks.
2. Season the filets with the salt and black pepper lightly.
3. Arrange the filet mignon onto a coking rack and spray with cooking spray.
4. Arrange the drip pan in the bottom of Instant Vortex Plus Air Fryer Oven cooking chamber.
5. Select "Air Fry" and then adjust the temperature to 375 degrees F.
6. Set the timer for 15 minutes and press the "Start".
7. When the display shows "Add Food" insert the cooking rack in the center position.
8. When the display shows "Turn Food" turn the filets.
9. When cooking time is complete, remove the rack from Vortex and serve hot.

Nutrition: Calories 360 Total Fat 19.6 g Saturated Fat 6.8 g Cholesterol 108 mg Sodium 737 mg Total Carbs 0.4 g Fiber 0 g Sugar 0 g Protein 42.6 g

423. Beef Burgers

Preparation Time: 15 minutes
Cooking Time: 18 minutes
Servings: 4
Ingredients:
For Burgers:
- 1-pound ground beef
- ½ cup panko breadcrumbs
- ¼ cup onion, chopped finely
- 3 tablespoons Dijon mustard
- 3 teaspoons low-sodium soy sauce
- 2 teaspoons fresh rosemary, chopped finely
- Salt, to taste

For Topping:
- 2 tablespoons Dijon mustard
- 1 tablespoon brown sugar
- 1 teaspoon soy sauce
- 4 Gruyere cheese slices

Directions:
1. In a large bowl, add all the ingredients and mix until well combined.
2. Make 4 equal-sized patties from the mixture.
3. Arrange the patties onto a cooking tray.
4. Arrange the drip pan in the bottom of Instant Vortex Plus Air Fryer Oven cooking chamber.
5. Select "Air Fry" and then adjust the temperature to 370 degrees F.
6. Set the timer for 15 minutes and press the "Start".
7. When the display shows "Add Food" insert the cooking rack in the center position.
8. When the display shows "Turn Food" turn the burgers.
9. Meanwhile, for sauce: in a small bowl, add the mustard, brown sugar and soy sauce and mix well.
10. When cooking time is complete, remove the tray from Vortex and coat the burgers with the sauce.
11. Top each burger with 1 cheese slice.
12. Return the tray to the cooking chamber and select "Broil".
13. Set the timer for 3 minutes and press the "Start".
14. When cooking time is complete, remove the tray from Vortex and serve hot.

Nutrition: Calories 402 Total Fat 18 g Saturated Fat 8.5 g Cholesterol 133mg Sodium 651 mg Total Carbs 6.3 g Fiber 0.8 g Sugar 3 g Protein 44.4 g

424. Beef Jerky

Preparation Time: 15 minutes
Cooking Time: 3 hours
Servings: 4
Ingredients:
- 1½ pounds beef round, trimmed
- ½ cup Worcestershire sauce
- ½ cup low-sodium soy sauce
- 2 teaspoons honey
- 1 teaspoon liquid smoke
- 2 teaspoons onion powder
- ½ teaspoon red pepper flakes
- Ground black pepper, as required

Directions:
1. In a zip-top bag, place the beef and freeze for 1-2 hours to firm up.
2. Place the meat onto a cutting board and cut against the grain into 1/8-¼-inch strips.
3. In a large bowl, add the remaining ingredients and mix until well combined.
4. Add the steak slices and coat with the mixture generously.
5. Refrigerate to marinate for about 4-6 hours.
6. Remove the beef slices from bowl and with paper towels, pat dry them.
7. Divide the steak strips onto the cooking trays and arrange in an even layer.
8. Select "Dehydrate" and then adjust the temperature to 160 degrees F.
9. Set the timer for 3 hours and press the "Start".
10. When the display shows "Add Food" insert 1 tray in the top position and another in the center position.
11. After 1½ hours, switch the position of cooking trays.
12. Meanwhile, in a small pan, add the remaining ingredients over medium heat and cook for about 10 minutes, stirring occasionally.
13. When cooking time is complete, remove the trays from Vortex.

Nutrition: Calories 372 Total Fat 10.7 g Saturated Fat 4 g Cholesterol 152 mg Sodium 2000 mg Total Carbs 12 g Fiber 0.2 g Sugar 11.3 g Protein 53.8 g

425. Sweet & Spicy Meatballs

Preparation Time: 20 minutes
Cooking Time: 30 minutes
Servings: 8
Ingredients:
For Meatballs:
- 2 pounds lean ground beef
- 2/3 cup quick-cooking oats
- ½ cup Ritz crackers, crushed
- 1 (5-ounce) can evaporated milk
- 2 large eggs, beaten lightly
- 1 teaspoon honey
- 1 tablespoon dried onion, minced
- 1 teaspoon garlic powder
- 1 teaspoon ground cumin
- Salt and ground black pepper, as required

For Sauce:
- 1/3 cup orange marmalade
- 1/3 cup honey
- 1/3 cup brown sugar
- 2 tablespoons cornstarch
- 2 tablespoons soy sauce
- 1-2 tablespoons hot sauce
- 1 tablespoon Worcestershire sauce

Directions:
1. For meatballs: in a large bowl, add all the ingredients and mix until well combined.
2. Make 1½-inch balls from the mixture.
3. Arrange half of the meatballs onto a cooking tray in a single layer.
4. Arrange the drip pan in the bottom of Instant Vortex Plus Air Fryer Oven cooking chamber.
5. Select "Air Fry" and then adjust the temperature to 380 degrees F.
6. Set the timer for 15 minutes and press the "Start".
7. When the display shows "Add Food" insert the cooking tray in the center position.
8. When the display shows "Turn Food" turn the meatballs.
9. When cooking time is complete, remove the tray from Vortex.
10. Repeat with the remaining meatballs.
11. Meanwhile, for sauce: in a small pan, add all the ingredients over medium heat and cook until thickened, stirring continuously.

MEAT RECIPES

12. Serve the meatballs with the topping of sauce.

Nutrition: Calories 411 Total Fat 11.1 g Saturated Fat 4.1 g Cholesterol 153 mg Sodium 448 mg Total Carbs 38.8 g Fiber 1 g Sugar 28.1 g Protein 38.9 g

426. Spiced Pork Shoulder

Preparation Time: 15 minutes
Cooking Time: 55 minutes
Servings: 6
Ingredients:
- 1 teaspoon ground cumin
- 1 teaspoon cayenne pepper
- 1 teaspoon garlic powder
- Salt and ground black pepper, as required
- 2 pounds skin-on pork shoulder

Directions:
1. In a small bowl, mix together the spices, salt and black pepper.
2. Arrange the pork shoulder onto a cutting board, skin-side down.
3. Season the inner side of pork shoulder with salt and black pepper.
4. With kitchen twines, tie the pork shoulder into a long round cylinder shape.
5. Season the outer side of pork shoulder with spice mixture.
6. Insert the rotisserie rod through the pork shoulder.
7. Insert the rotisserie forks, one on each side of the rod to secure the pork shoulder.
8. Arrange the drip pan in the bottom of Instant Vortex Plus Air Fryer Oven cooking chamber.
9. Select "Roast" and then adjust the temperature to 350 degrees F.
10. Set the timer for 55 minutes and press the "Start".
11. When the display shows "Add Food" press the red lever down and load the left side of the rod into the Vortex.
12. Now, slide the rod's left side into the groove along the metal bar so it doesn't move.
13. Then, close the door and touch "Rotate".
14. When cooking time is complete, press the red lever to release the rod.
15. Remove the pork from Vortex and place onto a platter for about 10 minutes before slicing.
16. With a sharp knife, cut the pork shoulder into desired sized slices and serve.

Nutrition: Calories 445 Total Fat 32.5 g Saturated Fat 11.9 g Cholesterol 136 mg Sodium 131 mg Total Carbs 0.7 g Fiber 0.2 g Sugar 0.2 g Protein 35.4 g

427. Seasoned Pork Tenderloin

Preparation Time: 10 minutes
Cooking Time: 45 minutes
Servings: 5
Ingredients:
- 1½ pounds pork tenderloin
- 2-3 tablespoons BBQ pork seasoning

Directions:
1. Rub the pork with seasoning generously.
2. Insert the rotisserie rod through the pork tenderloin.
3. Insert the rotisserie forks, one on each side of the rod to secure the pork tenderloin.
4. Arrange the drip pan in the bottom of Instant Vortex Plus Air Fryer Oven cooking chamber.
5. Select "Roast" and then adjust the temperature to 360 degrees F.
6. Set the timer for 45 minutes and press the "Start".
7. When the display shows "Add Food" press the red lever down and load the left side of the rod into the Vortex.
8. Now, slide the rod's left side into the groove along the metal bar so it doesn't move.
9. Then, close the door and touch "Rotate".
10. When cooking time is complete, press the red lever to release the rod.
11. Remove the pork from Vortex and place onto a platter for about 10 minutes before slicing.
12. With a sharp knife, cut the roast into desired sized slices and serve.

Nutrition: Calories 195 Total Fat 4.8 g Saturated Fat 1.6 g Cholesterol 99 mg Sodium 116 mg Total Carbs 0 g Fiber 0 g Sugar 0 g Protein 35.6 g

428. Garlicky Pork Tenderloin

Preparation Time: 15 minutes
Cooking Time: 20 minutes
Servings: 5
Ingredients:
- 1½ pounds pork tenderloin
- Nonstick cooking spray
- 2 small heads roasted garlic
- Salt and ground black pepper, as required

Directions:
1. Lightly, spray all the sides of pork with cooking spray and then, season with salt and black pepper.
2. Now, rub the pork with roasted garlic.
3. Arrange the roast onto the lightly greased cooking tray.
4. Arrange the drip pan in the bottom of Instant Vortex Plus Air Fryer Oven cooking chamber.
5. Select "Air Fry" and then adjust the temperature to 400 degrees F.
6. Set the timer for 20 minutes and press the "Start".
7. When the display shows "Add Food" insert the cooking tray in the center position.
8. When the display shows "Turn Food" turn the pork.
9. When cooking time is complete, remove the tray from Vortex and place the roast onto a platter for about 10 minutes before slicing.
10. With a sharp knife, cut the roast into desired sized slices and serve.

Nutrition: Calories 202 Total Fat 4.8 g Saturated Fat 1.6 g Cholesterol 99 mg Sodium 109 mg Total Carbs 1.7 g Fiber 0.1 g Sugar 0.1 g Protein 35.9 g

429. Glazed Pork Tenderloin

Preparation Time: 15 minutes
Cooking Time: 20 minutes
Servings: 3
Ingredients:
- 1-pound pork tenderloin
- 2 tablespoons Sriracha
- 2 tablespoons honey
- Salt, as required

Directions:
1. Insert the rotisserie rod through the pork tenderloin.
2. Insert the rotisserie forks, one on each side of the rod to secure the pork tenderloin.
3. In a small bowl, add the Sriracha, honey and salt and mix well.
4. Brush the pork tenderloin with honey mixture evenly.
5. Arrange the drip pan in the bottom of Instant Vortex Plus Air Fryer Oven cooking chamber.
6. Select "Air Fry" and then adjust the temperature to 350 degrees F.
7. Set the timer for 20 minutes and press the "Start".

8. When the display shows "Add Food" press the red lever down and load the left side of the rod into the Vortex.
9. Now, slide the rod's left side into the groove along the metal bar so it doesn't move.
10. Then, close the door and touch "Rotate".
11. When cooking time is complete, press the red lever to release the rod.
12. Remove the pork from Vortex and place onto a platter for about 10 minutes before slicing.
13. With a sharp knife, cut the roast into desired sized slices and serve.

Nutrition: Calories 269 Total Fat 5.3 g Saturated Fat 1.8 g Cholesterol 110 mg Sodium 207 mg Total Carbs 13.5 g Fiber 0 g Sugar 11.6 g Protein 39.7 g

430. Honey Mustard Pork Tenderloin

Preparation Time: 15 minutes
Cooking Time: 25 minutes
Servings: 3
Ingredients:
- 1-pound pork tenderloin
- 1 tablespoon garlic, minced
- 2 tablespoons soy sauce
- 2 tablespoons honey
- 1 tablespoon Dijon mustard
- 1 tablespoon grain mustard
- 1 teaspoon Sriracha sauce

Directions:
1. In a large bowl, add all the ingredients except pork and mix well.
2. Add the pork tenderloin and coat with the mixture generously.
3. Refrigerate to marinate for 2-3 hours.
4. Remove the pork tenderloin from bowl, reserving the marinade.
5. Place the pork tenderloin onto the lightly greased cooking tray.
6. Arrange the drip pan in the bottom of Instant Vortex Plus Air Fryer Oven cooking chamber.
7. Select "Air Fry" and then adjust the temperature to 380 degrees F.
8. Set the timer for 25 minutes and press the "Start".
9. When the display shows "Add Food" insert the cooking tray in the center position.
10. When the display shows "Turn Food" turn the pork and oat with the reserved marinade.
11. When cooking time is complete, remove the tray from Vortex and place the pork tenderloin onto a platter for about 10 minutes before slicing.
12. With a sharp knife, cut the pork tenderloin into desired sized slices and serve.

Nutrition: Calories 277 Total Fat 5.7 g Saturated Fat 1.8 g Cholesterol 110 mg Sodium 782 mg Total Carbs 14.2 g Fiber 0.4 g Sugar 11.8 g Protein 40.7 g

431. Seasoned Pork Chops

Preparation Time: 10 minutes
Cooking Time: 12 minutes
Servings: 4
Ingredients:
- 4 (6-ounce) boneless pork chops
- 2 tablespoons pork rub
- 1 tablespoon olive oil

Directions:
1. Coat both sides of the pork chops with the oil and then, rub with the pork rub.
2. Place the pork chops onto the lightly greased cooking tray.
3. Arrange the drip pan in the bottom of Instant Vortex Plus Air Fryer Oven cooking chamber.
4. Select "Air Fry" and then adjust the temperature to 400 degrees F.
5. Set the timer for 12 minutes and press the "Start".
6. When the display shows "Add Food" insert the cooking tray in the center position.
7. When the display shows "Turn Food" turn the pork chops.
8. When cooking time is complete, remove the tray from Vortex and serve hot.

Nutrition: Calories 285 Total Fat 9.5 g Saturated Fat 2.5 g Cholesterol 124 mg Sodium 262 mg Total Carbs 1.5 g Fiber 0 g Sugar 0.8 g Protein 44.5 g

432. Breaded Pork Chops

Preparation Time: 15 minutes
Cooking Time: 28 minutes
Servings: 2
Ingredients:
- 2 (5-ounce) boneless pork chops
- 1 cup buttermilk
- ½ cup flour
- 1 teaspoon garlic powder
- Salt and ground black pepper, as required
- Olive oil cooking spray

Directions:
1. In a bowl, place the chops and buttermilk and refrigerate, covered for about 12 hours.
2. Remove the chops from the bowl of buttermilk, discarding the buttermilk.
3. In a shallow dish, mix together the flour, garlic powder, salt, and black pepper.
4. Coat the chops with flour mixture generously.
5. Place the pork chops onto the cooking tray and spray with the cooking spray.
6. Arrange the drip pan in the bottom of Instant Vortex Plus Air Fryer Oven cooking chamber.
7. Select "Air Fry" and then adjust the temperature to 380 degrees F.
8. Set the timer for 28 minutes and press the "Start".
9. When the display shows "Add Food" insert the cooking tray in the center position.
10. When the display shows "Turn Food" turn the pork chops.
11. When cooking time is complete, remove the tray from Vortex and serve hot.

Nutrition: Calories 370 Total Fat 6.4 g Saturated Fat 2.4 g Cholesterol 108 mg Sodium 288 mg Total Carbs 30.7 g Fiber 1 g Sugar 6.3 g Protein 44.6 g

433. Crusted Rack Of Lamb

Preparation Time: 15 minutes
Cooking Time: 19 minutes
Servings: 4
Ingredients:
- 1 rack of lamb, trimmed all fat and frenched
- Salt and ground black pepper, as required
- 1/3 cup pistachios, chopped finely
- 2 tablespoons panko breadcrumbs
- 2 teaspoons fresh thyme, chopped finely
- 1 teaspoon fresh rosemary, chopped finely

MEAT RECIPES

- 1 tablespoon butter, melted
- 1 tablespoon Dijon mustard

Directions:
1. Insert the rotisserie rod through the rack on the meaty side of the ribs, right next to the bone.
2. Insert the rotisserie forks, one on each side of the rod to secure the rack.
3. Season the rack with salt and black pepper evenly.
4. Arrange the drip pan in the bottom of Instant Vortex Plus Air Fryer Oven cooking chamber.
5. Select "Air Fry" and then adjust the temperature to 380 degrees F.
6. Set the timer for 12 minutes and press the "Start".
7. When the display shows "Add Food" press the red lever down and load the left side of the rod into the Vortex.
8. Now, slide the rod's left side into the groove along the metal bar so it doesn't move.
9. Then, close the door and touch "Rotate".
10. Meanwhile, in a small bowl, mix together the remaining ingredients except the mustard.
11. When cooking time is complete, press the red lever to release the rod.
12. Remove the rack from Vortex and brush the meaty side with the mustard.
13. Then, coat the pistachio mixture on all sides of the rack and press firmly.
14. Now, place the rack of lamb onto the cooking tray, meat side up.
15. Select "Air Fry" and adjust the temperature to 380 degrees F.
16. Set the timer for 7 minutes and press the "Start".
17. When the display shows "Add Food" insert the cooking tray in the center position.
18. When the display shows "Turn Food" do nothing.
19. When cooking time is complete, remove the tray from Vortex and place the rack onto a cutting board for at least 10 minutes.
20. Cut the rack into individual chops and serve.

Nutrition: Calories 824 Total Fat 39.3 g Saturated Fat 14.2 g Cholesterol 233 mg Sodium 373 mg Total Carbs 10.3 g Fiber 1.2 g Sugar 0.2 g Protein 72 g

434. Lamb Burgers
Preparation Time: 15 minutes
Cooking Time: 8 minutes
Servings: 6
Ingredients:
- 2 pounds ground lamb
- 1 tablespoon onion powder
- Salt and ground black pepper, as required

Directions:
1. In a bowl, add all the ingredients and mix well.
2. Make 6 equal-sized patties from the mixture.
3. Arrange the patties onto a cooking tray.
4. Arrange the drip pan in the bottom of Instant Vortex Plus Air Fryer Oven cooking chamber.
5. Select "Air Fry" and then adjust the temperature to 360 degrees F.
6. Set the timer for 8 minutes and press the "Start".
7. When the display shows "Add Food" insert the cooking rack in the center position.
8. When the display shows "Turn Food" turn the burgers.
9. When cooking time is complete, remove the tray from Vortex and serve hot.

Nutrition: Calories 285 Total Fat 11.1 g Saturated Fat 4 g Cholesterol 136 mg Sodium 143 mg Total Carbs 0.9 g Fiber 0.1 g Sugar 0.4 g Protein 42.6 g

435. Pork Taquitos
Preparation Time: 10 minutes
Cooking Time: 16 minutes
Servings: 8
Ingredients:
- 1 juiced lime
- 10 whole wheat tortillas
- 2 ½ C. shredded mozzarella cheese
- 30 ounces of cooked and shredded pork tenderloin

Directions:
1. Preparing the Ingredients. Ensure your air fryer is preheated to 380 degrees.
2. Drizzle pork with lime juice and gently mix.
3. Heat up tortillas in the microwave with a dampened paper towel to soften.
4. Add about 3 ounces of pork and ¼ cup of shredded cheese to each tortilla. Tightly roll them up.
5. Spray the Pro Breeze air fryer basket with a bit of olive oil.
6. Air Frying. Set temperature to 380°F, and set time to 10 minutes. Air fry taquitos 7-10 minutes till tortillas turn a slight golden color, making sure to flip halfway through cooking process.

Nutrition: Calories: 309; Fat: 11g; Protein:21g;Sugar:2g

436. Cajun Bacon Pork Loin Fillet
Preparation Time: 10 minutes
Cooking Time: 20 minutes
Servings: 6
Ingredients:
- 1½ pounds pork loin fillet or pork tenderloin
- 3 tablespoons olive oil
- 2 tablespoons Cajun Spice Mix
- Salt
- 6 slices bacon
- Olive oil spray

Directions:
1. Preparing the Ingredients. Cut the pork in half so that it will fit in the air fryer basket.
2. Place both pieces of meat in a resealable plastic bag. Add the oil, Cajun seasoning, and salt to taste, if using. Seal the bag and massage to coat all of the meat with the oil and seasonings. Marinate in the refrigerator for at least 1 hour or up to 24 hours.
3. Air Frying. Remove the pork from the bag and wrap 3 bacon slices around each piece. Spray the Pro Breeze air fryer basket with olive oil spray. Place the meat in the air fryer. Set the Pro Breeze air fryer to 350°F for 15 minutes. Increase the temperature to 400°F for 5 minutes. Use a meat thermometer to ensure the meat has reached an internal temperature of 145°F.
4. Let the meat rest for 10 minutes. Slice into 6 medallions and serve.

Nutrition: Calories: 355 kcal Protein: 34.83 g Fat: 22.88 g Carbohydrates: 0.6 g

437. Panko-Breaded Pork Chops
Preparation Time: 5 minutes
Cooking Time: 12 minutes
Servings: 6
Ingredients:
- 5 (3½- to 5-ounce) pork chops (bone-in or boneless)
- Seasoning salt
- Pepper
- ¼ cup all-purpose flour
- 2 tablespoons panko bread crumbs

- Cooking oil

Directions:
1. Preparing the Ingredients. Season the pork chops with the seasoning salt and pepper to taste.
2. Sprinkle the flour on both sides of the pork chops, then coat both sides with panko bread crumbs.
3. Place the pork chops in the air fryer. Stacking them is okay.
4. Air Frying. Spray the pork chops with cooking oil. Cook for 6 minutes.
5. Open the Air fryer and flip the pork chops. Cook for an additional 6 minutes
6. Cool before serving.
7. Typically, bone-in pork chops are juicier than boneless. If you prefer really juicy pork chops, use bone-in.

Nutrition: Calories: 246 Fat: 13g Protein:26g Fiber:0g

438. Porchetta-Style Pork Chops

Preparation Time: 10 minutes
Cooking Time: 15 minutes
Servings: 2

Ingredients:
- 1 tablespoon extra-virgin olive oil
- Grated zest of 1 lemon
- 2 cloves garlic, minced
- 2 teaspoons chopped fresh rosemary
- 1 teaspoon finely chopped fresh sage
- 1 teaspoon fennel seeds, lightly crushed
- ¼ to ½ teaspoon red pepper flakes
- 1 teaspoon kosher salt
- 1 teaspoon black pepper
- (8-ounce) center-cut bone-in pork chops, about 1 inch thick

Directions:
1. Preparing the Ingredients. In a small bowl, combine the olive oil, zest, garlic, rosemary, sage, fennel seeds, red pepper, salt, and black pepper. Stir, crushing the herbs with the back of a spoon, until a paste forms. Spread the seasoning mix on both sides of the pork chops.
2. Air Frying. Place the chops in the air fryer basket. Set the Pro Breeze air fryer to 375°F for 15 minutes. Use a meat thermometer to ensure the chops have reached an internal temperature of 145°F.

Nutrition: Calories: 200 kcal Protein: 23.45 g Fat: 9.69 g Carbohydrates: 4.46 g

439. Apricot Glazed Pork Tenderloins

Preparation Time: 5 minutes
Cooking Time: 30 minutes
Servings: 3

Ingredients:
- 1 teaspoon salt
- 1/2 teaspoon pepper
- 1-lb pork tenderloin
- 2 tablespoons minced fresh rosemary or 1 tablespoon dried rosemary, crushed
- 2 tablespoons olive oil, divided
- 1 garlic cloves, minced
- Apricot Glaze Ingredients
- 1 cup apricot preserves
- 3 garlic cloves, minced
- 4 tablespoons lemon juice

Directions:

1. Preparing the Ingredients. Mix well pepper, salt, garlic, oil, and rosemary. Brush all over pork. If needed cut pork crosswise in half to fit in air fryer. Lightly grease baking pan of air fryer with cooking spray. Add pork.
2. Air Frying. For 3 minutes per side, brown pork in a preheated 390°F air fryer. Meanwhile, mix well all glaze Ingredients in a small bowl. Baste pork every 5 minutes. Cook for 20 minutes at 330°F. Serve and enjoy.

Nutrition: Calories: 454 kcal Protein: 43.76 g Fat: 16.71 g Carbohydrates: 33.68 g

440. Sweet & Spicy Country-Style Ribs

Preparation Time: 10 minutes
Cooking Time: 25 minutes
Servings: 4

Ingredients:
- 2 tablespoons brown sugar
- 2 tablespoons smoked paprika
- 1 teaspoon garlic powder
- 1 teaspoon onion powder
- 1 teaspoon dry mustard
- 1 teaspoon ground cumin
- 1 teaspoon kosher salt
- 1 teaspoon black pepper
- ¼ to ½ teaspoon cayenne pepper
- 1½ pounds boneless country-style pork ribs
- 1 cup barbecue sauce

Directions:
1. Preparing the Ingredients. In a small bowl, stir together the brown sugar, paprika, garlic powder, onion powder, dry mustard, cumin, salt, black pepper, and cayenne. Mix until well combined.
2. Pat the ribs dry with a paper towel. Generously sprinkle the rub evenly over both sides of the ribs and rub in with your fingers.
3. Air Frying. Place the ribs in the air fryer basket. Set the Pro Breeze air fryer to 350°F for 15 minutes. Turn the ribs and brush with ½ cup of the barbecue sauce. Cook for an additional 10 minutes. Use a meat thermometer to ensure the pork has reached an internal temperature of 145°F. Serve with remaining barbecue sauce.

Nutrition: Calories: 416 kcal Protein: 38.39 g Fat: 12.19 g Carbohydrates: 36.79 g

441. Pork Tenders With Bell Peppers

Preparation Time: 5 minutes
Cooking Time: 15 minutes
Servings: 4

Ingredients:
- 11 Oz Pork Tenderloin
- 1 Bell Pepper, in thin strips
- 1 Red Onion, sliced
- 2 Tsps. Provencal Herbs
- Black Pepper to taste
- 1 tbsp. Olive Oil
- 1/2 tbsp. Mustard

Directions:
1. Preparing the Ingredients. Preheat the Pro Breeze air fryer to 390 degrees.
2. In the oven dish, mix the bell pepper strips with the onion, herbs, and some salt and pepper to taste.
3. Add half a tablespoon of olive oil to the mixture

MEAT RECIPES

4. Cut the pork tenderloin into four pieces and rub with salt, pepper and mustard.
5. Thinly coat the pieces with remaining olive oil and place them upright in the oven dish on top of the pepper mixture
6. Air Frying. Place the bowl into the Air fryer. Set the timer to 15 minutes and roast the meat and the vegetables
7. Turn the meat and mix the peppers halfway through
8. Serve with a fresh salad

Nutrition: Calories: 220 kcal Protein: 23.79 g Fat: 12.36 g Carbohydrates: 2.45 g

442. Wonton Meatballs
Preparation Time: 15 minutes
Cooking Time: 10 minutes
Servings: 4
Ingredients:
- 1-pound ground pork
- 2 large eggs
- ¼ cup chopped green onions (white and green parts)
- ¼ cup chopped fresh cilantro or parsley
- 1 tablespoon minced fresh ginger
- 3 cloves garlic, minced
- 2 teaspoons soy sauce
- 1 teaspoon oyster sauce
- ½ teaspoon kosher salt
- 1 teaspoon black pepper

Directions:
1. Preparing the Ingredients. In the bowl of a stand mixer fitted with the paddle attachment, combine the pork, eggs, green onions, cilantro, ginger, garlic, soy sauce, oyster sauce, salt, and pepper. Mix on low speed until all of the ingredients are incorporated, 2 to 3 minutes.
2. Form the mixture into 12 meatballs and arrange in a single layer in the air fryer basket.
3. Air Frying. Set the Pro Breeze air fryer to 350°F for 10 minutes. Use a meat thermometer to ensure the meatballs have reached an internal temperature of 145°F.
4. Transfer the meatballs to a bowl and serve.

Nutrition: Calories: 402 kcal Protein: 32.69 g Fat: 27.91 g Carbohydrates: 3.1 g

443. Barbecue Flavored Pork Ribs
Preparation Time: 5 minutes
Cooking Time: 15 minutes
Servings: 6
Ingredients:
- ¼ cup honey, divided
- ¾ cup BBQ sauce
- 2 tablespoons tomato ketchup
- 1 tablespoon Worcestershire sauce
- 1 tablespoon soy sauce
- ½ teaspoon garlic powder
- Freshly ground white pepper, to taste
- 1¾ pound pork ribs

Directions:
1. Preparing the Ingredients. In a large bowl, mix together 3 tablespoons of honey and remaining ingredients except pork ribs. Refrigerate to marinate for about 20 minutes. Preheat the Pro Breeze air fryer to 355 degrees F. Place the ribs in an Air fryer basket.
2. Air Frying. Cook for about 13 minutes. Remove the ribs from the Air fryer and coat with remaining honey. Serve hot.

Nutrition: Calories: 265 kcal Protein: 29.47 g Fat: 9.04 g Carbohydrates: 15.87 g

444. Easy Air Fryer Marinated Pork Tenderloin
Preparation Time: 1 hour & 10 minutes
Cooking Time: 30 minutes
Servings: 4 to 6
Ingredients:
- ¼ cup olive oil
- ¼ cup soy sauce
- ¼ cup freshly squeezed lemon juice
- 1 garlic clove, minced
- 1 tablespoon Dijon mustard
- 1 teaspoon salt
- ½ teaspoon freshly ground black pepper
- 2 pounds pork tenderloin

Directions:
1. Preparing the Ingredients. In a large mixing bowl, make the marinade. Mix together the olive oil, soy sauce, lemon juice, minced garlic, Dijon mustard, salt, and pepper. Reserve ¼ cup of the marinade.
2. Place the tenderloin in a large bowl and pour the remaining marinade over the meat. Cover and marinate in the refrigerator for about 1 hour. Place the marinated pork tenderloin into the air fryer basket.
3. Air Frying. Set the temperature of your Pro Breeze AF to 400°F. Set the timer and roast for 10 minutes. Using tongs, flip the pork and baste it with half of the reserved marinade. Reset the timer and roast for 10 minutes more.
4. Using tongs, flip the pork, then baste with the remaining marinade.
5. Reset the timer and roast for another 10 minutes, for a total cooking time of 30 minutes.

Nutrition: Calories: 345 kcal Protein: 41.56 g Fat: 17.35 g Carbohydrates: 3.66 g

445. Balsamic Glazed Pork Chops
Preparation Time: 5 minutes
Cooking Time: 50
Servings: 4
Ingredients:
- ¾ cup balsamic vinegar
- 1 ½ tablespoons sugar
- 1 tablespoon butter
- 3 tablespoons olive oil
- 3 tablespoons salt
- 3 pork rib chops

Directions:
1. Preparing the Ingredients. Place all ingredients in bowl and allow the meat to marinate in the fridge for at least 2 hours. Preheat the Pro Breeze air fryer to 390°F. Place the grill pan accessory in the air fryer.
2. Air Frying. Grill the pork chops for 20 minutes making sure to flip the meat every 10 minutes for even grilling. Meanwhile, pour the balsamic vinegar on a saucepan and allow to simmer for at least 10 minutes until the sauce thickens. Brush the meat with the glaze before serving.

Nutrition: Calories: 274 Fat: 18g Protein: 17g

446. Perfect Air Fried Pork Chops
Preparation Time: 5 minutes
Cooking Time: 17 minutes
Servings: 4
Ingredients:
- 3 cups bread crumbs
- ½ cup grated Parmesan cheese
- 2 tablespoons vegetable oil

- 2 teaspoons salt
- 2 teaspoons sweet paprika
- ½ teaspoon onion powder
- ¼ teaspoon garlic powder
- 6 (½-inch-thick) bone-in pork chops

Directions:
1. Preparing the Ingredients. Spray the Pro Breeze air fryer basket with olive oil. In a large resealable bag, combine the bread crumbs, Parmesan cheese, oil, salt, paprika, onion powder, and garlic powder. Seal the bag and shake it a few times in order for the spices to blend together. Place the pork chops, one by one, in the bag and shake to coat.
2. Air Frying. Place the pork chops in the greased Pro Breeze air fryer basket in a single layer. Be careful not to overcrowd the basket. Spray the chops generously with olive oil to avoid powdery, uncooked breading.
3. Set the temperature of your Pro Breeze AF to 360°F. Set the timer and roast for 10 minutes.
4. Using tongs, flip the chops. Spray them generously with olive oil.
5. Reset the timer and roast for 7 minutes more.
6. Check that the pork has reached an internal temperature of 145°F. Add cooking time if needed.

Nutrition: Calories: 513 Fat: 23g Saturated fat: 8g Carbohydrate: 22g Fiber: 2g Sugar: 3g Protein: 50g Iron: 3mg; Sodium: 1521mg

447. Rustic Pork Ribs

Preparation Time: 5 minutes
Cooking Time: 15 minutes
Servings: 4

Ingredients:
- 1 rack of pork ribs
- 3 tablespoons dry red wine
- 1 tablespoon soy sauce
- 1/2 teaspoon dried thyme
- 1/2 teaspoon onion powder
- 1/2 teaspoon garlic powder
- 1/2 teaspoon ground black pepper
- 1 teaspoon smoke salt
- 1 tablespoon cornstarch
- 1/2 teaspoon olive oil

Directions:
1. Preparing the Ingredients. Begin by preheating your Air fryer to 390 degrees F. Place all ingredients in a mixing bowl and let them marinate at least 1 hour.
2. Air Frying. Cook the marinated ribs approximately 25 minutes at 390 degrees F. Serve hot.

Nutrition: Calories: 119 kcal Protein: 12.26 g Fat: 5.61 g Carbohydrates: 3.64 g

448. Air Fryer Baby Back Ribs

Preparation Time: 5 minutes
Cooking Time: 25 minutes
Servings: 4

Ingredients:
- 1 rack baby back ribs
- 1 tablespoon garlic powder
- 1 teaspoon freshly ground black pepper
- 2 tablespoons salt
- 1 cup barbecue sauce (any type)

Directions:
1. Preparing the Ingredients
2. Dry the ribs with a paper towel.
3. Season the ribs with the garlic powder, pepper, and salt.
4. Place the seasoned ribs into the air fryer.
5. Air Frying.
6. Set the temperature of your Pro Breeze AF to 400°F. Set the timer and grill for 10 minutes.
7. Using tongs, flip the ribs.
8. Reset the timer and grill for another 10 minutes.
9. Once the ribs are cooked, use a pastry brush to brush on the barbecue sauce, then set the timer and grill for a final 3 to 5 minutes.

Nutrition: Calories: 422 Fat: 27g Saturated fat: 10g Carbohydrate: 25g Fiber: 1g Sugar: 17g Protein: 18g Iron: 1mg Sodium: 4273mg

449. Parmesan Crusted Pork Chops

Preparation Time: 10 minutes
Cooking Time: 15 minutes
Servings: 8

Ingredients:
- 3 tbsp. grated parmesan cheese
- 1 C. pork rind crumbs
- 2 beaten eggs
- ¼ tsp. chili powder
- ½ tsp. onion powder
- 1 tsp. smoked paprika
- ¼ tsp. pepper
- ½ tsp. salt
- 4-6 thick boneless pork chops

Directions:
1. Preparing the Ingredients. Ensure your air fryer is preheated to 400 degrees.
2. With pepper and salt, season both sides of pork chops.
3. In a food processor, pulse pork rinds into crumbs. Mix crumbs with other seasonings.
4. Beat eggs and add to another bowl.
5. Dip pork chops into eggs then into pork rind crumb mixture.
6. Air Frying. Spray down air fryer with olive oil and add pork chops to the basket. Set temperature to 400°F, and set time to 15 minutes.

Nutrition: Calories: 422 Fat: 19g Protein:38g Sugar:2g

450. Pork Joint

Preparation Time: 10 minutes
Cooking Time: 20 minutes
Servings: 10

Ingredients:
- 3 cups Cooked shredded pork tenderloin or chicken
- 2.5 cups Fat-free shredded mozzarella
- 10 small Flour tortillas
- Lime juice

Directions:
1. Set the Air Fryer at 380° Fahrenheit.
2. Sprinkle the juice over the pork.
3. Microwave five of the tortillas at a time (putting a damp paper towel over them for 10 seconds). Add three ounces of pork and ¼ of a cup of cheese to each tortilla.
4. Tightly roll the tortillas. Line the tortillas onto a greased foil-lined pan.
5. Spray an even coat of cooking oil spray over the tortillas.
6. Air Fry for 7 to 10 minutes or until the tortillas are a golden color, flipping halfway through.

Nutrition: Calories: 334 kcal Protein: 32.03 g Fat: 6.87 g Carbohydrates: 33.92 g

VEGETABLES RECIPES

451. Air Fryer Asparagus
Preparation Time: 5 minutes
Cooking Time: 8 minutes
Servings: 2
Ingredients:
- Nutrition yeast
- Olive oil non-stick spray
- One bunch of asparagus

Directions:
1. Wash asparagus and then trim off thick, woody ends.
2. Spray asparagus with olive oil spray and sprinkle with yeast.
3. In your air fryer, lay asparagus in a singular layer.
4. Cook 8 minutes at 360 degrees.

Nutrition: Calories: 17 Fat: 4g Protein: 9g Sugar: 0g

452. Spicy Sweet Potato Fries
Preparation Time: 20 minutes
Cooking Time: 20 minutes
Servings: 4
Ingredients:
- 2 tbsp. sweet potato fry seasoning mix
- 2 tbsp. olive oil
- 2 sweet potatoes
- Seasoning Mix:
- 2 tbsp. salt
- 1 tbsp. cayenne pepper
- 1 tbsp. dried oregano
- 1 tbsp. fennel
- 2 tbsp. coriander

Directions:
1. Slice both ends off sweet potatoes and peel. Slice lengthwise in half and again crosswise to make four pieces from each potato.
2. Slice each potato piece into 2-3 slices, then slice into fries.
3. Grind together all of seasoning mix ingredients and mix in the salt.
4. Ensure air fryer is preheated to 350 degrees.
5. Toss potato pieces in olive oil, sprinkling with seasoning mix and tossing well to coat thoroughly.
6. Add fries to air fryer basket and set time for 27 minutes. Press start and cook 15 minutes.
7. Take out the basket and turn fries. Turn off air fryer and let cook 10-12 minutes till fries are golden.

Nutrition: Calories: 89 Fat: 14g Protein: 8g Sugar: 3g

453. Air Fryer Cauliflower Rice
Preparation Time: 20 minutes
Cooking Time: 20 minutes
Servings: 2 to 4
Ingredients:
- Round 1:
- 1 tsp. turmeric
- 1 C. diced carrot
- ½ C. diced onion
- 2 tbsp. low-sodium soy sauce
- ½ block of extra firm tofu
- Round 2:
- ½ C. frozen peas
- 2 minced garlic cloves
- ½ C. chopped broccoli
- 1 tbsp. minced ginger
- 1 tbsp. rice vinegar
- 1 ½ tsp. toasted sesame oil
- 2 tbsp. reduced-sodium soy sauce
- 3 C. riced cauliflower

Directions:
1. Crumble tofu in a large bowl and toss with all the Round one ingredients.
2. Preheat air fryer to 370 degrees and cook 10 minutes, making sure to shake once.
3. In another bowl, toss ingredients from Round 2 together.
4. Add Round 2 mixture to air fryer and cook another 10 minutes, ensuring to shake 5 minutes in.
5. Enjoy!

Nutrition: Calories: 67 Fat: 8g Protein: 3g Sugar: 0g

454. Air Fried Carrots, Yellow Squash & Zucchini
Preparation Time: 7 minutes
Cooking Time: 30 minutes
Servings: 4
Ingredients:
- 1 tbsp. chopped tarragon leaves
- ½ tsp. white pepper
- 1 tsp. salt
- 1-pound yellow squash
- 1-pound zucchini
- 6 tsp. olive oil
- ½ pound carrots

Directions:
1. Stem and root the end of squash and zucchini and cut in ¾-inch half-moons. Peel and cut carrots into 1-inch cubes
2. Combine carrot cubes with 2 teaspoons of olive oil, tossing to combine. Pour into air fryer basket and cook 5 minutes at 400 degrees.
3. As carrots cook, drizzle remaining olive oil over squash and zucchini pieces, then season with pepper and salt. Toss well to coat.
4. Add squash and zucchini when the timer for carrots goes off. Cook 30 minutes, making sure to toss 2-3 times during the cooking process.
5. Once done, take out veggies and toss with tarragon. Serve up warm!

Nutrition: Calories: 122 Fat: 9g Protein: 6g Sugar: 0g

455. Air Fried Kale Chips
Preparation Time: 5 minutes
Cooking Time: 5 minutes
Servings: 4 to 6
Ingredients:
- ¼ tsp. Himalayan salt
- 3 tbsp. yeast
- Avocado oil
- 1 bunch of kale

Directions:
1. Rinse kale and with paper towels, dry well.
2. Tear kale leaves into large pieces. Remember they will shrink as they cook so good sized pieces are necessary.
3. Place kale pieces in a bowl and spritz with avocado oil till shiny. Sprinkle with salt and yeast.
4. With your hands, toss kale leaves well to combine.

5. Pour half of the kale mixture into air fryer. Cook 5 minutes at 350 degrees. Remove and repeat with another half of kale.

Nutrition: Calories: 55 Fat: 10g Protein: 1g Sugar: 0g

456. Cheesy Cauliflower Fritters

Preparation Time: 5 minutes
Cooking Time: 14 minutes
Servings: 8

Ingredients:
- ½ C. chopped parsley
- 1 C. Italian breadcrumbs
- 1/3 C. shredded mozzarella cheese
- 1/3 C. shredded sharp cheddar cheese
- 1 egg
- 2 minced garlic cloves
- 3 chopped scallions
- 1 head of cauliflower

Directions:
1. Cut cauliflower up into florets. Wash well and pat dry. Place into a food processor and pulse 20-30 seconds till it looks like rice.
2. Place cauliflower rice in a bowl and mix with pepper, salt, egg, cheeses, breadcrumbs, garlic, and scallions.
3. With hands, form 15 patties of the mixture. Add more breadcrumbs if needed.
4. With olive oil, spritz patties, and place into your air fryer in a single layer.
5. Cook 14 minutes at 390 degrees, flipping after 7 minutes.

Nutrition: Calories: 209 Fat: 17g Protein: 6g Sugar: 0.5g

457. Avocado Fries

Preparation Time: 5 minutes
Cooking Time: 5 minutes
Servings: 6

Ingredients:
- 1 avocado
- ½ tsp. salt
- ½ C. panko breadcrumbs
- Bean liquid (aquafaba) from a 15-ounce can of white or garbanzo beans

Directions:
1. Peel, pit, and slice up avocado.
2. Toss salt and breadcrumbs together in a bowl. Place aquafaba into another bowl.
3. Dredge slices of avocado first in aquafaba and then in panko, making sure you get an even coating.
4. Place coated avocado slices into a single layer in the air fryer.
5. Cook 5 minutes at 390 degrees, shaking at 5 minutes.
6. Serve with your favorite dipping sauce!

Nutrition: Calories: 102 Fat: 22g Protein: 9g Sugar: 1g

458. Zucchini Parmesan Chips

Preparation Time: 5 minutes
Cooking Time: 8 minutes
Servings: 10

Ingredients:
- ½ tsp. paprika
- ½ C. grated parmesan cheese
- ½ C. Italian breadcrumbs
- 1 lightly beaten egg
- 2 thinly sliced zucchinis

Directions:
1. Use a very sharp knife or mandolin slicer to slice zucchini as thinly as you can. Pat off extra moisture.
2. Beat egg with a pinch of pepper and salt and a bit of water.
3. Combine paprika, cheese, and breadcrumbs in a bowl.
4. Dip slices of zucchini into the egg mixture and then into breadcrumb mixture. Press gently to coat.
5. With olive oil cooking spray, mist coated zucchini slices. Place into your air fryer in a single layer.
6. Cook 8 minutes at 350 degrees.
7. Sprinkle with salt and serve with salsa.

Nutrition: Calories: 211 Fat: 16g Protein: 8g Sugar: 0g

459. Crispy Roasted Broccoli

Preparation Time: 45 minutes
Cooking Time: 15 minutes
Servings: 2

Ingredients:
- ¼ tsp. Masala
- ½ tsp. red chili powder
- ½ tsp. salt
- ¼ tsp. turmeric powder
- 1 tbsp. chickpea flour
- 2 tbsp. yogurt
- 1-pound broccoli

Directions:
1. Cut broccoli up into florets. Soak in a bowl of water with 2 teaspoons of salt for at least half an hour to remove impurities.
2. Take out broccoli florets from water and let drain. Wipe down thoroughly.
3. Mix all other ingredients together to create a marinade.
4. Toss broccoli florets in the marinade. Cover and chill 15-30 minutes.
5. Preheat air fryer to 390 degrees. Place marinated broccoli florets into the fryer. Cook 10 minutes.
6. 5 minutes into cooking shake the basket. Florets will be crispy when done.

Nutrition: Calories: 96 Fat: 1.3g Protein: 7g Sugar: 4.5g

460. Crispy Jalapeno Coins

Preparation Time: 10 minutes
Cooking Time: 10 minutes
Servings: 8 to 10

Ingredients:
- 1 egg
- 2-3 tbsp. coconut flour
- 1 sliced and seeded jalapeno
- Pinch of garlic powder
- Pinch of onion powder
- Pinch of Cajun seasoning (optional)
- Pinch of pepper and salt

Directions:
1. Ensure your air fryer is preheated to 400 degrees.
2. Mix together all dry ingredients.
3. Pat jalapeno slices dry. Dip coins into egg wash and then into dry mixture. Toss to thoroughly coat.
4. Add coated jalapeno slices to air fryer in a singular layer. Spray with olive oil.
5. Cook just till crispy.

Nutrition: Calories: 128 Fat: 8g Protein: 7g Sugar: 0g

461. Buffalo Cauliflower

Preparation Time: 15 minutes
Cooking Time: 14 to 17 minutes
Servings: 6 to 8

Ingredients:
- Cauliflower:
- 1 C. panko breadcrumbs

VEGETABLES RECIPES

- 1 tsp. salt
- 4 C. cauliflower florets
- Buffalo Coating:
- ¼ C. Vegan Buffalo sauce
- ¼ C. melted vegan butter

Directions:
1. Melt butter in microwave and whisk in buffalo sauce.
2. Dip each cauliflower floret into buffalo mixture, ensuring it gets coated well. Hold over a bowl till floret is done dripping.
3. Mix breadcrumbs with salt.
4. Dredge dipped florets into breadcrumbs and place into air fryer.
5. Cook 14-17 minutes at 350 degrees. When slightly browned, they are ready to eat!
6. Serve with your favorite keto dipping sauce!

Nutrition: Calories: 194 Fat: 17g Protein: 10g Sugar: 3g

462. Jicama Fries

Preparation Time: 10 minutes
Cooking Time: 20 minutes
Servings: 8

Ingredients:
- 1 tbsp. dried thyme
- ¾ C. arrowroot flour
- ½ large Jicama
- 2 eggs

Directions:
1. Sliced jicama into fries.
2. Whisk eggs together and pour over fries. Toss to coat.
3. Mix a pinch of salt, thyme, and arrowroot flour together. Toss egg-coated jicama into dry mixture, tossing to coat well.
4. Spray air fryer basket with olive oil and add fries. Cook 20 minutes on CHIPS setting. Toss halfway into the cooking process.

Nutrition: Calories: 211 Fat: 19g Protein: 9g Sugar: 1g

463. Air Fryer Brussels Sprouts

Preparation Time: 5 minutes
Cooking Time: 10 minutes
Servings: 5

Ingredients:
- ¼ tsp. salt
- 1 tbsp. balsamic vinegar
- 1 tbsp. olive oil
- 2 C. Brussels sprouts

Directions:
1. Cut Brussels sprouts in half lengthwise. Toss with salt, vinegar, and olive oil till coated thoroughly.
2. Add coated sprouts to air fryer, cooking 8-10 minutes at 400 degrees. Shake after 5 minutes of cooking.
3. Brussels sprouts are ready to devour when brown and crisp!

Nutrition: Calories: 118 Fat: 9g Protein: 11g Sugar: 1g

464. Spaghetti Squash Tots

Preparation Time: 5 minutes
Cooking Time: 15 minutes
Servings: 8 to 10

Ingredients:
- ¼ tsp. pepper
- ½ tsp. salt
- 1 thinly sliced scallion
- 1 spaghetti squash

Directions:
1. Wash and cut the squash in half lengthwise. Scrape out the seeds.
2. With a fork, remove spaghetti meat by strands and throw out skins.
3. In a clean towel, toss in squash and wring out as much moisture as possible. Place in a bowl and with a knife slice through meat a few times to cut up smaller.
4. Add pepper, salt, and scallions to squash and mix well.
5. Create "tot" shapes with your hands and place in air fryer. Spray with olive oil.
6. Cook 15 minutes at 350 degrees until golden and crispy!

Nutrition: Calories: 231 Fat: 18g Protein: 5g Sugar: 0g

465. Cinnamon Butternut Squash Fries

Preparation Time: 10 minutes
Cooking Time: 10 minutes
Servings: 2

Ingredients:
- 1 pinch of salt
- 1 tbsp. powdered unprocessed sugar
- ½ tsp. nutmeg
- 2 tsp. cinnamon
- 1 tbsp. coconut oil
- 10 ounces pre-cut butternut squash fries

Directions:
1. In a plastic bag, pour in all ingredients. Coat fries with other components till coated and sugar is dissolved.
2. Spread coated fries into a single layer in the air fryer. Cook 10 minutes at 390 degrees until crispy.

Nutrition: Calories: 175 Fat: 8g Protein: 1g Sugar: 5g

466. Sweet Potato Chips

Preparation Time: 5 minutes
Cooking Time: 10 minutes
Servings: 4

Ingredients:
- 2 large sweet potatoes, cut into strips 25 mm thick
- 3 tsp of oil
- 2 tsp of salt
- ½ tsp black pepper
- ½ tsp of paprika
- ½ tsp garlic powder
- ½ tsp onion powder

Directions:
1. Cut the sweet potatoes into strips 25 mm thick.
2. Preheat the air fryer for a few minutes.
3. Add the cut sweet potatoes in a large bowl and mix with the oil until the potatoes are all evenly coated.
4. Sprinkle salt, black pepper, paprika, garlic powder and onion powder. Mix well.
5. Place the French fries in the preheated baskets and cook for 10 minutes at 4000F. Be sure to shake the baskets halfway through cooking.

Nutrition: Calories: 130 Fat: 0g Carbohydrates: 29g Protein: 2g Sugar: 9g Cholesterol: 0mg

467. Fried Zucchini

Preparation Time: 10 minutes
Cooking Time: 8 minutes
Servings: 4

Ingredients:
- 2 medium zucchinis, cut into strips 19 mm thick
- 2 oz. all-purpose flour
- ½ oz. of salt
- ½ tsp. black pepper

VEGETABLES RECIPES

- 2 beaten eggs
- 3 tsp of milk
- 3 oz. Italian seasoned breadcrumbs
- 0.8 oz. grated Parmesan cheese
- Nonstick Spray Oil
- Ranch sauce, to serve

Directions:
1. Cut the zucchini into strips 19 mm thick.
2. Mix with the flour, salt, and pepper on a plate. Mix the eggs and milk in a separate dish. Put breadcrumbs and Parmesan cheese in another dish.
3. Cover each piece of zucchini with flour, then dip them in egg and pass them through the crumbs. Leave aside.
4. Preheat the air fryer, set it to 3400F.
5. Place the covered zucchini in the preheated air fryer and spray with oil spray. Set the timer to 8 minutes and press Start/Pause.
6. Be sure to shake the baskets in the middle of cooking.
7. Serve with tomato sauce or ranch sauce.

Nutrition: Calories: 67 Fat: 4.1g Carbohydrates: 4.5g Protein: 3.3g Sugar: 1.47g Cholesterol: 20.7mg

468. Fried Avocado

Preparation Time: 15 minutes
Cooking Time: 10 minutes
Servings: 2

Ingredients:
- 2 avocados cut into wedges 25 mm thick
- 1.7 oz. Pan crumbs bread
- ½ tsp garlic powder
- ½ tsp onion powder
- ¼ tsp smoked paprika
- ¼ tsp cayenne pepper
- Salt and pepper to taste
- 2 oz. all-purpose flour
- 2 eggs, beaten
- Nonstick Spray Oil
- Tomato sauce or ranch sauce, to serve

Directions:
1. Cut the avocados into 25 mm thick pieces.
2. Combine the crumbs, garlic powder, onion powder, smoked paprika, cayenne pepper and salt in a bowl.
3. Separate each wedge of avocado in the flour, then dip the beaten eggs and stir in the breadcrumb mixture.
4. Preheat the air fryer.
5. Place the avocados in the preheated air fryer baskets, spray with oil spray and cook at 4000F for 10 minutes. Turn the fried avocado halfway through cooking and sprinkle with cooking oil.
6. Serve with tomato sauce or ranch sauce.

Nutrition: Calories: 96 Fat: 8.8g Carbohydrates: 5.12g Protein: 1.2g Sugar: 0.4g Cholesterol: 0mg

469. Vegetables In Air Fryer

Preparation Time: 20 minutes
Cooking Time: 30 minutes
Servings: 2

Ingredients:
- 2 potatoes
- 1 zucchini
- 1 onion
- 1 red pepper
- 1 green pepper

Directions:
1. Cut the potatoes into slices.
2. Cut the onion into rings.
3. Cut the zucchini slices.
4. Cut the peppers into strips.
5. Put all the ingredients in the bowl and add a little salt, ground pepper and some extra virgin olive oil.
6. Mix well.
7. Pass to the basket of the air fryer.
8. Select 3200F, 30 minutes.
9. Check that the vegetables are to your liking.

Nutrition: Calories: 135 Fat: 11g Carbohydrates: 8g Protein: 1g Sugar: 2g Cholesterol: 0mg

470. Crispy Rye Bread Snacks With Guacamole And Anchovies

Preparation Time: 10 minutes
Cooking Time: 10 minutes
Servings: 4

Ingredients:
- 4 slices of rye bread
- Guacamole
- Anchovies in oil

Directions:
1. Cut each slice of bread into 3 strips of bread.
2. Place in the basket of the air fryer, without piling up, and we go in batches giving it the touch you want to give it. You can select 3500F, 10 minutes.
3. When you have all the crusty rye bread strips, put a layer of guacamole on top, whether homemade or commercial.
4. In each bread, place 2 anchovies on the guacamole.

Nutrition: Calories: 180 Fat: 11.6g Carbohydrates: 16g Protein: 6.2g Sugar: 0g Cholesterol: 19.6mg

471. Mushrooms Stuffed With Tomato

Preparation Time: 5 minutes
Cooking Time: 50 minutes
Servings: 4

Ingredients:
- 8 large mushrooms
- ½ lb of minced meat
- 4 cloves of garlic
- Extra virgin olive oil
- Salt
- Ground pepper
- Flour, beaten egg and breadcrumbs
- Frying oil
- Fried Tomato Sauce

Directions:
1. Remove the stem from the mushrooms and chop it. Peel the garlic and chop. Put some extra virgin olive oil in a pan and add the garlic and mushroom stems.
2. Sauté and add the minced meat. Sauté well until the meat is well cooked and season.
3. Fill the mushrooms with the minced meat.
4. Press well and take the freezer for 30 minutes.
5. Pass the mushrooms with flour, beaten egg and breadcrumbs. Beaten egg and breadcrumbs.
6. Place the mushrooms in the basket of the air fryer.
7. Select 20 minutes, 3500F.
8. Distribute the mushrooms once cooked in the dishes.
9. Heat the tomato sauce and cover the stuffed mushrooms.

Nutrition: Calories: 160 Fat: 7.96g Carbohydrates: 19.41g Protein: 7.94g Sugar: 9.19g Cholesterol: 0mg

472. Spiced Potato Wedges

Preparation Time: 15 minutes

Cooking Time: 40 minutes
Servings: 4
Ingredients:
- 8 medium potatoes
- Salt
- Ground pepper
- Garlic powder
- Aromatic herbs, the one we like the most
- 2 tbsp. extra virgin olive oil
- 4 tbsp. breadcrumbs or chickpea flour

Directions:
1. Put the unpeeled potatoes in a pot with boiling water and a little salt.
2. Let cook 5 minutes. Drain and let cool. Cut into thick segments, without peeling.
3. Put the potatoes in a bowl and add salt, pepper, garlic powder, the aromatic herb that we have chosen oil and breadcrumbs or chickpea flour.
4. Stir well and leave 15 minutes. Pass to the basket of the air fryer and select 20 minutes, 3500F.
5. From time to time shake the basket so that the potatoes mix and change position. Check that they are tender.

Nutrition: Calories: 121 Fat: 3g Carbohydrates: 19g Protein: 2g Sugar: 0g Cholesterol: 0mg

473. Egg Stuffed Zucchini Balls

Preparation Time: 15 minutes
Cooking Time: 45 to 60 minutes
Servings: 4

Ingredients:
- 2 zucchinis
- 1 onion
- 1 egg
- 4 ¼ oz. of grated cheese
- 4 eggs
- Salt
- Ground pepper
- Flour

Directions:
1. Chop the zucchini and onion in the Thermomix, 10 seconds speed 8, in the Cuisine with the kneader chopper at speed 10 about 15 seconds or we can chop the onion by hand and the zucchini grate. No matter how you do it, the important thing is that the zucchini and onion are as small as possible.
2. Put in a bowl and add the cheese and the egg. Pepper and bind well.
3. Incorporate the flour, until you have a very brown dough with which you can wrap the eggs without problems.
4. Cook the eggs and peel.
5. Cover the eggs with the zucchini dough and pass through the flour.
6. Place the four balls in the basket of the air fryer and paint with oil.
7. Select 3500F and leave for 45 to 60 minutes or until you see that the balls are crispy on the outside.
8. Serve over a layer of mayonnaise or aioli.

Nutrition: Calories: 23 Fat: 0.5g Carbohydrates: 2g Protein: 1.8g Sugar: 0g Cholesterol: 15mg

474. Vegetables With Provolone

Preparation Time: 10 minutes
Cooking Time: 30 minutes
Servings: 4

Ingredients:
- 1 bag of 1 lb of frozen tempura vegetables
- Extra virgin olive oil
- Salt
- 1 slice of provolone cheese

Directions:
1. Put the vegetables in the basket of the air fryer. Add some strands of extra virgin olive oil and close.
2. Select 20 minutes, 3920F.
3. Pass the vegetables to a clay pot and place the provolone cheese on top.
4. Take to the oven, 3500F, about 10 minutes or so or until you see that the cheese has melted to your liking.

Nutrition: Calories: 104 Fat: 8g Carbohydrates: 0g Protein: 8g Sugar: 0g Cholesterol: 0mg

475. Spicy Potatoes

Preparation Time: 10 minutes
Cooking Time: 30 minutes
Servings: 4

Ingredients:
- 1 lb. potatoes
- 2 tbsp. spicy paprika
- 1 tbsp. olive oil
- Catupiry or cottage cheese
- Salt to taste

Directions:
1. Wash the potatoes with a brush. Unpeeled, cut vertically in a crescent shape, about 1 finger thick Place the potatoes in a bowl and cover with water. Let stand for about half an hour.
2. Preheat the air fryer. Set the timer of 5 minutes and the temperature to 3920F.
3. Drain the water from the potatoes and dry with paper towels or a clean cloth. Put them back in the bowl and pour the oil, salt and paprika over them. Mix well with your hands so that all of them are covered evenly with the spice mixture. Pour the spiced potatoes in the basket of the air fryer. Set the timer for 30 minutes and press the power button. Stir the potatoes in half the time.
4. Remove the potatoes from the air fryer, place on a plate.
5. Serve with cheese and sauce.

Nutrition: Calories: 153 Fat: 4g Carbohydrates: 26 Protein: 3g Sugar: 0g Cholesterol: 5mg

476. Scrambled Eggs With Beans, Zucchini, Potatoes And Onions

Preparation Time: 30 minutes
Cooking Time: 35 minutes
Servings: 4

Ingredients:
- ½ lb of beans
- 2 onions
- 1 zucchini
- 4 potatoes
- 8 eggs
- Extra virgin olive oil
- Salt
- Ground pepper
- A splash of soy sauce

Directions:
1. Put the beans taken from their pod to cook in abundant saltwater. Drain when they are tender and reserve.
2. Peel the potatoes and cut into dice. Season and put some threads of oil. Mix and take to the air fryer. Select 3500F, 15 minutes.

3. After that time, add together with the potatoes, diced zucchini, and onion in julienne, mix and select 3500F, 20 minutes.
4. From time to time mix and stir.
5. Pass the contents of the air fryer together with the beans to a pan.
6. Add a little soy sauce and salt to taste.
7. Sauté and peel the eggs.
8. Do the scrambled.

Nutrition: Calories: 65 Fat: 0.4g Carbohydrates: 8.6g Proteins: 4.6g Sugar: 0g Cholesterol: 0mg

477. French Toast

Preparation Time: 5 minutes
Cooking Time: 15 minutes
Servings: 8
Ingredients:
For the bread:
- 1 lb of flour
- 0.8 oz. of oil
- ½ lb. of water
- 0.8 oz. of fresh bread yeast
- 3 tsp of salt

For French toast:
- Milk and cinnamon or milk and sweet wine
- Eggs
- Honey

Directions:
1. The first thing is to make bread a day before. Put in the MasterChef Gourmet the ingredients of the bread and knead 1 minute at speed 1. Let the dough rise 1 hour and knead 1 minute at speed 1 again. Remove the dough and divide into 4 portions. Make a ball and spread like a pizza. Roll up to make a small loaf of bread and let rise 1 hour or so.
2. Take to the oven and bake 40 minutes, 3920F. Let the bread cool on a rack and reserve for the next day. Cut the bread into slices and reserve. Prepare the milk to wet the slices of bread. To do so, put the milk to heat, like 500 ml or so with a cinnamon stick or the same milk with a glass of sweet wine, as you like. When the milk has started to boil, remove from heat, and let cool.
3. Beat the eggs. Place a rack on a plate and we dip the slices of bread in the cold milk, then in the beaten egg and pass to the rack with the plate underneath to release the excess liquid. Put the slices of bread in the bucket of the air fryer, in batches, not piled up, and we take the air fryer, 3500F, 10 minutes each batch.
4. When you have all the slices passed through the air fryer, put the honey in a casserole, like 500g, next to 1 small glass of water and 4 tablespoons of sugar. When the honey starts to boil, lower the heat, and pass the bread slices through the honey. Place in a fountain and the rest of the honey we put it on top, bathing again the French toast. Ready our French toast, when they cool, they can already be eaten.

Nutrition: Calories: 224 Fat: 15.2g Carbohydrates: 17.39g Protein: 4.81g Sugar: 5.76g Cholesterol: 84mg

478. Sweet Potato Salt And Pepper

Preparation Time: 5 minutes
Cooking Time: 20 minutes
Servings: 4
Ingredients:
- 1 large sweet potato
- Extra virgin olive oil
- Salt
- Ground pepper

Directions:
1. Peel the sweet potato and cut into thin strips, if you have a mandolin it will be easier for you.
2. Wash well and put salt.
3. Add a little oil to impregnate the sweet potato in strips and place in the air fryer basket.
4. Select 3500F, 30 minutes or so. From time to time, shake the basket so that the sweet potato moves.
5. Pass to a tray or plate and sprinkle with fine salt and ground pepper.

Nutrition: Calories: 107 Fat: 0.6g Carbohydrates: 24.19g Protein: 1.61g Sugar: 5.95g Cholesterol: 0mg

479. Basil Tomatoes

Preparation Time: 10 minutes
Cooking Time: 10 minutes
Servings: 2
Ingredients:
- 3 tomatoes, halved
- Olive oil cooking spray
- Salt and ground black pepper, as required
- 1 tablespoon fresh basil, chopped

Directions:
1. Drizzle cut sides of the tomato halves with cooking spray evenly.
2. Sprinkle with salt, black pepper and basil.
3. Press "Power Button" of Air Fry Oven and turn the dial to select the "Air Fry" mode.
4. Press the Time button and again turn the dial to set the cooking time to 10 minutes.
5. Now push the Temp button and rotate the dial to set the temperature at 320 degrees F.
6. Press "Start/Pause" button to start.
7. When the unit beeps to show that it is preheated, open the lid.
8. Arrange the tomatoes in "Air Fry Basket" and insert in the oven.
9. Serve warm.

Nutrition: Calories 34 Total Fat 0.4 g Saturated Fat 0.1 g Cholesterol 0 mg Sodium 87 mg Total Carbs 7.2 g Fiber 2.2 g Sugar 4.9 g Protein 1.7 g

480. Pesto Tomatoes

Preparation Time: 15 minutes
Cooking Time: 14 minutes
Servings: 4
Ingredients:
- 3 large heirloom tomatoes, cut into ½ inch thick slices.
- 1 cup pesto
- 8 oz. feta cheese, cut into ½ inch thick slices.
- ½ cup red onions, sliced thinly
- 1 tablespoon olive oil

Directions:
1. Spread some pesto on each slice of tomato.
2. Top each tomato slice with a feta slice and onion and drizzle with oil.
3. Press "Power Button" of Air Fry Oven and turn the dial to select the "Air Fry" mode.
4. Press the Time button and again turn the dial to set the cooking time to 14 minutes.
5. Now push the Temp button and rotate the dial to set the temperature at 390 degrees F.
6. Press "Start/Pause" button to start.
7. When the unit beeps to show that it is preheated, open the lid.

8. Arrange the tomatoes in greased "Air Fry Basket" and insert in the oven.
9. Serve warm.

Nutrition: Calories 480 Total Fat 41.9 g Saturated Fat 14 g Cholesterol 65 mg Sodium 1000 mg Total Carbs 13 g Fiber 3 g Sugar 10.5 g Protein 15.4 g

481. Stuffed Tomatoes

Preparation Time: 15 minutes
Cooking Time: 15 minutes
Servings: 2

Ingredients:
- 2 large tomatoes
- ½ cup broccoli, chopped finely
- ½ cup Cheddar cheese, shredded
- Salt and ground black pepper, as required
- 1 tablespoon unsalted butter, melted
- ½ teaspoon dried thyme, crushed

Directions:
1. Carefully, cut the top of each tomato and scoop out pulp and seeds.
2. In a bowl, mix together chopped broccoli, cheese, salt and black pepper.
3. Stuff each tomato with broccoli mixture evenly.
4. Press "Power Button" of Air Fry Oven and turn the dial to select the "Air Fry" mode.
5. Press the Time button and again turn the dial to set the cooking time to 15 minutes.
6. Now push the Temp button and rotate the dial to set the temperature at 355 degrees F.
7. Press "Start/Pause" button to start.
8. When the unit beeps to show that it is preheated, open the lid.
9. Arrange the tomatoes in greased "Air Fry Basket" and insert in the oven.
10. Serve warm with the garnishing of thyme.

Nutrition: Calories 206 Total Fat 15.6 g Saturated Fat 9.7 g Cholesterol 45 mg Sodium 310 mg Total Carbs 9 g Fiber 2.9 g Sugar 5.3 g Protein 9.4 g

482. Parmesan Asparagus

Preparation Time: 10 minutes
Cooking Time: 10 minutes
Servings: 3

Ingredients:
- 1 lb. fresh asparagus, trimmed
- 1 tablespoon Parmesan cheese, grated
- 1 tablespoon butter, melted
- 1 teaspoon garlic powder
- Salt and ground black pepper, as required

Directions:
1. In a bowl, mix together the asparagus, cheese, butter, garlic powder, salt, and black pepper.
2. Press "Power Button" of Air Fry Oven and turn the dial to select the "Air Fry" mode.
3. Press the Time button and again turn the dial to set the cooking time to 10 minutes.
4. Now push the Temp button and rotate the dial to set the temperature at 400 degrees F.
5. Press "Start/Pause" button to start.
6. When the unit beeps to show that it is preheated, open the lid.
7. Arrange the veggie mixture in greased "Air Fry Basket" and insert in the oven.
8. Serve hot.

Nutrition: Calories 73 Total Fat 4.4 g Saturated Fat 2.7 g Cholesterol 12 mg Sodium 95 mg Total Carbs 6.6 g Fiber 3.3 g Sugar 3.1 g Protein 4.2 g

483. Almond Asparagus

Preparation Time: 15 minutes
Cooking Time: 6 minutes
Servings: 3

Ingredients:
- 1 lb. asparagus
- 2 tablespoons olive oil
- 2 tablespoons balsamic vinegar
- Salt and ground black pepper, as required
- 1/3 cup almonds, sliced

Directions:
1. In a bowl, mix together the asparagus, oil, vinegar, salt, and black pepper.
2. Press "Power Button" of Air Fry Oven and turn the dial to select the "Air Fry" mode.
3. Press the Time button and again turn the dial to set the cooking time to 6 minutes.
4. Now push the Temp button and rotate the dial to set the temperature at 400 degrees F.
5. Press "Start/Pause" button to start.
6. When the unit beeps to show that it is preheated, open the lid.
7. Arrange the veggie mixture in greased "Air Fry Basket" and insert in the oven.
8. Serve hot.

Nutrition: Calories 173 Total Fat 14.8 g Saturated Fat 1.8 g Cholesterol 0 mg Sodium 54 mg Total Carbs 8.2 g Fiber 4.5 g Sugar 3.3 g Protein 5.6 g

484. Spicy Butternut Squash

Preparation Time: 15 minutes
Cooking Time: 20 minutes
Servings: 4

Ingredients:
- 1 medium butternut squash, peeled, seeded and cut into chunk
- 2 teaspoons cumin seeds
- 1/8 teaspoon garlic powder
- 1/8 teaspoon chili flakes, crushed
- Salt and ground black pepper, as required
- 1 tablespoon olive oil
- 2 tablespoons pine nuts
- 2 tablespoons fresh cilantro, chopped

Directions:
1. In a bowl, mix together the squash, spices, and oil.
2. Press "Power Button" of Air Fry Oven and turn the dial to select the "Air Fry" mode.
3. Press the Time button and again turn the dial to set the cooking time to 20 minutes.
4. Now push the Temp button and rotate the dial to set the temperature at 375 degrees F.
5. Press "Start/Pause" button to start.
6. When the unit beeps to show that it is preheated, open the lid.
7. Arrange the squash chunks in greased "Air Fry Basket" and insert in the oven.
8. Serve hot with the garnishing of pine nuts and cilantro.

Nutrition: Calories 191 Total Fat 7 g Saturated Fat 0.8 g Cholesterol 0 mg Sodium 52 mg Total Carbs 34.3 g Fiber 6 g Sugar 6.4 g Protein 3.7 g

485. Sweet & Spicy Parsnips

Preparation Time: 15 minutes

Cooking Time: 44 minutes
Servings: 5
Ingredients:
- 1½ lbs. parsnip, peeled and cut into 1-inch chunks
- 1 tablespoon butter, melted
- 2 tablespoons honey
- 1 tablespoon dried parsley flakes, crushed
- ¼ teaspoon red pepper flakes, crushed
- Salt and ground black pepper, as required

Directions:
1. In a large bowl, mix together the parsnips and butter.
2. Press "Power Button" of Air Fry Oven and turn the dial to select the "Air Fry" mode.
3. Press the Time button and again turn the dial to set the cooking time to 44 minutes.
4. Now push the Temp button and rotate the dial to set the temperature at 355 degrees F.
5. Press "Start/Pause" button to start.
6. When the unit beeps to show that it is preheated, open the lid.
7. Arrange the squash chunks in greased "Air Fry Basket" and insert in the oven.
8. Meanwhile, in another large bowl, mix together the remaining ingredients.
9. After 40 minutes of cooking, press "Start/Pause" button to pause the unit.
10. Transfer the parsnips chunks into the bowl of honey mixture and toss to coat well.
11. Again, arrange the parsnip chunks in "Air Fry Basket" and insert in the oven.
12. Serve hot.

Nutrition: Calories 149 Total Fat 2.7 g Saturated Fat 1.5 g Cholesterol 6 mg Sodium 62 mg Total Carbs 31.5 g Fiber 6.7 g Sugar 13.5 g Protein 1.7 g

486. Caramelized Baby Carrots
Preparation Time: 10 minutes
Cooking Time: 15 minutes
Servings: 4
Ingredients:
- ½ cup butter, melted
- ½ cup brown sugar
- 1 lb. bag baby carrots

Directions:
1. In a bowl, mix together the butter, brown sugar and carrots.
2. Press "Power Button" of Air Fry Oven and turn the dial to select the "Air Fry" mode.
3. Press the Time button and again turn the dial to set the cooking time to 15 minutes.
4. Now push the Temp button and rotate the dial to set the temperature at 400 degrees F.
5. Press "Start/Pause" button to start.
6. When the unit beeps to show that it is preheated, open the lid.
7. Arrange the carrots in greased "Air Fry Basket" and insert in the oven.
8. Serve warm.

Nutrition: Calories 312 Total Fat 23.2 g Saturated Fat 14.5 g Cholesterol 61 mg Sodium 257 mg Total Carbs 27.1 g Fiber 3.3 g Sugar 23 g Protein 1 g

487. Carrot With Spinach
Preparation Time: 15 minutes
Cooking Time: 35 minutes
Servings: 4
Ingredients:
- 4 teaspoons butter, melted and divided
- ¼ lb. carrots, peeled and sliced
- 1 lb. zucchinis, sliced
- 1 tablespoon fresh basil, chopped
- Salt and ground black pepper, as required

Directions:
1. In a bowl, mix together 2 teaspoons of the butter and carrots.
2. Press "Power Button" of Air Fry Oven and turn the dial to select the "Air Fry" mode.
3. Press the Time button and again turn the dial to set the cooking time to 35 minutes.
4. Now push the Temp button and rotate the dial to set the temperature at 400 degrees F.
5. Press "Start/Pause" button to start.
6. When the unit beeps to show that it is preheated, open the lid.
7. Arrange the carrots in greased "Air Fry Basket" and insert in the oven.
8. Meanwhile, in a large bowl, mix together remaining butter, zucchini, basil, salt and black pepper.
9. After 5 minutes of cooking, place the zucchini mixture into the basket with carrots.
10. Toss the vegetable mixture 2-3 times during the cooking.
11. Serve hot.

Nutrition: Calories 64 Total Fat 4 g Saturated Fat 2.5 g Cholesterol 10 mg Sodium 97 mg Total Carbs 6.6 g Fiber 2 g Sugar 3.4 g Protein 1.7 g

488. Broccoli With Sweet Potatoes
Preparation Time: 15 minutes
Cooking Time: 20 minutes
Servings: 4
Ingredients:
- 2 medium sweet potatoes, peeled and cut in 1-inch cubes
- 1 head broccoli, cut in 1-inch florets
- 2 tablespoons vegetable oil
- Salt and ground black pepper, as required

Directions:
1. In a large bowl, add all the ingredients and toss to coat well.
2. Press "Power Button" of Air Fry Oven and turn the dial to select the "Air Roast" mode.
3. Press the Time button and again turn the dial to set the cooking time to 20 minutes.
4. Now push the Temp button and rotate the dial to set the temperature at 415 degrees F.
5. Press "Start/Pause" button to start.
6. When the unit beeps to show that it is preheated, open the lid.
7. Arrange the carrots in greased "Air Fry Basket" and insert in the oven.
8. Meanwhile, in a large bowl, mix together remaining butter, zucchini, basil, salt and black pepper.
9. After 5 minutes of cooking, place the zucchini mixture into the basket with carrots.
10. Serve hot.

Nutrition: Calories 170 Total Fat 7.1 g Saturated Fat 1.4 g Cholesterol 0 mg Sodium 67 mg Total Carbs 25.2 g Fiber 4.7 g Sugar 1.5 g Protein 2.9 g

489. Broccoli With Olives
Preparation Time: 15 minutes
Cooking Time: 15 minutes
Servings: 6
Ingredients:

- 1½ lbs. broccoli head, stemmed and cut into 1-inch florets
- 2 tablespoons olive oil
- Salt and ground black pepper, as required
- 1/3 cup Kalamata olives, halved and pitted
- 2 teaspoons fresh lemon zest, grated
- ¼ cup Parmesan cheese, grated

Directions:
1. In a pan of the boiling water, add the broccoli and cook for about 3-4 minutes.
2. Drain the broccoli well.
3. In a bowl, place the broccoli, oil, salt, and black pepper and toss to coat well.
4. Press "Power Button" of Air Fry Oven and turn the dial to select the "Air Fry" mode.
5. Press the Time button and again turn the dial to set the cooking time to 15 minutes.
6. Now push the Temp button and rotate the dial to set the temperature at 355 degrees F.
7. Press "Start/Pause" button to start.
8. When the unit beeps to show that it is preheated, open the lid.
9. Arrange the broccoli in greased "Air Fry Basket" and insert in the oven.
10. After 8 minutes of cooking, toss the broccoli florets.
11. Transfer the broccoli into a large bowl and immediately, stir in the olives, lemon zest and cheese.
12. Serve immediately.

Nutrition: Calories 100 Total Fat 6.6 g Saturated Fat 1.2 g Cholesterol 3 mg Sodium 158 mg Total Carbs 8.1 g Fiber 3.2 g Sugar 2 g Protein 4.6 g

490. **Broccoli With Cauliflower**

Preparation Time: 15 minutes
Cooking Time: 20 minutes
Servings: 4

Ingredients:
- 1½ cups broccoli, cut into 1-inch pieces
- 1½ cups cauliflower, cut into 1-inch pieces
- 1 tablespoon olive oil
- Salt, as required

Directions:
1. In a bowl, add the vegetables, oil, and salt and toss to coat well.
2. Press "Power Button" of Air Fry Oven and turn the dial to select the "Air Fry" mode.
3. Press the Time button and again turn the dial to set the cooking time to 20 minutes.
4. Now push the Temp button and rotate the dial to set the temperature at 375 degrees F.
5. Press "Start/Pause" button to start.
6. When the unit beeps to show that it is preheated, open the lid.
7. Arrange the veggie mixture in greased "Air Fry Basket" and insert in the oven.
8. Serve hot.

Nutrition: Calories 51 Total Fat 3.7 g Saturated Fat 0.5 g Cholesterol 0 mg Sodium 61 mg Total Carbs 4.3 g Fiber 1.8 g Sugar 1.5 g Protein 1.7 g

491. **Cauliflower In Buffalo Sauce**

Preparation Time: 13 minutes
Cooking Time: 12 minutes
Servings: 4

Ingredients:
- 1 large head cauliflower, cut into bite-size florets
- 1 tablespoon olive oil
- 2 teaspoons garlic powder
- Salt and ground black pepper, as required
- 1 tablespoon butter, melted
- 2/3 cup warm buffalo sauce

Directions:
1. In a large bowl, add cauliflower florets, olive oil, garlic powder, salt and pepper and toss to coat.
2. Press "Power Button" of Air Fry Oven and turn the dial to select the "Air Fry" mode.
3. Press the Time button and again turn the dial to set the cooking time to 12 minutes.
4. Now push the Temp button and rotate the dial to set the temperature at 375 degrees F.
5. Press "Start/Pause" button to start.
6. When the unit beeps to show that it is preheated, open the lid.
7. Arrange the cauliflower florets in "Air Fry Basket" and insert in the oven.
8. After 7 minutes of cooking, coat the cauliflower florets with buffalo sauce.
9. Serve hot.

Nutrition: Calories 183 Total Fat 17.1 g Saturated Fat 4.3 g Cholesterol 8 mg Sodium 826 mg Total Carbs 5.9 g Fiber 1.8 g Sugar 1.9 g Protein 1.6 g

492. **Curried Cauliflower**

Preparation Time: 15 minutes
Cooking Time: 10 minutes
Servings: 4

Ingredients:
- 2 tablespoons golden raisins
- ½ head cauliflower, cored and cut into 1-inch pieces
- ½ cup olive oil, divided
- ½ tablespoon curry powder
- Salt, to taste
- 2 tablespoons pine nuts, toasted

Directions:
1. Soak the raisins in boiling water and set aside.
2. In a bowl, mix together the cauliflower, oil, curry powder and salt.
3. Press "Power Button" of Air Fry Oven and turn the dial to select the "Air Fry" mode.
4. Press the Time button and again turn the dial to set the cooking time to 10 minutes.
5. Now push the Temp button and rotate the dial to set the temperature at 390 degrees F.
6. Press "Start/Pause" button to start.
7. When the unit beeps to show that it is preheated, open the lid.
8. Arrange the cauliflower florets in "Air Fry Basket" and insert in the oven.
9. Drain the golden raisins into a strainer.
10. In a bowl, add cauliflower, raisins and pine nuts and toss to coat.
11. Serve immediately.

Nutrition: Calories 269 Total Fat 28.3 g Saturated Fat 3.8 g Cholesterol 0 mg Sodium 50mg Total Carbs 6.4 g Fiber 1.4 g Sugar 3.7 g Protein 1.5 g

493. **Lemony Green Beans**

Preparation Time: 15 minutes
Cooking Time: 12 minutes
Servings: 4

Ingredients:
- 1 lb. green beans, trimmed
- 1 tablespoon butter, melted

VEGETABLES RECIPES

- 1 tablespoon fresh lemon juice
- ¼ teaspoon garlic powder
- Salt and ground black pepper, as required
- ½ teaspoon lemon zest, grated

Directions:
1. In a large bowl, add all the ingredients except the lemon zest and toss to coat well.
2. Press "Power Button" of Air Fry Oven and turn the dial to select the "Air Fry" mode.
3. Press the Time button and again turn the dial to set the cooking time to 12 minutes.
4. Now push the Temp button and rotate the dial to set the temperature at 400 degrees F.
5. Press "Start/Pause" button to start.
6. When the unit beeps to show that it is preheated, open the lid.
7. Arrange the green beans in "Air Fry Basket" and insert in the oven.
8. Serve warm with the garnishing of lemon zest.

Nutrition: Calories 62 Total Fat 3.1 g Saturated Fat 1.9 g Cholesterol 8 mg Sodium 67 mg Total Carbs 8.4 g Fiber 3.9 g Sugar 1.7 g Protein 2.2 g

494. Roasted Okra
Preparation Time: 10 minutes
Cooking Time: 10 minutes
Servings: 1

Ingredients:
- ½ lb. okra, ends trimmed and pods sliced
- ¼ tsp salt
- tsp olive oil
- 1/8 tsp ground black pepper

Directions:
1. Ensure that your air fryer is preheated to 350 F.
2. Get a clean bowl and in it, combine okra, salt, olive oil, and pepper. Stir the mixture gently.
3. Place in a single layer in the air fryer bas-ket.
4. Allow cooking in the air fryer for 5 minutes.
5. Toss and cook for an additional 5 minutes.
6. Toss again and allow cooking for an extra 2 minutes.
7. Withdraw and serve instantly.

Nutrition: Calories: 198 kcal Protein: 10.82 g Fat: 11.01 g Carbohydrates: 17.15 g

495. Artichoke Hearts
Preparation Time: 10 minutes
Cooking Time: 35 minutes
Servings: 1-2

Ingredients:
- cup arrowroot flour (gluten free & easily di-gestible)
- 1 tbsp. organic herb de provence
- 1-2 eggs
- 1 bag of frozen artichoke hearts
- Cooking spray

Directions:
1. Get a clean bowl, and in it, combine a cup of Arrowroot Flour alongside Herb de Provence. Mix well.
2. Get another bowl and make an egg wash by whisking 1-2 eggs.
3. Pick each artichoke and dip in the egg mixture before the flour mixture. Ensure generous coating in both instances, while avoiding the contamination of the egg wash by the excess flour mix from your hands.
4. Ensure that our air fryer basket remains non-sticky by coating oil.
5. Allow the chips to cook for 15 minutes under the chips feature.
6. Flip the artichokes after about 7 minutes using your thongs.

Nutrition: Calories: 405 kcal Protein: 12.77 g Fat: 10.45 g Carbohydrates: 65.71

496. Jalapeno Poppers
Preparation Time: 22 minutes
Cooking Time: 28 minutes
Servings: 2-3

Ingredients:
- 8 oz. of cream cheese
- ¾ cup gluten-free tortilla or bread crumbs
- ¼ cup fresh parsley
- 10 jalapeno peppers halved and deseeded

Directions:
1. Combine the cream cheese and half of the crumbs first before adding the parsley.
2. Fill each piece of pepper with this mixture.
3. Press the top of each pepper into the other ¼ cup of crumbs, thus creating the top coating.
4. Allow the peppers to cook in the air fryer at 370 F for 6-8 minutes. If you are using a conventional oven, just set the tempera-ture to 375 F and the time, 20 minutes.
5. Allow the peppers to cool before serving.

Nutrition: Calories: 289 kcal Protein: 8.85 g Fat: 24.15 g Carbohydrates: 10.33 g

497. Asparagus Fries
Preparation Time: 20 minutes
Cooking Time: 6 minutes
Servings: 6

Ingredients:
- large egg, beaten
- 1 tsp honey
- ½ cup Parmesan cheese, grated
- 1 cup panko bread crumbs
- 12 asparagus spears, trimmed
- 1 pinch cayenne pepper, optional
- ¼ cup Greek yogurt
- ¼ cup stone-ground mustard

Directions:
1. Ensure that your air fryer is preheated to 400 F.
2. Get a long, narrow dish, and in it combing egg and honey. Beat together and set aside.
3. In a separate plate, combine the Parmesan cheese and panko.
4. After coating each asparagus stalk in the egg mixture, roll it also in the panko mix and allow thorough coating.
5. Arrange six spears in the air fryer and allow cooking to the desired brownness - this takes 4 to 6 minutes. Do the same for the other spears.
6. Get a small bowl, and in it, mix the cayenne pepper, yogurt, and mustard.
7. Serve the asparagus spears with the dip-ping sauce.

Nutrition: Calories: 135 kcal Protein: 6.34 g Fat: 9.08 g Carbohydrates: 8.01 g

498. Vegan Veggie Balls
Preparation Time: 25 minutes
Cooking Time: 20 minutes
Servings: 6

Ingredients:
- 3 oz. parsnips
- 3 oz. carrot
- 4 oz. sweet potato

- 8 oz. cauliflower
- 2 tsp oregano
- 2 tsp garlic puree
- tsp mixed spice
- 1 tsp chives
- 1 tsp paprika
- 1 cup gluten free oats
- ½ cup desiccated coconut
- Salt and ground black pepper to taste

Directions:
1. Combine the vegetables in your food pro-cessor and blend until the raw vegetables appear like breadcrumbs.
2. Transfer them into a tea towel and get rid of the excess water by ringing out the towel, with the resulting mixture firm.
3. Place the dry vegetables in a mixing bowl, and combine it with the remaining ingre-dients.
4. Mix thoroughly and mold into medium-sized balls.
5. Transfer the balls into the fridge and allow them to stay for up to 2 hours. This will make them firmer.
6. From the fridge, move them into the air fryer and allow cooking for 10 minutes at 320 F.
7. After the first 10 minutes, roll over the balls to the other side and cook for 10 minutes more at 390 F.
8. Serve the cooked vegetable balls.

Nutrition: Calories: 104 kcal Protein: 5.68 g Fat: 2.49 g Carbohydrates: 21.88 g

499. Spinach Sauté

Preparation Time: 5 minutes
Cooking Time: 8 minutes
Servings: 4
Ingredients:
- 2 pounds baby spinach
- 1 tablespoon avocado oil
- 1 cup cherry tomatoes, halved
- 4 scallions, chopped
- Salt and black pepper to the taste
- 1 tablespoon chives, chopped

Directions:
1. Heat up the air fryer with oil at 350 degrees F, add the spinach, tomatoes and the other ingredients, toss and cook for 8 minutes.
2. Divide between plates and serve.

Nutrition: Calories 190 Fat 4 Fiber 2 Carbohydrates 13 Protein 9

500. Paprika Tomatoes

Preparation Time: 10 minutes
Cooking Time: 15 minutes
Servings: 4
Ingredients:
- 1-pound cherry tomatoes, halved
- 1 tablespoon sweet paprika
- 2 tablespoons olive oil
- 2 garlic cloves, minced
- 1 tablespoon lime juice
- 1 tablespoon chives, chopped

Directions:
1. In your air fryer's basket, combine the tomatoes with the paprika and the other ingredients, toss and cook at a temperature of 370 degrees F for 15 minutes.
2. Divide between plates and serve.

Nutrition: Calories 131 Fat 4 Fiber 7 Carbohydrates 10 Protein 8

501. Cilantro Beets

Preparation Time: 10 minutes
Cooking Time: 20 minutes
Servings: 4
Ingredients:
- 4 beets, peeled and cut into wedges
- 2 tablespoons cilantro, chopped
- 2 tablespoons avocado oil
- 2 tablespoons balsamic vinegar
- Salt and black pepper to the taste

Directions:
1. In your air fryer's basket, combine the beets with the oil and the other ingredients, toss and cook at 400 degrees F for 20 minutes.
2. Divide everything between plates and serve.

Nutrition: Calories 70 Fat 1 Fiber 1 Carbohydrates 6 Protein 4

502. Kale Sauté

Preparation Time: 10 minutes
Cooking Time: 12 minutes
Servings: 4
Ingredients:
- 1-pound baby kale
- 2 scallions, chopped
- 1 tablespoon olive oil
- 2 tablespoons balsamic vinegar
- ½ teaspoon chili powder
- 1 teaspoon coriander, ground
- Salt and black pepper to the taste

Directions:
1. Heat up air fryer with the oil at 370 degrees F, add the kale, scallions and the other ingredients, toss and cook for 12 minutes.
2. Divide the mix between plates and serve.

Nutrition: Calories 151 Fat 2 Fiber 3 Carbohydrates 9 Protein 4

503. Mustard Beets

Preparation Time: 5 minutes
Cooking Time: 25 minutes
Servings: 4
Ingredients:
- Peeled and cut into wedges 1-pound beets
- Salt and black pepper to the taste
- 1 tablespoon mustard
- 1 tablespoon olive oil
- 2 tablespoons chives, chopped
- 1 teaspoon sweet paprika

Directions:
1. In your air fryer's basket, combine the beets with the mustard, salt, pepper and the other ingredients, toss and cook at 380 degrees F for 25 minutes.
2. Divide the beets between plates and serve.

Nutrition: Calories 122 Fat 2 Fiber 2 Carbohydrates 9 Protein 4

504. Cabbage Sauté

Preparation Time: 5 minutes
Cooking Time: 15 minutes
Servings: 4
Ingredients:
- 1-pound red cabbage, shredded
- 1 tablespoon balsamic vinegar
- 2 red onions, sliced
- 1 tablespoon olive oil
- 1 tablespoon dill, chopped
- Salt and black pepper to the taste

Directions:

1. Heat up air fryer with oil at 380 degrees F, add the cabbage, onions and the other ingredients, toss and cook for 15 minutes.
2. Divide between plates and serve.

Nutrition: Calories 100 Fat 4 Fiber 2 Carbohydrates 7 Protein 2

505. Turmeric Carrots

Preparation Time: 10 minutes
Cooking Time: 20 minutes
Servings: 4
Ingredients:
- 1-pound baby carrots, peeled
- 3 tablespoons butter, melted
- 1 teaspoon turmeric powder
- 1 teaspoon rosemary, dried
- A pinch of salt and black pepper
- 1 tablespoon chives, chopped

Directions:
1. In your air fryer's basket, combine the carrots with the butter, turmeric and the other ingredients, toss and cook at 380 degrees F for 20 minutes.
2. Divide between plates and serve.

Nutrition: Calories 90 Fat 2 Fiber 3 Carbohydrates 4 Protein 4

506. Coriander Endives

Preparation Time: 5 minutes
Cooking Time: 15 minutes
Servings: 4
Ingredients:
- 2 endives, trimmed and halved
- 1 tablespoon coriander, chopped
- 1 teaspoon sweet paprika
- 2 tablespoons olive oil
- A pinch of salt and black pepper
- 2 tablespoons white vinegar
- ½ cup almonds, chopped

Directions:
1. Mix the endives with the coriander and the other ingredients in the air fryer's pan, toss, cook at 350 degrees F for 15 minutes, divide between plates and serve.

Nutrition: Calories 154 Fat 4 Fiber 3 Carbohydrates 6 Protein 7

507. Lemon Fennel

Preparation Time: 5 minutes
Cooking Time: 15 minutes
Servings: 4
Ingredients:
- 3 tablespoons butter, melted
- 2 fennel bulbs, sliced
- 1 teaspoon turmeric powder
- 1 teaspoon coriander, ground
- 1 tablespoon lemon zest, grated
- A pinch of salt and black pepper
- 1 tablespoon lemon juice

Directions:
1. In the air fryer's pan, mix the fennel with the melted butter and the other ingredients, toss and cook at 350 degrees F for 15 minutes.
2. Divide between plates and serve.

Nutrition: Calories 163 Fat 4 Fiber 3 Carbohydrates 5 Protein 6

508. Turmeric Kale

Preparation Time: 5 minutes
Cooking Time: 20 minutes
Servings: 4
Ingredients:
- 1 pound baby kale
- 1 teaspoon turmeric powder
- 1 red bell pepper, cut into strips
- 1 red onion, chopped
- 2 tablespoons butter, melted
- 1 tablespoon dill, chopped

Directions:
1. Mix the kale with the turmeric and the other ingredients in a pan that fits your air fryer, put the pan in the fryer and cook at 370 degrees F for 20 minutes.
2. Divide everything between plates and serve.

Nutrition: Calories 173 Fat 5 Fiber 3 Carbohydrates 6 Protein 7

509. Garlic Corn

Preparation Time: 5 minutes
Cooking time: 15 minutes
Servings: 4
Ingredients:
- 2 cups corn
- 3 garlic cloves, minced
- 1 tablespoon olive oil
- Juice of 1 lime
- 1 teaspoon sweet paprika
- Salt and black pepper to the taste
- 2 tablespoons dill, chopped

Directions:
1. Mix the corn with the garlic and the other ingredients in a pan that fits the air fryer, toss, put the pan in the machine and cook at 390 degrees F for 15 minutes.
2. Divide everything between plates and serve.

Nutrition: Calories 180 Fat 3 Fiber 2 Carbohydrates 4 Protein 6

510. Lemon Tomatoes

Preparation time: 5 minutes
Cooking time: 20 minutes
Servings: 4
Ingredients:
- 2 pounds cherry tomatoes, halved
- 1 teaspoon sweet paprika
- 1 teaspoon coriander, ground
- 2 teaspoons lemon zest, grated
- 2 tablespoons olive oil
- 2 tablespoons lemon juice
- A handful parsley, chopped

Directions:
1. Mix the tomatoes with the paprika and the other ingredients in the air fryer's pan, toss and cook at 370 degrees F for 20 minutes.
2. Divide between plates and serve.

Nutrition: Calories 151 Fat 2 Fiber 3 Carbohydrates 5 Protein 5

511. Garlic Carrots

Preparation time: 5 minutes
Cooking time: 20 minutes
Servings: 4
Ingredients:
- 1 tablespoon avocado oil
- 1 pound baby carrots, peeled
- Juice of 1 lime
- ½ teaspoon sweet paprika
- 6 garlic cloves, minced
- 1 tablespoon balsamic vinegar
- Salt and black pepper to the taste

Directions:
1. Combine the carrots with the oil and the other ingredients in a pan that fits the air fryer, toss gently, put

the pan in the air fryer and cook at 380 degrees F for 20 minutes.

2. Divide between plates and serve.

Nutrition: Calories 121 Fat 3 Fiber 2 Carbohydrates 4 Protein 6

SNACK RECIPES

512. Prosciutto-Wrapped Parmesan Asparagus

Preparation Time: 10 minutes
Cooking Time: 10 minutes
Servings: 4
Ingredients:
- 1-pound asparagus
- 12 (0.5-ounce) slices prosciutto
- 1 tablespoon coconut oil, melted
- 2 teaspoons lemon juice
- ⅛ teaspoon red pepper flakes
- ⅓ cup grated Parmesan cheese
- 2 tablespoons salted butter, melted

Directions:
1. On a clean work surface, place an asparagus spear onto a slice of prosciutto.
2. Drizzle with coconut oil and lemon juice. Sprinkle red pepper flakes and Parmesan across asparagus. Roll prosciutto around asparagus spear. Place into the air fryer basket.
3. Adjust the temperature to 375°F and set the timer for 10 minutes.
4. Drizzle the asparagus roll with butter before serving.

Nutrition: Calories: 263 Protein: 13.9 g Fiber: 2.4 g Net carbohydrates: 4.3 g Fat: 20.2 g Sodium: 368 mg Carbohydrates: 6.7 g Sugar: 2.2 g

513. Bacon-Wrapped Jalapeño Poppers

Preparation Time: 15 minutes
Cooking Time: 12 minutes
Servings: 4
Ingredients:
- jalapeños (about 4" long each)
- 3 ounces full-fat cream cheese
- ⅓ cup shredded medium Cheddar cheese
- ¼ teaspoon garlic powder
- 12 slices sugar-free bacon

Directions:
1. Cut the tops off of the jalapeños and slice down the center lengthwise into two pieces. Use a knife to carefully remove white membrane and seeds from peppers.
2. In a large microwave-safe bowl, place cream cheese, Cheddar, and garlic powder. Microwave for 30 seconds and stir. Spoon cheese mixture into hollow jalapeños.
3. Wrap a slice of bacon around each jalapeño half, completely covering pepper. Place into the air fryer basket.
4. Adjust the temperature to 400°F and set the timer for 12 minutes.
5. Turn the peppers halfway through the cooking time. Serve warm.

Nutrition: Calories: 246 Protein: 14.4 g Fiber: 0.6 g Net carbohydrates: 2.0 g Fat: 17.9 g Sodium: 625 mg Carbohydrates: 2.6 g Sugar: 1.6 g

514. Garlic Parmesan Chicken Wings

Preparation Time: 5 minutes
Cooking Time: 25 minutes
Servings: 4
Ingredients:
- 2 pounds raw chicken wings
- 1 teaspoon pink Himalayan salt
- ½ teaspoon garlic powder
- 1 tablespoon baking powder
- 4 tablespoons unsalted butter, melted
- ⅓ cup grated Parmesan cheese
- ¼ teaspoon dried parsley

Directions:
1. In a large bowl, place chicken wings, salt, ½ teaspoon garlic powder, and baking powder, then toss. Place wings into the air fryer basket.
2. Adjust the temperature to 400°F and set the timer for 25 minutes.
3. Toss the basket two or three times during the cooking time.
4. In a small bowl, combine butter, Parmesan, and parsley.
5. Remove wings from the fryer and place into a clean large bowl. Pour the butter mixture over the wings and toss until coated. Serve warm.

Nutrition: Calories: 565 Protein: 41.8 g Fiber: 0.1 g Net carbohydrates: 2.1 g Fat: 42.1 g Sodium: 1,067 mg Carbohydrates: 2.2 g Sugar: 0.0 g

515. Spicy Buffalo Chicken Dip

Preparation Time: 10 minutes
Cooking Time: 10 minutes
Servings: 4
Ingredients:
- 1 cup cooked, diced chicken breast
- 8 ounces full-fat cream cheese, softened
- ½ cup buffalo sauce
- ⅓ cup full-fat ranch dressing
- ⅓ cup chopped pickled jalapeños
- 1½ cups shredded medium Cheddar cheese, divided
- 2 scallions, sliced on the bias

Directions:
1. Place chicken into a large bowl. Add cream cheese, buffalo sauce, and ranch dressing. Stir until the sauces are well mixed and mostly smooth. Fold in jalapeños and 1 cup Cheddar.
2. Pour the mixture into a 4-cup round baking dish and place remaining Cheddar on top. Place dish into the air fryer basket.
3. Adjust the temperature to 350°F and set the timer for 10 minutes.
4. When done, the top will be brown and the dip bubbling. Top with sliced scallions. Serve warm.

Nutrition: Calories: 472 Protein: 25.6 g Fiber: 0.6 g Net carbohydrates: 8.5 g Fat: 32.0 g Sodium: 1,532 mg Carbohydrates: 9.1 g Sugar: 7.4 g

516. Bacon Jalapeño Cheese Bread

Preparation Time: 10 minutes
Cooking Time: 15 minutes
Servings: 8 sticks
Ingredients:
- 2 cups shredded mozzarella cheese
- ¼ cup grated Parmesan cheese
- ¼ cup chopped pickled jalapeños
- 2 large eggs
- slices sugar-free bacon, cooked and chopped

Directions:

1. Mix all ingredients in a large bowl. Cut a piece of parchment to fit your air fryer basket.
2. Dampen your hands with a bit of water and press out the mixture into a circle. You may need to separate this into two smaller cheese breads, depending on the size of your fryer.
3. Place the parchment and cheese bread into the air fryer basket.
4. Adjust the temperature to 320°F and set the timer for 15 minutes.
5. Carefully flip the bread when 5 minutes remain.
6. When fully cooked, the top will be golden brown. Serve warm.

Nutrition: Calories: 273 Protein: 20.1 g Fiber: 0.1 g Net carbohydrates: 2.1 g Fat: 18.1 g Sodium: 749 mg Carbohydrates: 2.3 g Sugar: 0.7 g

517. Pizza Rolls
Preparation Time: 15 minutes
Cooking Time: 10 minutes
Servings: 24
Ingredients:
- 2 cups shredded mozzarella cheese
- ½ cup almond flour
- 2 large eggs
- 72 slices pepperoni
- (1-ounce) mozzarella string cheese sticks, cut into 3 pieces each
- 2 tablespoons unsalted butter, melted
- ¼ teaspoon garlic powder
- ½ teaspoon dried parsley
- 2 tablespoons grated Parmesan cheese

Directions:
1. In a large microwave-safe bowl, place mozzarella and almond flour. Microwave for 1 minute. Remove bowl and mix until ball of dough forms. Microwave additional 30 seconds if necessary.
2. Crack eggs into the bowl and mix until smooth dough ball forms. Wet your hands with water and knead the dough briefly.
3. Tear off two large pieces of parchment paper and spray one side of each with nonstick cooking spray. Place the dough ball between the two sheets, with sprayed sides facing dough. Use a rolling pin to roll dough out to ¼" thickness.
4. Use a knife to slice into 24 rectangles. On each rectangle place 3 pepperoni slices and 1 piece string cheese.
5. Fold the rectangle in half, covering pepperoni and cheese filling. Pinch or roll sides closed. Cut a piece of parchment to fit your air fryer basket and place it into the basket. Put the rolls onto the parchment.
6. Adjust the temperature to 350°F and set the timer for 10 minutes.
7. After 5 minutes, open the fryer and flip the pizza rolls. Restart the fryer and continue cooking until pizza rolls are golden.
8. In a small bowl, place butter, garlic powder, and parsley. Brush the mixture over cooked pizza rolls and then sprinkle with Parmesan. Serve warm.

Nutrition: Calories: 333 Protein: 20.7 g Fiber: 0.8 g Net carbohydrates: 2.5 g Fat: 24.0 g Sodium: 708 mg Carbohydrates: 3.3 g Sugar: 0.9 g

518. Bacon Cheeseburger Dip
Preparation Time: 20 minutes
Cooking Time: 10 minutes
Servings: 6
Ingredients:
- ounces full-fat cream cheese
- ¼ cup full-fat mayonnaise
- ¼ cup full-fat sour cream
- ¼ cup chopped onion
- 1 teaspoon garlic powder
- 1 tablespoon Worcestershire sauce
- 1¼ cups shredded medium Cheddar cheese, divided
- ½ pound cooked 80/20 ground beef
- slices sugar-free bacon, cooked and crumbled
- 2 large pickle spears, chopped

Directions:
1. Place cream cheese in a large microwave-safe bowl and microwave for 45 seconds. Stir in mayonnaise, sour cream, onion, garlic powder, Worcestershire sauce, and 1 cup Cheddar. Add cooked ground beef and bacon. Sprinkle remaining Cheddar on top.
2. Place in 6" bowl and put into the air fryer basket.
3. Adjust the temperature to 400°F and set the timer for 10 minutes.
4. Dip is done when top is golden and bubbling. Sprinkle pickles over dish. Serve warm.

Nutrition: Calories: 457 Protein: 21.6 g Fiber: 0.2 g Net carbohydrates: 3.6 g Fat: 35.0 g Sodium: 589 mg Carbohydrates: 3.8 g Sugar: 2.2 g

519. Pork Rind Tortillas
Preparation Time: 10 minutes
Cooking Time: 5 minutes
Servings: 4
Ingredients:
- 1 ounce pork rinds
- ¾ cup shredded mozzarella cheese
- 2 tablespoons full-fat cream cheese
- 1 large egg

Directions:
1. Place pork rinds into food processor and pulse until finely ground.
2. Place mozzarella into a large microwave-safe bowl. Break cream cheese into small pieces and add them to the bowl. Microwave for 30 seconds, or until both cheeses are melted and can easily be stirred together into a ball. Add ground pork rinds and egg to the cheese mixture.
3. Continue stirring until the mixture forms a ball. If it cools too much and cheese hardens, microwave for 10 more seconds.
4. Separate the dough into four small balls. Place each ball of dough between two sheets of parchment and roll into ¼" flat layer.
5. Place tortillas into the air fryer basket in single layer, working in batches if necessary.
6. Adjust the temperature to 400°F and set the timer for 5 minutes.
7. Tortillas will be crispy and firm when fully cooked. Serve immediately.

Nutrition: Calories: 145 Protein: 10.7 g Fiber: 0.0 g Net carbohydrates: 0.8 g Fat: 10.0 g Sodium: 291 mg Carbohydrates: 0.8 g Sugar: 0.5 g

520. Mozzarella Sticks
Preparation Time: 1 hour
Cooking Time: 10 minutes
Servings: Yields 12 sticks (3 per serving)
Ingredients:
- (1-ounce) mozzarella string cheese sticks
- ½ cup grated Parmesan cheese

- ½ ounce pork rinds, finely ground
- 1 teaspoon dried parsley
- 2 large eggs

Directions:
1. Place mozzarella sticks on a cutting board and cut in half. Freeze 45 minutes or until firm. If freezing overnight, remove frozen sticks after 1 hour and place into airtight zip-top storage bag and place back in freezer for future use.
2. In a large bowl, mix Parmesan, ground pork rinds, and parsley.
3. In a medium bowl, whisk eggs.
4. Dip a frozen mozzarella stick into beaten eggs and then into Parmesan mixture to coat. Repeat with remaining sticks. Place mozzarella sticks into the air fryer basket.
5. Adjust the temperature to 400°F and set the timer for 10 minutes or until golden.
6. Serve warm.

Nutrition: Calories: 236 Protein: 19.2 g Fiber: 0.0 g Net carbohydrates: 4.7 g Fat: 13.8 g Sodium: 609 mg Carbohydrates: 4.7 g Sugar: 1.1 g

521. Bacon-Wrapped Onion Rings

Preparation Time: 5 minutes
Cooking Time: 10 minutes
Servings: 4

Ingredients:
- 1 large onion, peeled
- 1 tablespoon sriracha
- slices sugar-free bacon

Directions:
1. Slice onion into ¼"-thick slices. Brush sriracha over the onion slices. Take two slices of onion and wrap bacon around the rings. Repeat with remaining onion and bacon. Place into the air fryer basket.
2. Adjust the temperature to 350°F and set the timer for 10 minutes.
3. Use tongs to flip the onion rings halfway through the cooking time. When fully cooked, bacon will be crispy. Serve warm.

Nutrition: Calories: 105 Protein: 7.5 g Fiber: 0.6 g Net carbohydrates: 3.7 g Fat: 5.9 g Sodium: 401 mg Carbohydrates: 4.3 g Sugar: 2.3 g

522. Mini Sweet Pepper Poppers

Preparation Time: 15 minutes
Cooking Time: 8 minutes
Servings: 16

Ingredients:
- mini sweet peppers
- ounces full-fat cream cheese, softened
- slices sugar-free bacon, cooked and crumbled
- ¼ cup shredded pepper jack cheese

Directions:
1. Remove the tops from the peppers and slice each one in half lengthwise. Use a small knife to remove seeds and membranes.
2. In a small bowl, mix cream cheese, bacon, and pepper jack.
3. Place 3 teaspoons of the mixture into each sweet pepper and press down smooth. Place into the fryer basket.
4. Adjust the temperature to 400°F and set the timer for 8 minutes.
5. Serve warm.

Nutrition: Calories: 176 Protein: 7.4 g Fiber: 0.9 g Net carbohydrates: 2.7 g Fat: 13.4 g Sodium: 309 mg Carbohydrates: 3.6 g Sugar: 2.2 g

523. Spicy Spinach Artichoke Dip

Preparation Time: 10 minutes
Cooking Time: 10 minutes
Servings: 6

Ingredients:
- ounces frozen spinach, drained and thawed
- 1 (14-ounce) can artichoke hearts, drained and chopped
- ¼ cup chopped pickled jalapeños
- ounces full-fat cream cheese, softened
- ¼ cup full-fat mayonnaise
- ¼ cup full-fat sour cream
- ½ teaspoon garlic powder
- ¼ cup grated Parmesan cheese
- 1 cup shredded pepper jack cheese

Directions:
1. Mix all ingredients in a 4-cup baking bowl. Place into the air fryer basket.
2. Adjust the temperature to 320°F and set the timer for 10 minutes.
3. Remove when brown and bubbling. Serve warm.

Nutrition: Calories: 226 Protein: 10.0 g Fiber: 3.7 g Net carbohydrates: 6.5 g Fat: 15.9 g Sodium: 776 mg Carbohydrates: 10.2 g Sugar: 3.4 g

524. Personal Mozzarella Pizza Crust

Preparation Time: 5 minutes
Cooking Time: 10 minutes
Servings: 1

Ingredients:
- ½ cup shredded whole-milk mozzarella cheese
- 2 tablespoons blanched finely ground almond flour
- 1 tablespoon full-fat cream cheese
- 1 large egg white

Directions:
1. Place mozzarella, almond flour, and cream cheese in a medium microwave-safe bowl. Microwave for 30 seconds. Stir until smooth ball of dough forms. Add egg white and stir until soft round dough forms.
2. Press into a 6" round pizza crust.
3. Cut a piece of parchment to fit your air fryer basket and place crust on parchment. Place into the air fryer basket.
4. Adjust the temperature to 350°F and set the timer for 10 minutes.
5. Flip after 5 minutes and at this time place any desired toppings on the crust. Continue cooking until golden. Serve immediately.

Nutrition: Calories: 314 Protein: 19.9 g Fiber: 1.5 g Net carbohydrates: 3.6 g Fat: 22.7 g Sodium: 457 mg Carbohydrates: 5.1 g Sugar: 1.8 g

525. Garlic Cheese Bread

Preparation Time: 10 minutes
Cooking Time: 10 minutes
Servings: 2

Ingredients:
- 1 cup shredded mozzarella cheese
- ¼ cup grated Parmesan cheese
- 1 large egg
- ½ teaspoon garlic powder

Directions:
1. Mix all Ingredients in a large bowl. Cut a piece of parchment to fit your air fryer basket. Press the mixture into a circle on the parchment and place into the air fryer basket.

2. Adjust the temperature to 350°F and set the timer for 10 minutes.
3. Serve warm.

Nutrition: Calories: 258 Protein: 19.2 g Fiber: 0.1 g Net carbohydrates: 3.6 g Fat: 16.6 g Sodium: 612 mg Carbohydrates: 3.7 g Sugar: 0.7 g

526. Crustless Three-Meat Pizza

Preparation Time: 5 minutes
Cooking Time: 5 minutes
Servings: 1
Ingredients:
- ½ cup shredded mozzarella cheese
- slices pepperoni
- ¼ cup cooked ground sausage
- 2 slices sugar-free bacon, cooked and crumbled
- 1 tablespoon grated Parmesan cheese
- 2 tablespoons low-carb, sugar-free pizza sauce, for dipping

Directions:
1. Cover the bottom of a 6" cake pan with mozzarella. Place pepperoni, sausage, and bacon on top of cheese and sprinkle with Parmesan. Place pan into the air fryer basket.
2. Adjust the temperature to 400°F and set the timer for 5 minutes.
3. Remove when cheese is bubbling and golden. Serve warm with pizza sauce for dipping.

Nutrition: Calories: 466 Protein: 28.1 g Fiber: 0.5 g Net carbohydrates: 4.7 g Fat: 34.0 g Sodium: 1,446 mg Carbohydrates: 5.2 g Sugar: 1.6 g

527. Bacon Snack

Preparation Time: 15 minutes
Cooking Time: 10 minutes
Servings: 4
Ingredients:
- 1cup dark chocolate; melted
- 4bacon slices; halved
- A pinch of pink salt

Directions:
1. Dip each bacon slice in some chocolate, sprinkle pink salt over them.
2. Put them in your air fryer's basket and
3. cook at 350°F for 10 minutes

Nutrition: Calories: 151 Fat: 4g Fiber: 2g Carbs: 4g Protein: 8g

528. Shrimp Snack

Preparation Time: 15 minutes
Cooking Time: 10 minutes
Servings: 4
Ingredients:
- 1lb. shrimp; peeled and deveined
- ¼ cup olive oil
- 3garlic cloves; minced
- ¼ tsp. cayenne pepper
- Juice of ½ lemon
- A pinch of salt and black pepper

Directions:
1. In a pan that fits your air fryer, mix all the
2. ingredients, toss,
3. Introduce in the fryer and cook at 370°F for 10 minutes
4. Servings as a snack

Nutrition: Calories: 242 Fat: 14g Fiber: 2g Carbs: 3g Protein: 17g

529. Avocado Wraps

Preparation Time: : 20 minutes
Cooking Time: 15 minutes
Servings: 4
Ingredients:
- 2avocados, peeled, pitted and cut into 12 wedges
- 1tbsp. ghee; melted
- 12bacon strips

Directions:
1. Wrap each avocado wedge in a bacon strip, brush them with the ghee.
2. Put them in your air fryer's basket and cook at 360°F for 15 minutes
3. Servings as an appetizer

Nutrition: Calories: 161 Fat: 4g Fiber: 2g Carbs: 4g Protein: 6g

530. Cheesy Meatballs

Preparation Time: 30 minutes
Cooking Time: 30 minutes
Servings: 16
Ingredients:
- 1lb. 80/20 ground beef.
- 3oz.low-moisture, whole-milk mozzarella, cubed
- 1large egg.
- ½ cup low-carb, no-sugar-added pasta sauce.
- ¼ cup grated Parmesan cheese.
- ¼ cup blanched finely ground almond flour.
- ¼ tsp. onion powder.
- tsp. dried parsley.
- ½ tsp. garlic powder.

Directions:
1. Take a large bowl, add ground beef, almond flour, parsley, garlic powder, onion powder and egg. Fold ingredientstogether until fully combined
2. Form the mixture into 2-inch balls and use your thumb or a spoon to create an indent in the center of each meatball. Place a cube of cheese in the center and form the ball around it.
3. Place the meatballs into the air fryer, working in batches if necessary. Adjust the temperature to 350 Degrees F and set the timer for 15 minutes
4. Meatballs will be slightly crispy on the outside and fully cooked when at least 180 Degrees F internally.
5. When they are finished cooking, toss the meatballs in the sauce and sprinkle with grated Parmesan for serving.

Nutrition: Calories: 447 Protein: 29.6g Fiber: 1.8g Fat: 29.7g Carbs: 5.4g

531. Tuna Appetizer

Preparation Time: 15 minutes
Cooking Time: 10 minutes
Servings: 2
Ingredients:
- 1lb. tuna, skinless; boneless and cubed
- 3scallion stalks; minced
- 1chili pepper; minced
- 2tomatoes; cubed
- 1tbsp. coconut aminos
- 2tbsp. olive oil
- 1tbsp. coconut cream
- 1tsp. sesame seeds

Directions:
1. In a pan that fits your air fryer, mix all the ingredientsexcept the sesame seeds, toss, introduce in the fryer and cook at 360°F for 10 minutes
2. Divide into bowls and serve as an appetizer with sesame seeds sprinkled on top.

Nutrition: Calories: 231 Fat: 18g Fiber: 3g Carbs: 4g Protein: 18g

532. Cheese And Leeks Dip

Preparation Time: 17 minutes
Cooking Time: 12 minutes
Servings: 6

Ingredients:
- 2spring onions; minced
- 4leeks; sliced
- ¼ cup coconut cream
- 3tbsp. coconut milk
- 2tbsp. butter; melted
- Salt and white pepper to the taste

Directions:
1. In a pan that fits your air fryer, mix all the ingredients and whisk them well.
2. Introduce the pan in the fryer and cook at 390°F for 12 minutes. Divide into bowls and serve

Nutrition: Calories: 204 Fat: 12g Fiber: 2g Carbs: 4g Protein: 14g

533. Cucumber Salsa

Preparation Time: 10 minutes
Cooking Time: 5 minutes
Servings: 4

Ingredients:
- 1½ lb. cucumbers; sliced
- 2red chili peppers; chopped.
- 2tomatoes cubed
- 2spring onions; chopped.
- 1tbsp. balsamic vinegar
- 2tbsp. ginger; grated
- A drizzle of olive oil

Directions:
1. In a pan that fits your air fryer, mix all the ingredients, toss, introduce in the fryer and cook at 340°F for 5 minutes
2. Divide into bowls and serve cold as an appetizer.

Nutrition: Calories: 150 Fat: 2g Fiber: 1g Carbs: 2g Protein: 4g

534. Chicken Cubes

Preparation Time: 25 minutes
Cooking Time: 20 minutes
Servings: 4

Ingredients:
- 1lb. chicken breasts, skinless; boneless and cubed
- 2eggs
- ¾ cup coconut flakes
- 2tsp. garlic powder
- Cooking spray
- Salt and black pepper to taste.

Directions:
1. Put the coconut in a bowl and mix the eggs with garlic powder, salt and pepper in a second one.
2. Dredge the chicken cubes in eggs and then in coconut and arrange them all in your air fryer's basket
3. Grease with cooking spray, cook at 370°F for 20 minutes. Arrange the chicken bites on a platter and serve as an appetizer.

Nutrition: Calories: 202 Fat: 12g Fiber: 2g Carbs: 4g Protein: 7g

535. Salmon Spread

Preparation Time: 11 minutes
Cooking Time: 6 minutes
Servings: 4

Ingredients:
- 8oz. cream cheese, soft
- ½ cup coconut cream
- 4oz. smoked salmon, skinless; boneless and minced
- 2tbsp. lemon juice
- 1tbsp. chives; chopped.
- A pinch of salt and black pepper

Directions:
1. Take a bowl and mix all the ingredients
2. and whisk them really well.
3. Transfer the mix to a ramekin, place it in your air fryer's basket and cook at 360°F for 6 minutes

Nutrition: Calories: 180 Fat: 7g Fiber: 1g Carbs: 5g Protein: 7g

536. Crustless Pizza

Preparation Time: 10 minutes
Cooking Time: 5 minutes
Servings: 1

Ingredients:
- 2slices sugar-free bacon; cooked and crumbled
- 7slices pepperoni
- ½ cup shredded mozzarella cheese
- ¼ cup cooked ground sausage
- 2tbsp. low-carb, sugar-free pizza sauce, for dipping
- 1tbsp. grated Parmesan cheese

Directions:
1. Cover the bottom of a 6-inch cake pan with mozzarella. Place pepperoni, sausage and bacon on top of cheese and sprinkle with Parmesan
2. Place pan into the air fryer basket. Adjust the temperature to 400 Degrees F and set the timer for 5 minutes.
3. Remove when cheese is bubbling and golden. Serve warm with pizza sauce for dipping

Nutrition: Calories: 466 Protein: 28.1g Fiber: 0.5g Fat: 34.0g Carbs: 5.2g

537. Olives And Zucchini Cakes

Preparation Time: 17 minutes
Cooking Time: 6 minutes
Servings: 6

Ingredients:
- 3spring onions; chopped.
- ½ cup kalamata olives, pitted and minced
- 3zucchinis; grated
- ½ cup parsley; chopped.
- ½ cup almond flour
- 1egg
- Cooking spray
- Salt and black pepper to taste.

Directions:
1. Take a bowl and mix all the ingredients except the cooking spray, stir well and shape medium cakes out of this mixture
2. Place the cakes in your air fryer's basket, grease them with cooking spray and cook at 380°F for 6 minutes on each side. Serve as an appetizer.

Nutrition: Calories: 165 Fat: 5g Fiber: 2g Carbs: 3g Protein: 7g

538. Fluffy Strawberry Muffins

Preparation Time: 10 minutes
Cooking Time: 25 minutes
Servings: 12

Ingredients:
- 1 ½ cups almond flour
- 1 tsp baking powder
- ½ tsp xanthan gum
- ½ cup Lakanto monk fruit sweetener
- 2 eggs, beaten
- 1 tsp vanilla extract

SNACK RECIPES

- ½ tsp almond extract
- 3 tbsps. unsalted butter
- 3 tbsps. unsweetened vanilla almond milk
- ½ cup chopped strawberries

Directions:
1. Preheat the oven to 350° F.
2. Take the 2 eggs and beat them with vanilla extract, melted butter, almond extract, and unsweetened almond milk until creamy and smooth. This should take around 2 minutes.
3. In another bowl, mix sweetener, xanthan gum, baking powder, and almond flour.
4. Combine the dry and wet ingredients and mix well; you should not have any lumps.
5. Add the chopped strawberries to the batter and use a plastic spatula to fold them in.
6. Take a muffin tin and put cupcake liners in each of the molds. Fill ¾ of each mold with the batter.
7. Bake for 20-25 minutes. You can check if they are done by inserting a toothpick into the center of a muffin; the toothpick will come out clean if they are done.

Nutrition: Calories 144 Carbs 2g Protein 5g Fat 13g Fiber 2g

539. Paleo Blueberry Muffins
Preparation Time: 10 minutes
Cooking Time: 20 minutes
Servings: 12
Ingredients:
- ½ cup coconut flour
- 4 ½ tbsps. coconut oil
- 6 organic eggs
- 4 tbsps. milk
- ½ tsp apple cider vinegar
- ½ tsp baking soda
- ¼ tsp baking powder
- 1 tsp cinnamon
- ¼ tsp sea salt
- 2 tbsps. raw honey
- ½ cup blueberries

Directions:
1. Preheat the oven to 400° F.
2. Combine all wet ingredients(coconut oil, eggs, milk, apple cider vinegar, honey) in a medium-sized bowl.
3. In another bowl, mix all the dry ingredients(coconut flour, baking soda, baking powder, cinnamon, sea salt).
4. Add dry ingredientsto the bowl of the wet ingredients and combine them well.
5. Add blueberries to the batter and stir thoroughly. The blueberries should be evenly spread throughout the batter.
6. Pour batter into baking cups or a muffin tin. If you are using a muffin tin, make sure to use cupcake liners.
7. Bake for 10-15 minutes, or until golden brown.

Nutrition: Calories 210 Carbs 6g Sugar 2g Protein 7g Fat 19g Fiber 3g

540. Orange Cardamom Muffins With Coconut Butter Glaze
Preparation Time: 10 minutes
Cooking Time: 30 minutes
Servings: 6
Ingredients:
- 2 cups blanched almond flour
- 3 large eggs
- 1 tbsp orange zest
- ¼ cup fresh orange juice
- ½ tsp cardamom
- ¼ tsp salt
- 1 tsp baking powder
- 2 tsp Stevia sweetener
- 2 tbsps. coconut oil, melted
- For coconut butter glaze:
- 1 tbsp coconut oil
- ¼ cup coconut butter
- ½ tbsp Stevia sweetener

Directions:
1. Preheat the oven to 350° F.
2. In a medium-sized bowl, whisk eggs, orange zest, and orange juice.
3. In another bowl, combine the dry ingredients(almond flour, cardamom, salt, baking powder, sweetener).
4. Combine dry ingredientswith the wet ingredientsby folding them in gently, then stir to form an even better.
5. After this, add the coconut oil and fold through again.
6. Line muffin tin with paper liners and pour ⅓ cup of batter into each muffin cup.
7. Bake for 25-30 minutes.
8. When done, let the cupcakes cool down for at least 10 minutes.
9. While your cupcakes are cooling, start working on the glaze. Start by melting the coconut oil and coconut butter on the stove.
10. Stir this mixture until it is smooth and take it off the stove, then add the sweetener.
11. Once your cupcakes have fully cooled, drizzle the glaze on top of them.

Nutrition: Calories 219 Carbs 7g Sugar 2g Protein 5.5g Fat 20g Fiber 2.5g

541. Bacon And Egg Cups
Preparation Time: 10 minutes
Cooking Time: 20 minutes
Servings: 6
Ingredients:
- 6 eggs
- 2 tbsps. fresh parsley
- 3 ounces of cheddar cheese
- 6 slices regular-cut bacon
- Salt and pepper to taste

Directions:
1. Preheat the oven to 350° F.
2. Spray or grease your muffin pan with coconut oil.
3. Line the sides of each muffin cup with a bacon slice.
4. Crack an egg into each bacon-lined muffin cup.
5. Add salt and pepper, and sprinkle with cheese.
6. Bake for 20 minutes; the eggs need this much time to cook fully.
7. Garnish with chopped parsley and serve.

Nutrition: Calories 210 Carbs 0g Sugar 0g Protein 15g Fat 16g

542. Breadsticks
Preparation Time: 20 minutes
Cooking Time: 10 minutes
Servings: 12
Ingredients:
- 1 ½ cups part skim low moisture shredded mozzarella cheese
- 1 ounce of cream cheese
- ½ cup almond flour
- 3 tbsps. coconut flour
- 1 large egg

- For topping:
- ½ cup part skim low moisture shredded mozzarella cheese
- ½ cup shredded Parmesan cheese
- 1 tsp finely chopped parsley

Directions:
1. Preheat the oven to 425° F.
2. Melt the cheese you will use in your batter. Put the cream cheese and mozzarella in a microwaveable bowl and microwave for 1 minute. Stir, then put it back in for another 30 seconds. Keep repeating this process until you end up with a smooth and even mixture.
3. Use a food processor on a high speed to combine the cheese mixture with coconut flour, almond flour, and egg. The end result should be a uniform mixture without any lumps.
4. The dough will be a little sticky at this stage and will need to cool down a bit. Cooling the dough will help you roll it out easier.
5. Between 2 pieces of parchment paper, roll the dough to around ¼ inch thick, then remove top piece of parchment paper.
6. Transfer dough and parchment paper to a baking sheet and spread ¼ cup mozzarella cheese over the top of the dough.
7. Bake for 5-6 minutes, or until the edges are golden and puffy.
8. Sprinkle Parmesan cheese and the rest of the mozzarella on the dough and bake for another 4-5 minutes, or until cheese is melted.
9. Once baked, garnish with parsley and serve.

Nutrition: Calories 207 Carbs 7g Sugar 2g Protein 13g Fat 14g

543. Butter Crackers

Preparation Time: 5 minutes
Cooking Time: 15 minutes
Servings: 25

Ingredients:
- 8 tbsps. salted butter, softened
- 2 egg whites
- 2 ¼ cups almond flour
- Salt to taste

Directions:
1. Preheat the oven to 350° F.
2. Combine butter and almond flour in a medium bowl and mix on low-medium speed with an electric mixer.
3. Add egg whites and salt to this mixture and combine them with the mixer. You should expect to have smooth dough within 5-10 minutes.
4. Roll the dough between 2 pieces of parchment paper to a thickness of around ⅛ inch.
5. Remove the top parchment paper and place the dough and bottom parchment paper onto the baking sheet.
6. Use a pizza cutter or knife to divide the dough into 2-inch squares. You can sprinkle the dough with salt if you prefer.
7. Bake for 10-15 minutes, or until golden brown; the time will vary according to the width of the dough squares.
8. Serve immediately, while they are still crunchy. However, if you want to store them, keep them in an airtight container rather than in the refrigerator; the refrigerator causes the crackers to lose their crunch.

Nutrition: Calories 90 Carbs 8g Protein 2g Fat 8g Fiber 1g

544. Homemade Almond Crackers

Preparation Time: 15 minutes
Cooking Time: 30 minutes
Servings: 12

Ingredients:
- 1 cup almond flour
- 3 tbsps. water
- 1 tbsp ground flaxseed
- ½ tsp fine sea salt
- Flaked sea salt to garnish (optional)

Directions:
1. Preheat the oven to 350° F.
2. Combine almond flour, water, ground flaxseed, and salt in a large bowl and stir the mixture to form dough.
3. Place the dough between 2 pieces of parchment paper and roll it to ⅛ inch thick.
4. Dispose of top piece of parchment paper, then sprinkle flaked sea salt on the dough. Press the salt into the dough with your fingers.
5. With a knife, cut the dough into small 1-inch by 1-inch squares. You can also use a toothpick to create little holes in the crackers.
6. Place the parchment paper with the dough pieces into the oven and bake for 25-30 minutes, or until golden brown.
7. Allow the crackers to cool down before serving. If you are not eating them immediately, make sure to use an airtight container to store them.

Nutrition: Calories 173 Carbs 7g Sugar 1g Protein 6g Fat 15g Fiber 4g

545. Pepperoni Chips

Preparation Time: 2 minutes
Cooking Time: 6 minutes
Servings: 6

Ingredients:
- 6 ounces of pepperoni

Directions:
1. Preheat the oven to 400° F.
2. Thinly slice the pepperoni.
3. Place a piece of parchment paper on a baking sheet, then place all the pepperoni slices at an equal distance from each other on the sheet.
4. Bake for 5 minutes, then use a power towel to sponge off the excess oil from the slices.
5. To crisp them up, put the slices back in the oven for 1 more minute. However, depending on how crisp you want them to be, you can keep them in for a bit longer. Remember, don't burn them!
6. Let them cool before serving.

Nutrition: Calories 140 Carbs 0g Sugar 0g Protein 5g Fat 12g

546. 3-Ingredient Flourless Cheesy Breadsticks

Preparation Time: 15 minutes
Cooking Time: 25 minutes
Servings: 10

Ingredients:
- 1 ½ cups shredded mozzarella cheese
- 2 large eggs
- ½ tsp Italian seasoning
- For topping:
- ½ cup shredded mozzarella cheese
- 2 tbsps. shredded parmesan cheese (optional)
- 1 tsp finely chopped parsley (optional)

Directions:
1. Preheat the oven to 350° F.
2. Line a 9-inch by 9-inch baking pan with parchment paper.

SNACK RECIPES

3. Blend the eggs and shredded mozzarella cheese until everything is combined evenly. Add Italian seasoning at this stage. An electric mixer is recommended.
4. Mixture needs to be evenly spread out in the baking pan and baked for 20 minutes. Once done, the crust should be firm.
5. Allow it to cool for at least 5 minutes.
6. Increase oven temperature to 425° F.
7. Remove crust from parchment paper and place it on a cooling rack. Add the remaining cheese on top of the crust. You can use parmesan or cheddar instead of mozzarella, depending on what you prefer.
8. Bake crust on cooling rack in oven for about 5 more minutes so it crisps up.
9. Garnish with parsley, then serve.

Nutrition: Calories 142 Carbs 3g Sugar 1g Protein 11g Fat 9g

547. Cauliflower Breadsticks
Preparation Time: 10 minutes
Cooking Time: 32 minutes
Servings: 8-10
Ingredients:
- 2 cups cauliflower rice
- 2 eggs
- ½ tsp granulated garlic
- ½ tsp ground pepper
- 1 cup shredded mozzarella or Mexican blend cheese
- ¼ cup grated Parmesan cheese
- 1 tsp Italian Seasoning
- ½ tsp salt

Directions:
1. Preheat the oven to 350° F.
2. Grease a baking sheet with oil or butter. If you are not greasing, then remember to place a piece of parchment paper on the baking sheet.
3. Combine cauliflower rice, eggs, garlic, pepper, and cheese to a food processor. Add salt and Italian seasoning at this stage. Work at low or medium speeds to break down the cauliflower as much as possible so that a smooth mixture is formed.
4. Pour mixture onto the baking sheet. The dough should have a thickness of around ¼ inch.
5. Bake for 30 minutes.
6. Add more cheese on top after you have taken it out of the oven.
7. Bake for another 2-3 minutes to melt the added cheese.
8. Cut into 8-10 breadstick slices and serve.

Nutrition: Calories 165 Carbs 5g Sugar 1g Protein 13g Fat 10g

548. Breadsticks With Mozzarella Dough
Preparation Time: 10 minutes
Cooking Time: 10 minutes
Servings: 10
Ingredients:
- ⅔ cup almond flour
- 1 ¾ cups shredded mozzarella cheese
- 2 tbsps. full-fat cream cheese
- Pinch of salt to taste
- 1 medium egg
- 1 tbsp garlic, crushed
- 1 tsp dried rosemary
- 1 tbsp parsley, fresh or dried

Directions:
1. Preheat the oven to 425° F.
2. In a large microwavable bowl, combine almond flour, mozzarella, cream cheese, and salt, and microwave for 1 minute.
3. Stir the mixture and microwave for another 30 seconds.
4. Add the egg to create a cheesy dough.
5. Make dough balls and roll them into long, thin breadsticks. The smaller the dough balls, the more breadsticks you will be able to make.
6. Bake for 10 minutes, or until golden brown. Check after 5 minutes and see whether they are golden brown or not. If they are too light, put them back into the oven for another 5 minutes. If they are already done, take them out. The baking time can vary depending on the thickness of the breadsticks.

Nutrition: Calories 58 Carbs 1.2 g Sugar 0.3g Protein 2g Fat 5g Fiber 0.5g

549. Bacon Onion Cookies
Preparation Time: 15 minutes
Cooking Time: 15 minutes
Servings: 12
Ingredients:
- 4 slices bacon, crisped and crumbled
- 1 tbsp onion powder
- ½ tsp sea salt or pink Himalayan rock salt
- Pinch of freshly ground pepper
- 1 ½ cups almond flour
- 1 tbsp psyllium husk powder
- ⅓ cup flax meal
- 1 large egg

Directions:
1. Preheat the oven to 375° F.
2. Put a piece of parchment paper on a baking sheet. Carefully line the bacon slices on the sheet and put it in the oven for around 10 minutes, or until it reaches your preferred crispiness.
3. In a bowl, mix onion powder, salt, pepper, almond flour, psyllium husk powder, and flax meal.
4. Add the egg to the dry ingredients and work the dough with your hands.
5. Crumble your bacon slices and add them to the dough.
6. Put a fresh piece of parchment paper on your baking sheet.
7. Form small or medium dough balls and space them equally on your baking sheet.
8. Use a fork to press the dough balls down and flatten them.
9. Bake for 10-12 minutes, or until golden brown. Keep a close eye on the cookies as they bake since almond flour can burn easily.
10. Cool before serving. Use an airtight container for storage.

Nutrition: Calories 109 Carbs 4.3 g Protein 4.8 g Fat 9g Fiber 2.7 g

550. Cinnamon Swirl Cookies
Preparation Time: 30 minutes
Cooking Time: 50 minutes
Servings: 8
Ingredients:
- 3 cups almond flour
- ½ cup low-carb sweetener
- 2 tsps. gluten-free baking powder
- ¼ tsp salt
- 1 egg
- 2 tbsps. butter, melted
- 2 tsps. cinnamon

Directions:

SNACK RECIPES

1. In a large bowl, mix almond flour, sweetener, baking powder, and salt.
2. Add butter and egg to the dry ingredients. You will see the dough forming as you mix and combine.
3. Divide the dough into 2 equal parts. Add cinnamon to one and leave the other one plain.
4. Keep both doughs in the bowl and cover with plastic wrap or a kitchen towel. Put in the refrigerator for at least 30 minutes.
5. Preheat the oven to 280° F.
6. Roll both types of dough to ¼ inch thick between 2 pieces of parchment paper.
7. Place cinnamon dough on top of plain dough and roll into a tight log.
8. Cut dough log into cookies that are about ½ inch thick.
9. Place cookies on a baking sheet lined with parchment paper and bake for 30 minutes, or until golden brown.
10. Cool before serving.

Nutrition: Nutrition Facts Serving size: 1 cookie Calories 106 Carbs 2g Sugar 1g Protein 4g Fat 9g Fiber 2g

551. **Peanut Butter Cookies**

Preparation Time: 5 minutes
Cooking Time: 15 minutes
Servings: 12
Ingredients:
- ½ cup peanut butter
- ¼ cup powdered erythritol sweetener
- 1 egg

Directions:
1. Preheat the oven to 350° F.
2. Use a spatula to combine peanut butter, powdered sweetener, and egg.
3. Use a cookie scoop to scoop cookie dough into balls of a uniform size.
4. Line a baking sheet with parchment paper and place the cookie dough balls on it in a vertical line.
5. Bake for 12-15 minutes, or until crisp and golden brown.
6. Cool for at least 10 minutes before serving.

Nutrition: Calories 82 Carbs 3g Protein 4g Fat 7g Fiber 1g

552. **Cranberry Pistachio Vegan Shortbread Cookies**

Preparation Time: 20 minutes
Cooking Time: 10 minutes
Servings: 12
Ingredients:
- 2 cups ground almond flour
- ⅓ cup coconut sugar
- ½ tsp baking soda
- ½ tsp sea salt
- ½ cup pistachios, shelled and chopped
- ½ cup dried cranberries
- ½ cup coconut oil
- For dipping the cookies (optional):
- ⅔ cup chocolate chips

Directions:
1. Use a mixer to combine all the ingredients for the shortbread. Keep beating until a crumbly dough has formed.
2. Place the dough onto a piece of plastic wrap and shape it into a cylinder.
3. Wrap the dough in plastic wrap and put it into the freezer for a minimum of 2 hours. When you are ready to bake it, let it thaw for a little bit; chilling the dough makes it easier to cut when you are ready.
4. Preheat the oven to 350° F and line a baking sheet with parchment paper.
5. Use a knife to cut the dough into ¼-inch to ½-inch thick disks and lay these on the parchment paper.
6. Bake the cookies for 10-15 minutes, or until golden brown.
7. Let them cool for at least 30 minutes.
8. If you want to drizzle chocolate on your cookies or dip them in chocolate, melt the chocolate chips in the microwave for 10 seconds. Stir chocolate and repeat until it has reached a smooth consistency.

Nutrition: Calories 192 Carbs 13g Sugar 11g Protein 2g Fat 15.5g Fiber 1g

553. **Garlic Edamame**

Preparation Time: 5 minutes
Cooking Time: 10 minutes
Servings: 4
Ingredients:
- Olive oil
- 1 (16-ounce) bag frozen edamame in pods
- ½ teaspoon salt
- ½ teaspoon garlic salt
- ¼ teaspoon freshly ground black pepper
- ½ teaspoon red pepper flakes (optional)

Directions:
1. Spray a fryer basket lightly with olive oil.
2. In a medium bowl, add the frozen edamame and lightly spray with olive oil. Toss to coat.
3. In a small bowl, mix together the salt, garlic salt, black pepper, and red pepper flakes (if using). Add the mixture to the edamame and toss until evenly coated.
4. Place half the edamame in the fryer basket. Do not overfill the basket.
5. Air fry for 5 minutes. Shake the basket and cook until the edamame is starting to brown and get crispy, 3 to 5 more minutes.
6. Repeat with the remaining edamame and serve immediately.
7. Pair It With: These make a nice side dish to almost any meal.
8. Air Fry Like a Pro: If you use fresh edamame, reduce the air fry time by 2 to 3 minutes to avoid overcooking. Air-fried edamame do not retain their crisp texture, so it's best to eat them right after cooking.

Nutrition: Calories: 100 Total Fat: 3g Saturated Fat: 0g Cholesterol: 0mg Carbohydrates: 9g Protein: 8g Fiber: 4g Sodium: 496mg

554. **Spicy Chickpeas**

Preparation Time: 5 minutes
Cooking Time: 20 minutes
Servings: 4
Ingredients:
- Olive oil
- ½ teaspoon ground cumin
- ½ teaspoon chili powder
- ¼ teaspoon cayenne pepper
- ¼ teaspoon salt
- 1 (19-ounce) can chickpeas, drained and rinsed

Directions:
1. Spray a fryer basket lightly with olive oil.
2. In a small bowl, combine the cumin, chili powder, cayenne pepper, and salt.
3. In a medium bowl, add the chickpeas and lightly spray them with olive oil. Add the spice mixture and toss until coated evenly.

SNACK RECIPES

4. Transfer the chickpeas to the fryer basket. Air fry until the chickpeas reach your desired level of crunchiness, 15 to 20 minutes, making sure to shake the basket every 5 minutes.
5. Air Fry Like a Pro: I find 20 minutes to be the sweet spot for very crunchy chickpeas. If you prefer them less crispy, cook for about 15 minutes. These make a great vehicle for experimenting with different seasoning mixes such as Chinese 5-spice, a mixture of curry and turmeric, or herbes de Provence.

Nutrition: Calories: 122 Total Fat: 1g Saturated Fat: 0g Cholesterol: 0mg Carbohydrates: 22g Protein: 6g Fiber: 6g Sodium: 152mg

555. Black Bean Corn Dip

Preparation Time: 10 minutes
Cooking Time: 10 minutes
Servings: 4
Ingredients:
- ½ (15-ounce) can black beans, drained and rinsed
- ½ (15-ounce) can corn, drained and rinsed
- ¼ cup chunky salsa
- 2 ounces reduced-fat cream cheese, softened
- ¼ cup shredded reduced-fat Cheddar cheese
- ½ teaspoon ground cumin
- ½ teaspoon paprika
- Salt
- Freshly ground black pepper

Directions:
1. In a medium bowl, mix together the black beans, corn, salsa, cream cheese, Cheddar cheese, cumin, and paprika. Season with salt and pepper and stir until well combined.
2. Spoon the mixture into an air fryer–safe baking dish.
3. Place baking dish in the fryer basket and air fry until heated through, about 10 minutes.
4. Serve hot.
5. Pair It With: If you're really craving chips, serve the dip with Crunchy Tex-Mex Tortilla Chips.

Nutrition: Calories: 129 Total Fat: 4g Saturated Fat: 2g Cholesterol: 11mg Carbohydrates: 18g Protein: 6g Fiber: 4g Sodium: 200mg

556. Crunchy Tex-Mex Tortilla Chips

Preparation Time: 5 minutes
Cooking Time: 5 minutes
Servings: 4
Ingredients:
- Olive oil
- ½ teaspoon salt
- ½ teaspoon ground cumin
- ½ teaspoon chili powder
- ½ teaspoon paprika
- Pinch cayenne pepper
- 8 (6-inch) corn tortillas, each cut into 6 wedges

Directions:
1. Spray fryer basket lightly with olive oil.
2. In a small bowl, combine the salt, cumin, chili powder, paprika, and cayenne pepper.
3. Place the tortilla wedges in the fryer basket in a single layer. Spray the tortillas lightly with oil and sprinkle with some of the seasoning mixture. You will need to cook the tortillas in batches.
4. Air fry for 2 to 3 minutes. Shake the basket and cook until the chips are light brown and crispy, an additional 2 to 3 minutes. Watch the chips closely so they do not burn.
5. Pair It With: Serve with a simple salsa or the Black Bean Corn Dip for an even heartier snack.

Nutrition: Calories: 116 Total Fat: 2g Saturated Fat: 1g Cholesterol: 0mg Carbohydrates: 24g Protein: 3g Fiber: 4g Sodium: 321mg

557. Egg Roll Pizza Sticks

Preparation Time: 10 minutes
Cooking Time: 5 minutes
Servings: 4
Ingredients:
- Olive oil
- 8 pieces reduced-fat string cheese
- 8 egg roll wrappers
- 24 slices turkey pepperoni
- Marinara sauce, for dipping (optional)

Directions:
1. Olive oil
2. 8 pieces reduced-fat string cheese
3. 8 egg roll wrappers
4. 24 slices turkey pepperoni
5. Marinara sauce, for dipping (optional)
6. Spray a fryer basket lightly with olive oil. Fill a small bowl with water.
7. Place each egg roll wrapper diagonally on a work surface. It should look like a diamond.
8. .Place 3 slices of turkey pepperoni in a vertical line down the center of the wrapper.
9. Place 1 mozzarella cheese stick on top of the turkey pepperoni.
10. Fold the top and bottom corners of the egg roll wrapper over the cheese stick.
11. Fold the left corner over the cheese stick and roll the cheese stick up to resemble a spring roll. Dip a finger in the water and seal the edge of the roll
12. Repeat with the rest of the pizza sticks.
13. Place them in the fryer basket in a single layer, making sure to leave a little space between each one. Lightly spray the pizza sticks with oil. You may need to cook these in batches.
14. Air fry until the pizza sticks are lightly browned and crispy, about 5 minutes.
15. These are best served hot while the cheese is melted. Accompany with a small bowl of marinara sauce, if desired.

Nutrition: Calories: 362 Total Fat: 8g Saturated Fat: 4g Cholesterol: 43mg Carbohydrates: 40g Protein: 23g Fiber: 1g Sodium: 1,026mg

558. Cajun Zucchini Chips

Preparation Time: 10 minutes
Cooking Time: 15 minutes
Servings: 4
Ingredients:
- Olive oil
- 2 large zucchini, cut into ⅛-inch-thick slices
- 2 teaspoons Cajun seasoning

Directions:
1. Spray a fryer basket lightly with olive oil.
2. Put the zucchini slices in a medium bowl and spray them generously with olive oil.
3. Sprinkle the Cajun seasoning over the zucchini and stir to make sure they are evenly coated with oil and seasoning.
4. Place slices in a single layer in the fryer basket, making sure not to overcrowd. You will need to cook these in several batches.
5. Air fry for 8 minutes. Flip the slices over and air fry until they are as crisp and brown as you prefer, an additional 7 to 8 minutes.

Nutrition: Calories: 26 Total Fat: <1g Saturated Fat: <1g Cholesterol: 0mg Carbohydrates: 5g Protein: 2g Fiber: 2g Sodium: 286mg

559. Mexican Potato Skins
Preparation Time: 10 minutes
Cooking Time: : 55 minutes
Servings: 6
Ingredients:
- Olive oil
- 6 medium russet potatoes, scrubbed
- Salt
- Freshly ground black pepper
- 1 cup fat-free refried black beans
- 1 tablespoon taco seasoning
- ½ cup salsa
- ¾ cup reduced-fat shredded Cheddar cheese

Directions:
1. Spray a fryer basket lightly with olive oil.
2. Spray the potatoes lightly with oil and season with salt and pepper. Pierce each potato a few times with a fork.
3. Place the potatoes in the fryer basket. Air fry until fork tender, 30 to 40 minutes. The cooking time will depend on the size of the potatoes. You can cook the potatoes in the microwave or a standard oven, but they won't get the same lovely crispy skin they will get in the air fryer.
4. While the potatoes are cooking, in a small bowl, mix together the beans and taco seasoning. Set aside until the potatoes are cool enough to handle.
5. Cut each potato in half lengthwise. Scoop out most of the insides, leaving about ¼ inch in the skins so the potato skins hold their shape.
6. Season the insides of the potato skins with salt and black pepper. Lightly spray the insides of the potato skins with oil. You may need to cook them in batches.
7. Place them into the fryer basket, skin side down, and air fry until crisp and golden, 8 to 10 minutes.
8. Transfer the skins to a work surface and spoon ½ tablespoon of seasoned refried black beans into each one. Top each with 2 teaspoons salsa and 1 tablespoon shredded Cheddar cheese.
9. Place filled potato skins in the fryer basket in a single layer. Lightly spray with oil.
10. Air fry until the cheese is melted and bubbly, 2 to 3 minutes.

Nutrition: Calories: 245 Total Fat: 3g Saturated Fat: 2g Cholesterol: 10mg Carbohydrates: 46g Protein: 10g Fiber: 5g Sodium: 461mg

560. Crispy Old Bay Chicken Wings
Preparation Time: 10 minutes
Cooking Time: 15 minutes
Servings: 4
Ingredients:
- Olive oil
- 2 tablespoons Old Bay seasoning
- 2 teaspoons baking powder
- 2 teaspoons salt
- 2 pounds chicken wings

Directions:
1. Spray a fryer basket lightly with olive oil.
2. In a large zip-top plastic bag, mix together the Old Bay seasoning, baking powder, and salt.
3. Pat the wings dry with paper towels.
4. Place the wings in the zip-top bag, seal, and toss with the seasoning mixture until evenly coated.
5. Place the seasoned wings in the fryer basket in a single layer. Lightly spray with olive oil. You may need to cook them in batches.
6. Air fry for 7 minutes. Turn the wings over, lightly spray them with olive oil, and air fry until the wings are crispy and lightly browned, 5 to 8 more minutes. Using a meat thermometer, check to make sure the internal temperature is 165°F or higher.

Nutrition: Calories: 501 Total Fat: 36g Saturated Fat: 10g Cholesterol: 170mg Carbohydrates: 1g Protein: 42g Fiber: 0g Sodium: 2,527mg

561. Cinnamon Apple Chips
Preparation Time: 10 minutes
Cooking Time: 10 minutes
Servings: 4
Ingredients:
- Olive oil
- 2 apples, any variety, cored, cut in half, and cut into thin slices

Directions:
1. Spray a fryer basket lightly with oil.
2. Place the apple slices in the fryer basket in a single layer. You may need to cook them in batches.
3. Air fry for 4 to 5 minutes. Shake the basket and cook until crispy, another 4 to 5 minutes.

Nutrition: Calories: 39 Total Fat: 1g Saturated Fat: 0g Cholesterol: 0mg Carbohydrates: 11g Protein: 1g Fiber: 2g Sodium: 1mg

562. Cinnamon and Sugar Peaches
Preparation Time: 10 minutes
Cooking Time: 13 minutes
Servings: 4
Ingredients:
- Olive oil
- 2 tablespoons sugar
- ¼ teaspoon ground cinnamon
- 4 peaches, cut into wedges

Directions:
1. Spray a fryer basket lightly with olive oil.
2. In a medium bowl, combine the sugar and cinnamon. Add the peaches and toss to coat evenly.
3. Place the peaches in a single layer in the fryer basket on their sides. You may need to cook them in batches.
4. Air fry for 5 minutes. Turn the peaches skin side down, lightly spray them with oil, and air fry until the peaches are lightly brown and caramelized, 5 to 8 more minutes.
5. Make it Even Lower Calorie: Use a zero calorie sugar substitute such as Nutrisweet or monk fruit sweetener instead of granulated sugar.
6. Air Fry Like a Pro: These do not get truly crispy, but rather they remain soft, sweet, and caramelized. They are truly delightful and make a wonderful dessert option.

Nutrition: Calories: 67 Total Fat: 1g Saturated Fat: 0g Cholesterol: 0mg Carbohydrates: 17g Protein: 1g Fiber: 2g Sodium: 0mg

563. Spicy Dill Pickle Fries
Preparation Time: 15 minutes
Cooking Time: 15 minutes
Servings: 4
Ingredients:
- Olive oil
- 1 cup whole-wheat flour
- 1 teaspoon paprika
- 1 egg
- 1⅓ cups whole-wheat panko bread crumbs
- 1 (24-ounce) jar spicy dill pickle spears

Directions:
1. Spray a fryer basket lightly with olive oil.
2. In a small, shallow bowl, combine the whole-wheat flour and paprika.
3. In another small, shallow bowl, whisk the egg.
4. Put the panko bread crumbs in another small.
5. Pat the pickle spears dry with paper towels.
6. Dip each pickle spear in the flour mixture, coat in the egg, and dredge in the panko bread crumbs.
7. Place each pickle spear in the fryer basket in a single layer, leaving a little space between each one. Spray the pickles lightly with olive oil. You may need to cook them in batches.
8. Air fry for 7 minutes. Turn the pickles over and cook until lightly browned and crispy, another 5 to 8 minutes.

Nutrition: Calories: 233 Total Fat: 2g Saturated Fat: 1g Cholesterol: 47mg Carbohydrates: 45g Protein: 10g Fiber: 7g Sodium: 1,249mg

564. Carrot Chips
Preparation Time: 15 minutes
Cooking Time: 10 minutes
Servings: 4
Ingredients:
- 1 tablespoon olive oil plus more for spraying
- 4 to 5 medium carrots, trimmed
- 1 teaspoon seasoned salt

Directions:
1. Spray a fryer basket lightly with olive oil.
2. Using a mandolin slicer set to the smallest setting or a sharp knife, cut the carrots into very thin slices.
3. In a medium bowl, toss the carrot slices with 1 tablespoon of olive oil and the seasoned salt.
4. Put half the carrots the fryer basket. Do not overcrowd the basket.
5. Air fry for 5 minutes. Shake the basket and cook until crispy, 3 to 5 additional minutes. The longer you cook the carrot slices, the crispier they will become. Watch closely because smaller slices could burn.
6. Repeat with the remaining carrots.

Nutrition: Calories: 55 Total Fat: 4g Saturated Fat: 1g Cholesterol: 0mg Carbohydrates: 6g Protein: 1g Fiber: 2g Sodium: 422mg

565. Spicy Corn On The Cob
Preparation Time: 10 minutes
Cooking Time: 16 minutes
Servings: 4
Ingredients:
- Olive oil
- 2 tablespoons grated Parmesan cheese
- 1 teaspoon chili powder
- 1 teaspoon garlic powder
- 1 teaspoon ground cumin
- 1 teaspoon paprika
- 1 teaspoon salt
- ¼ teaspoon cayenne pepper, optional
- 4 ears fresh corn, shucked

Directions:
1. Spray a fryer basket lightly with olive oil.
2. In a small bowl, mix together the Parmesan cheese, chili powder, garlic powder, cumin, paprika, salt, and cayenne pepper.
3. Lightly spray the ears of corn with olive oil. Sprinkle them with the seasoning mixture.
4. Place the ears of corn in the fryer basket in a single layer. You may need to cook them in more than one batch.
5. Air fry for 7 minutes. Turn the corn over and air fry until lightly browned, 7 to 9 more minutes.
6. Make It Even Lower Calorie: This recipe is just as tasty without Parmesan, especially when the corn is super fresh and sweet.

Nutrition: Calories: 116 Total Fat: 2g Saturated Fat: 1g Cholesterol: 2mg Carbohydrates: 23g Protein: 5g Fiber: 4g Sodium: 652mg

566. Pickle Chips
Preparation Time: 5 minutes
Cooking Time: 12 hours
Servings: 12
Ingredients:
- 1 jar large dill pickles

Directions:
1. Remove pickles from the jar and pat dry with paper towels. Slice the pickles length-wise into long, thin slabs about 1/4 inch thick.
2. Lay the pickle slices on the racks of your Nesco Snack Master and set to 125F. Dehydrate for 12 hours or until the pickles are completely dried.
3. Remove from the racks and eat like chips or store and rehydrate when needed. To rehydrate simply place the dried pickle slices in a bowl of lukewarm water and wait 5 to 10 minutes.

Nutrition: Calories: 1 Fat: 0 gram Carbs: 0.3 grams Protein: 0.1 gram

567. Potato Chips
Preparation Time: 10 minutes
Cooking Time: 6 hours
Servings: 6
Ingredients:
- 2 russet potatoes, peeled
- Vegetable oil spray
- Salt

Directions:
1. Rinse and peel the potatoes and use a mandolin to slice them into thin rounds. Lay the rounds on a baking sheet and spray with cooking oil on both sides.
2. Sprinkle the rounds with salt and place on the racks of your SnackMaster. Set to 110F and dehydrate for 6 hours or until the chips are dried and crispy.
3. Store in a large zip-lock bag until ready to use.

Nutrition: Calories: 49 Fat: 0.1 gram Carbs: 11.2 grams Protein: 1.2 grams

568. Dehydrated Coconut Wrap
Preparation Time: 15 minutes
Cooking Time: 16 hours
Servings: 1 to 2
Ingredients:
- 1 – 2 tablespoons of raw coconut water
- 2 cups raw coconut meat
- 1/2 teaspoon unrefined sea salt

Directions:
1. Put the coconut meat in a grinder or food processor and pulse to a mushy consistency.
2. Now add the salt and then alternate the pulsing with small quantities of coconut water until the mixture becomes spreadable in consistency but not too thin.
3. Spread the mixture to about 1/4-inch thickness on the dehydrator sheet and dry at 105 degrees. When it dries up on the top, flip it and dry the other side for a few hours.

Nutrition: Calories: 70 Fat: 5 grams Carbs: 6 grams Protein: 1 gram

569. Dehydrated Banana Chips
Preparation Time: 10 minutes
Cooking Time: 20 hours
Servings: 6

Ingredients:
- 2 – 4 ripe bananas

Directions:
1. Cut the bananas into 1/8-inch-thick slices.
2. Prepare the dehydrator as per manufacturer's instructions and line it with parchment paper.
3. Spread out the banana slices on the parchment paper and dry them for 18 – 20 hours or until they are completely dry.

Nutrition: Calories: 60 Fat: 0 gram Carbs: 15 grams Protein: 1 gram

570. Dehydrated Banana Candy

Preparation Time: 10 minutes
Cooking Time: 15 hours
Servings: 6

Ingredients:
- 2 – 4 ripe bananas

Directions:
1. Cut the bananas into 1/4-inch-thick slices.
2. Prepare the dehydrator as per manufacturer's instructions and line it with parchment paper.
3. Spread out the banana slices on the parchment paper and dry them for 15 hours.

Nutrition: Calories: 14 Fat: 0 gram Carbs: 3 grams Protein: 0 gram

571. Garlic Jerky

Preparation Time: 15 minutes
Cooking Time: 4 hours
Servings: 8

Ingredients:
- 3 lbs. flank steak, cut into ¼ inch thick slices
- 2 tablespoon garlic powder
- ¼ cup coconut amino

Directions:
1. In a bowl, mix together garlic powder and coconut amino.
2. Add meat slices to the bowl and mix until well coated. Cover bowl and place in refrigerator for overnight.
3. Remove marinated meat slices from marinade and arrange meat slices on dehydrator racks.
4. Arrange dehydrator tray according to the manufacturer's instructions and dehydrate at 145 F/ 63 C for 4 hours.

Nutrition: Calories: 344 Fat: 14.2 grams Carbs: 3 grams Protein: 47.7 grams

572. Sweet & Tangy Mango Slices

Preparation Time: 15 minutes
Cooking Time: 12 hours
Servings: 6

Ingredients:
- 4 mangoes
- 1 tablespoon honey
- ¼ cup lemon juice

Directions:
1. In a bowl, mix together lemon juice and honey and set aside.
2. Peel the mangoes and cut into ¼ inch thick slices.
3. Add mango slices in lemon honey mixture and coat well.
4. Arrange mango slices on dehydrator racks and dehydrate at 135 F/ 58 C for 12 hours.

Nutrition: Calories: 147 Fat: 0.9 grams Carbs: 36.7 grams Protein: 1.9 grams

573. Dehydrated Bananas

Preparation Time: 15 minutes
Cooking Time: 8 hours
Servings: 4

Ingredients:
- 2 bananas, cut into 1/8-inch-thick slices
- ½ cup fresh lemon juice

Directions:
1. Add sliced bananas and lemon juice in a bowl and toss well.
2. Arrange sliced bananas on dehydrator racks and dehydrate at 135 F/ 58 C for 6-8 hours.

Nutrition: Calories: 60 Fat: 0.4 grams Carbs: 14.1 grams Protein: 0.9 grams

574. Canned Peaches

Preparation Time: 10 minutes
Cooking Time: 8 hours
Servings: 4

Ingredients:
- 2 canned peaches

Directions:
1. Arrange peach slices on dehydrator racks and dehydrate at 135 F/ 58 C for 4 hours.
2. Turn peach slices to other side and dehydrate for 4 hours more.
3. Store in air-tight container.

Nutrition: Calories: 30 Fat: 0.2 grams Carbs: 7 grams Protein: 0.7 grams

575. Peach Wedges

Preparation Time: 15 minutes
Cooking Time: 8 hours
Servings: 4

Ingredients:
- 3 peaches, cut and remove pits and sliced
- ½ cup lemon juice

Directions:
1. Add lemon juice and peach slices into the bowl and toss well.
2. Arrange peach slices on dehydrator racks and dehydrate at 135 F/ 58 C for 6-8 hours.

Nutrition: Calories: 52 Fat: 0.5 grams Carbs: 11.1 grams Protein: 1.3 grams

576. Cinnamon & Vinegar Apple Chips

Preparation Time: 15 minutes
Cooking Time: 12 hours
Servings: 4

Ingredients:
- 4 apples, cored, sliced 1/8 inch thick
- 1 teaspoon ground cinnamon
- 2 cups water
- 1 tablespoon lemon juice
- 1 tablespoon vinegar

Directions:
1. In a bowl, add water, lemon juice, and vinegar and mix well.
2. Add apple slices in the water and let sit for 5 minutes.
3. Remove apple slices from water and pat dry with paper towel.
4. Arrange apple slices on a dehydrator tray and sprinkle with cinnamon and dehydrate at 135 F/ 58 C for 12 hours.

Nutrition: Calories: 119 Fat: 0.4 grams Carbs: 31.4 grams Protein: 0.7 grams

577. Green Apple Chips

Preparation Time: 10 minutes
Cooking Time: 8 hours
Servings: 4

Ingredients:

- 4 green apples, cored and sliced 1/8 inch thick
- ½ lime juice

Directions:
1. Add apple slices and lime juice in a bowl and toss well and set aside for 5 minutes.
2. Arrange apple slices on dehydrator trays and dehydrate at 145 F/ 63 C for 8 hours.
3. Store in air-tight container.

Nutrition: Calories: 117 Fat: 0.4 g Carbs: 31.3 g Protein: 0.6 g

578. Sliced Strawberries

Preparation Time: 10 minutes
Cooking Time: 12 hours
Servings: 4

Ingredients:
- 2 cups strawberries, sliced ¼ inch thick

Directions:
1. Arrange strawberry slices on dehydrator trays and dehydrate at 135 F/ 58 C for 8-12 hours.
2. Store dried strawberries in air-tight container.

Nutrition: Calories: 23 Fat: 0.2 g Carbs: 5.5 g Protein: 0.5 g

579. Dried Raspberries

Preparation Time: 10 minutes
Cooking Time: 18 hours
Servings: 4

Ingredients:
- 4 cups raspberries, wash and dry
- ¼ cup lemon juice

Directions:
1. Add raspberries and lemon juice in a bowl and toss well.
2. Arrange raspberries on dehydrator trays and dehydrate at 135 F/58 C for 15-18 hours.
3. Store in air-tight container.

Nutrition: Calories: 68 Fat: 0.9 grams Carbs: 15 grams Protein: 1.6 grams

580. Bite-Sized Blooming Onions

Preparation Time: 20 minutes
Cooking Time: 14 minutes
Servings: 5

Ingredients:
- 10 ounces raw yellow pearl onions (about 20)
- 1/2 cup all-purpose flour
- 1 teaspoon salt, plus more for sprinkling
- 1/2 teaspoon ground dry mustard
- 1/2 teaspoon chili powder
- 1 large egg
- 1/2 cup whole milk
- 1 cup panko bread crumbs, crushed fine
- 1/2 cup cornmeal

Directions:
1. Shallowly cut the root end off of each onion so it can sit flat but the sections remain attached. Peel and discard the skins. Using a sharp knife, gently slice about three-quarters of the way down through the onion into fifths, as if you were cutting a pie, revealing a total of ten sections, keeping the base intact. Soak the onions in a bowl of ice water 30 minutes to help spread the sections. Transfer onions to a paper towel and remove excess water.discuss
2. Add flour, salt, mustard, and chili powder to a small bowl.
3. In a separate small bowl, whisk together egg and milk.
4. Combine bread crumbs and cornmeal in a shallow dish.
5. Preheat air fryer at 375°F for 3 minutes.
6. Roll onions in flour and spice mixture. Shake off excess flour. Dredge onions in egg mixture. Shake off excess. Roll in bread crumb mixture. Transfer to a plate. Repeat with remaining onions.
7. Add half of onions to fryer basket. Cook 7 minutes. Transfer to a plate and repeat with remaining onions. Sprinkle with salt. Serve warm.

Nutrition: Calories: 192 Fat: 2.1 g Protein: 5.4 g Sodium: 416 mg Fiber: 1.7 g Carbohydrates: 36.0 g Sugar: 4.5 g

581. Mini Scotch Eggs

Preparation Time: 15 minutes
Cooking Time: 10 minutes
Servings: 4

Ingredients:
- 12 quail eggs
- 1 cup ice
- 1 cup water
- 1/2-pound lean ground pork
- 1 teaspoon fresh thyme leaves
- 1/4 teaspoon salt
- 1/4 teaspoon freshly ground black pepper
- 1 large egg
- 1/2 cup panko bread crumbs

Directions:
1. Preheat air fryer at 250°F for 3 minutes.
2. Place eggs in air fryer basket. Cook 4 minutes.
3. Add ice and water to a medium bowl. Transfer eggs to this water bath immediately to stop the cooking process. After 5 minutes, peel eggs.
4. In a medium bowl, combine pork, thyme, salt, and pepper. Form a thin layer of pork around each egg.
5. Preheat air fryer at 375°F for 3 minutes.
6. In a small bowl, whisk large egg. In another bowl, add bread crumbs.
7. Dip covered eggs in whisked egg and then dredge in bread crumbs.
8. Place eggs in air fryer basket. Cook 3 minutes. Turn. Cook an additional 3 minutes. Serve warm.

Nutrition: Calories: 168 Fat: 5.8 g Protein: 17.7 g Sodium: 250 mg Fiber: 0.1 g Carbohydrates: 8.3 g Sugar: 0.5 g

582. Pimiento Cheese-Stuffed Jalapeños

Preparation Time: 10 minutes
Cooking Time: 16 minutes
Servings: 4

Ingredients:
- 6 medium jalapeño peppers
- 1/2 cup pimiento cheese

Directions:
1. Cut jalapeño peppers lengthwise and discard seeds. (If you like the heat, stir the seeds into the pimiento cheese.)
2. Press equal amounts pimiento cheese into each jalapeño half.
3. Preheat air fryer at 350°F for 3 minutes.
4. Lay six stuffed peppers into air fryer basket. Cook 8 minutes. Transfer cooked peppers to a serving plate. Repeat with remaining peppers.
5. Transfer to a serving plate and serve warm.
6. How to Make Pimiento Cheese
7. although prepared pimiento cheese can be purchased in the deli section of most grocery stores, making it couldn't be any easier! simply combine the following ingredients and then refrigerate covered until ready to use. combine: 16 ounces finely shredded sharp cheddar cheese, 1 (4-ounce) jar pimientos including juice, 1/2 cup mayonnaise,

1/4 teaspoon salt, and 1/4 teaspoon freshly ground black pepper. stir. refrigerate 15 minutes.

Nutrition: Calories: 71 Fat: 5.2 g Protein: 4.1 g Sodium: 160 mg Fiber: 0.6 g Carbohydrates: 1.7 g Sugar: 1.0 g

583. Jalapeño Popper Bombs

Preparation Time: 10 minutes
Cooking Time: 12 minutes
Servings: 3

Ingredients:
- 1/3 cup all-purpose flour
- 1/4 teaspoon salt
- 1/4 teaspoon baking powder
- 2 tablespoons diced jalapeño pepper, seeds removed
- 2 ounces cream cheese, at room temperature
- 1 tablespoon shredded Monterey jack cheese
- 2 tablespoons shredded Cheddar cheese
- 2 tablespoons whole milk
- 1/2 teaspoon olive oil

Directions:
1. In a medium bowl, combine flour, salt, and baking powder.
2. In a small bowl, combine remaining ingredients.
3. Pour mixture from small bowl into dry ingredients in medium bowl.
4. Preheat air fryer at 325°F for 3 minutes.
5. Form mixture into nine (1") balls. Place in lightly greased pizza pan (accessory). It's all right if the poppers are touching. Cook 12 minutes.
6. Transfer to a plate. Serve warm.

Nutrition: Calories: 155 Fat: 8.7 g Protein: 4.6 g Sodium: 350 mg Fiber: 0.5 g Carbohydrates: 12.3 g Sugar: 1.3 g

584. Cheddar Biscuit-Breaded Green Olives

Preparation Time: 15 minutes
Cooking Time: 8 minutes
Servings: 5

Ingredients:
- 2/3 cup all-purpose flour
- 1/2 teaspoon baking powder
- 1/2 cup finely grated sharp Cheddar cheese
- 4 tablespoons butter, melted
- 25 pimiento-stuffed standard Manzanilla green olives

Directions:
1. In a food processor, pulse flour, baking powder, cheese, and melted butter until a doughy ball forms.
2. Drain olives and pat dry with a paper towel.
3. Form just enough flour mixture around an olive to cover it. Roll between your hands to form a smooth ball. Repeat with remaining olives.
4. Preheat air fryer at 375°F for 3 minutes.
5. Place olives in lightly greased air fryer basket. Cook 3 minutes. Gently shake. Cook an additional 3 minutes. Gently shake. Cook an additional 2 minutes. Check to see if lightly browned. Give more time if needed; otherwise, transfer to a serving dish and let rest 5 minutes before serving warm.

Nutrition: Calories: 207 Fat: 14.0 g Protein: 4.7 g Sodium: 332 mg Fiber: 0.9 g Carbohydrates: 13.5 g Sugar: 0.2 g

585. Fried Feta-Dill-Breaded Kalamata Olives

Preparation Time: 15 minutes
Cooking Time: 8 minutes
Servings: 5

Ingredients:
- 2/3 cup all-purpose flour
- 1/2 teaspoon baking powder
- 1/2 cup crumbled feta cheese
- 1/2 teaspoon dried dill
- 4 tablespoons butter, melted
- 25 pitted standard Kalamata olives

Directions:
1. In a food processor, pulse flour, baking powder, feta cheese, dill, and melted butter until a doughy ball forms.
2. Drain olives and pat dry with a paper towel.
3. Form just enough flour mixture around an olive to cover it. Roll between your hands to form a smooth ball. Repeat with remaining olives.
4. Preheat air fryer at 375°F for 3 minutes.
5. Place olives in lightly greased air fryer basket. Cook 3 minutes. Gently shake. Cook an additional 3 minutes. Gently shake. Cook an additional 2 minutes. Check to see if lightly browned. Give more time if needed; otherwise, transfer to a serving dish and let rest 5 minutes before serving warm.

Nutrition: Calories: 225 Fat: 16.7 g Protein: 4.0 g Sodium: 475 mg Fiber: 0.5 g Carbohydrates: 13.5 g Sugar: 0.7 g

586. Buffalo-Honey Chicken Wings

Preparation Time: 15 minutes
Cooking Time: 44 minutes
Servings: 6

Ingredients:
- 1 tablespoon water
- 2 pounds chicken wings, split at the joint, tips removed
- 1 tablespoon butter
- 1/2 cup buffalo sauce
- 2 tablespoons honey

Directions:
1. Place 1 tablespoon water in the bottom of the air fryer to ensure minimum smoke from fat drippings.
2. Preheat air fryer at 250°F for 3 minutes.
3. Place half of wings in air fryer basket. Cook 6 minutes. Flip wings. Cook an additional 6 minutes.
4. While wings are cooking, combine butter, wing sauce, and honey in a large bowl. The chicken wings will melt the butter, so don't worry about melting it beforehand.
5. Raise temperature on air fryer to 400°F. Flip wings and cook 5 minutes. Flip wings and cook an additional 5 minutes. Transfer to bowl with sauce and toss.
6. Repeat process with remaining wings and transfer all to a serving dish.

Nutrition: Calories: 368 Fat: 22.9 g Protein: 31.0 g Sodium: 741 mg Fiber: 0.0 g Carbohydrates: 5.8 g Sugar: 5.8 g

587. Peanut Butter And Strawberry Jelly Wings

Preparation Time: 15 minutes
Cooking Time: 44 minutes
Servings: 6

Ingredients:
- 1 tablespoon water
- 2 pounds chicken wings, split at the joint, tips removed
- 2 teaspoons butter
- 1/4 cup creamy peanut butter
- 1/2 cup strawberry jelly
- 2 tablespoons apple cider vinegar
- 1 teaspoon hot sauce

Directions:

1. Place 1 tablespoon water in the bottom of the air fryer to ensure minimum smoke from fat drippings.
2. Preheat air fryer at 250°F for 3 minutes.
3. Place half of wings in air fryer basket. Cook 6 minutes. Flip wings. Cook an additional 6 minutes.
4. While wings are cooking, combine butter, peanut butter, jelly, vinegar, and hot sauce in a large bowl. The chicken wings will melt the butter, so don't worry about melting it beforehand.
5. Raise temperature on air fryer to 400°F. Flip wings and cook 5 minutes. Flip wings and cook an additional 5 minutes. Transfer to bowl with sauce and toss.
6. Repeat process with remaining wings and transfer all to a serving dish.

Nutrition: Calories: 480 Fat: 27.6 g Protein: 33.4 g Sodium: 142 mg Fiber: 0.8 g Carbohydrates: 20.8 g Sugar: 14.1 g

588. Thai Sweet Chili Wings

Preparation Time: 15 minutes
Cooking Time: 44 minutes
Servings: 6
Ingredients:
- 1 tablespoon water
- 2 pounds chicken wings, split at the joint, tips removed
- 1/2 cup Sweet Chili Sauce

Directions:
1. Place 1 tablespoon water in the bottom of the air fryer to ensure minimum smoke from fat drippings.
2. Preheat air fryer at 250°F for 3 minutes.
3. Place half of wings in air fryer basket. Cook 6 minutes. Flip wings. Cook an additional 6 minutes.
4. While wings are cooking, add sauce to a large bowl.
5. Raise temperature on air fryer to 400°F. Flip wings and cook 5 minutes. Flip wings and cook an additional 5 minutes. Transfer to bowl with sauce and toss.
6. Repeat process with remaining wings and transfer all to a serving dish.

Nutrition: Calories: 472 Fat: 21.1 g Protein: 31.1 g Sodium: 238 mg Fiber: 0.0 g Carbohydrates: 35.2 g Sugar: 33.6 g

589. Salmon Croquettes

Preparation Time: 15 minutes
Cooking Time: 24 minutes
Servings: 4
Ingredients:
- 1 (14.75-ounce) can wild-caught salmon, drained
- 1/3 cup mayonnaise
- 1 tablespoon minced celery
- 2 teaspoons dried dill, divided
- 1 teaspoon lime juice
- 1/2 cup panko bread crumbs, divided
- 1 large egg
- 1 teaspoon prepared horseradish
- 1/4 cup cornmeal
- 1 teaspoon salt

Directions:
1. In a medium bowl, combine salmon, mayonnaise, celery, 1 teaspoon dill, lime juice, 1/4 cup bread crumbs, egg, and horseradish.
2. In a shallow dish, combine 1/4 cup bread crumbs, cornmeal, remaining dill, and salt.
3. Preheat air fryer at 375°F for 3 minutes.
4. Form 2 tablespoons salmon mixture into sixteen tots or egg shapes. Roll in bread crumb mixture. Continue with remainder of salmon.
5. Place eight tots in lightly greased air fryer basket. Cook 4 minutes. Gently turn tots a third of the way around. Cook an additional 4 minutes. Gently turn tots another third. Cook an additional 4 minutes. Transfer to a serving dish. Repeat with remaining tots. Let rest 5 minutes before serving warm.

Nutrition: Calories: 395 Fat: 20.1 g Protein: 31.6 g Sodium: 1,154 mg Fiber: 0.5 g Carbohydrates: 18.6 g Sugar: 1.0 g

590. Pepperoni Pizza Bites

Preparation Time: 10 minutes
Cooking Time: 12 minutes
Servings: 2
Ingredients:
- 1/3 cup all-purpose flour
- 1/4 teaspoon salt
- 1/4 teaspoon baking powder
- 1/2 cup small-diced pepperoni
- 2 ounces cream cheese, at room temperature
- 1/4 cup shredded mozzarella cheese
- 1/2 teaspoon Italian seasoning
- 2 tablespoons whole milk
- 1 teaspoon olive oil

Directions:
1. In a small bowl, combine flour, salt, and baking powder.
2. In a medium bowl, combine remaining ingredients until smooth. Add dry ingredients until well combined.
3. Preheat air fryer at 325°F for 5 minutes.
4. Form mixture into nine (1") balls and add to pizza pan (accessory). It's all right if the pizza bites are touching. Cook 12 minutes.
5. Transfer to a plate. Serve warm.

Nutrition: Calories: 366 Fat: 22.8 g Protein: 13.1 g Sodium: 987 mg Fiber: 0.6 g Carbohydrates: 18.2 g Sugar: 1.9 g

591. Broccoli Snackers

Preparation Time: 10 minutes
Cooking Time: 12 minutes
Servings: 4
Ingredients:
- 1 large head of broccoli, chopped into florets
- 1 tablespoon olive oil
- 1/2 teaspoon salt

Directions:
1. Preheat air fryer at 350°F for 3 minutes.
2. In a large bowl, toss broccoli florets with olive oil.
3. Place half of broccoli in fryer basket. Cook 3 minutes. Shake. Cook an additional 3 minutes. Transfer to a serving bowl. Season with salt.
4. Repeat with remaining broccoli and serve warm.

Nutrition: Calories: 81 Fat: 3.4 g Protein: 4.3 g Sodium: 340 mg Fiber: 4.0 g Carbohydrates: 10.1 g Sugar: 2.6 g

592. Bite-Sized Pork Egg Rolls

Preparation Time: 30 minutes
Cooking Time: 24 minutes
Servings: 10
Ingredients:
- 1/2-pound lean ground pork
- 2 cups coleslaw mix (shredded cabbage and carrots)
- 3 scallions, trimmed and minced
- 1 tablespoon hoisin sauce
- 1 tablespoon soy sauce
- 1/4 teaspoon sriracha
- 1/2 teaspoon lime juice
- 30 wonton wrappers

- 2 teaspoons olive oil

Directions:
1. In a large skillet, heat ground pork over medium-high heat. Stir-fry 5–6 minutes until no longer pink. Add coleslaw mix and stir into pork. Add scallions, hoisin sauce, soy sauce, sriracha, and lime juice. Stir-fry an additional 2 minutes. Remove from heat and let rest 5 minutes off the burner.
2. Place a wonton wrapper on a cutting board. Place a small bowl of water near the board. Spoon approximately 2 teaspoons mixture in a line in the middle of the wrapper. Dip your finger into the water and lightly run it around the perimeter of the wonton wrapper. Fold 1/4" of the perimeter of wonton toward the middle. Roll up the length to form an egg roll. Repeat for each wonton wrapper.
3. Preheat air fryer at 325°F for 3 minutes.
4. Place half of the egg rolls in the air fryer basket. Cook 3 minutes. Lightly brush the tops of egg rolls with olive oil. Cook an additional 5 minutes. Repeat with second batch.
5. Transfer to a plate. Serve warm.

Nutrition: Calories: 106 Fat: 1.2 g Protein: 7.5 g Sodium: 268 mg Fiber: 0.9 g Carbohydrates: 15.7 g Sugar: 1.0 g

593. Green Chili Crispy Wonton Squares

Preparation Time: 15 minutes
Cooking Time: 35 minutes
Servings: 6

Ingredients:
- 30 wonton wrappers
- 1 cup refried beans
- 2 (4-ounce) cans diced green chilies
- 1 cup grated queso fresco

Directions:
1. Place a wonton wrapper on a cutting board. Place approximately 1 1/2 teaspoons beans in the middle of wrapper. Add approximately 1 1/2 teaspoons green chilies and approximately 1 1/2 teaspoons queso fresco.
2. Place a small bowl of water near the working area. Dip your finger in the water bowl and run it around the perimeter of the wonton. Bring all corners to the center and press the straight edges together. Set aside. Repeat with remaining wontons.
3. Preheat air fryer at 325°F for 3 minutes.
4. Place six wontons in air fryer basket. Cook 7 minutes. Transfer to a plate and cook the remaining batches. Serve warm.

Nutrition: Calories: 220 Fat: 4.8 g Protein: 9.7 g Sodium: 680 mg Fiber: 3.9 g Carbohydrates: 31.7 g Sugar: 2.0 g

594. Brie And Red Pepper Jelly Triangles

Preparation Time: 10 minutes
Cooking Time: 16 minutes
Servings: 4

Ingredients:
- 20 wonton wrappers
- 10 teaspoons Brie cheese
- 10 teaspoons red pepper jelly
- 40 almond slivers
- 1 tablespoon olive oil

Directions:
1. Place a wonton wrapper on a cutting board. Place approximately 1/2 teaspoon Brie and then 1/2 teaspoon red pepper jelly in the middle of wrapper. Place 2 almond slivers on top.
2. Place a small bowl of water near the working area. Dip your finger in the water bowl and run it around the perimeter of the wonton. Fold one corner to the opposite corner, forming a triangle. Press down edges to seal. Set aside. Repeat with remaining wontons.
3. Preheat air fryer at 325°F for 3 minutes.
4. Place half of the triangles in the air fryer basket. Cook 3 minutes. Lightly brush the tops of triangles with olive oil. Cook an additional 5 minutes. Repeat with second batch.
5. Transfer to a plate. Serve warm.

Nutrition: Calories: 239 Fat: 8.9 g Protein: 6.9 g Sodium: 292 mg Fiber: 1.6 g Carbohydrates: 32.2 g Sugar: 7.8 g

595. Reuben Pizza For One

Preparation Time: 10 minutes
Cooking Time: 17 minutes
Servings: 1

Ingredients:
- 1/4-pound fresh pizza dough, about the size of a tennis ball
- 1/4 teaspoon caraway seeds
- 2 tablespoons Thousand Island dressing (or Russian dressing)
- 1/4 cup chopped corned beef
- 1/4 cup shredded Swiss cheese
- 1/4 cup sauerkraut, drained

Directions:
1. Preheat air fryer at 200°F for 6 minutes.
2. Press out dough to fit pizza pan (accessory). Sprinkle caraway seeds evenly over dough. Cook 7 minutes.
3. Turn up the heat to 275°F.
4. Remove basket and spread dressing over dough, leaving 1/4" outer crust uncovered. Evenly add corned beef. Sprinkle cheese over meat. Cook an additional 10 minutes.
5. Gently transfer pizza to a cutting board. Evenly add sauerkraut. Cut into six slices and serve.

Nutrition: Calories: 848 Fat: 42.5 g Protein: 41.3 g Sodium: 2,409 mg Fiber: 3.1 g Carbohydrates: 62.7 g Sugar: 12.8 g

596. Parsnip Sticks

Preparation Time: 10 minutes
Cooking Time: 20 minutes
Servings: 4

Ingredients:
- 1 pound parsnips, peeled and cut into sticks
- Salt and black pepper to the taste
- 2 tablespoons butter, melted
- Juice of 1 lime
- 1 teaspoon mint, dried
- 1 teaspoon rosemary, dried

Directions:
1. In the air fryer's basket, mix the parsnip sticks with the melted butter and the other ingredients, toss, cook at 320 degrees F for 20 minutes and serve as a snack.

Nutrition: Calories 40 Fat 3 Fiber 7 Carbs 3 Protein 7

597. Turmeric Sweet Potato Bites

Preparation Time: 10 minutes
Cooking Time: 25 minutes
Servings: 4

Ingredients:
- 2 sweet potatoes, peeled and roughly cubed
- 1 tablespoon olive oil
- ½ teaspoon sweet paprika

- 1 teaspoon turmeric powder
- 1 tablespoon chives, chopped
- Salt and black pepper to the taste

Directions:
1. In the air fryer's basket, mix the potato bites with the oil, paprika and the other ingredients, toss and cook at 380 degrees F for 25 minutes, shaking the fryer from time to time.
2. Serve as a snack right away.

Nutrition: Calories 161 Fat 1 Fiber 2 Carbs 5 Protein 3

598. Avocado Balls

Preparation Time: 10 minutes
Cooking Time: 16 minutes
Servings: 6

Ingredients:
- 10 oz. ground beef
- 1/3 teaspoon salt
- 1 onion, diced
- 1 avocado, pitted, peeled
- ½ teaspoon ground black pepper
- 1 tablespoon avocado oil

Directions:
1. Blend the avocado and put it in the bowl.
2. Add ground beef and salt.
3. After this, add the diced onion and ground black pepper.
4. Stir the ground beef mixture until homogenous.
5. Make the medium balls from the mixture and put them in the air fryer basket.
6. Sprinkle the avocado balls with the oil and cook them for 16 minutes at 365 F.
7. Stir the avocado balls time to time with the help of a spatula.
8. Serve it!

Nutrition: Calories 164 Fat 9.5 Fiber 2.7 Carbs 4.7 Protein 15.2

599. Hard-Boiled Egg Halves with Bacon

Preparation Time: 10 minutes
Cooking Time: 15 minutes
Servings: 6

Ingredients:
- 3 eggs
- 6 oz. bacon, chopped, cooked
- 1 teaspoon fresh parsley, chopped
- 1 teaspoon fresh dill, chopped
- 1 teaspoon olive oil
- 1 cherry tomato

Directions:
1. Put the eggs in the air fryer basket.
2. Cook the eggs for 15 minutes at 250 F.
3. Meanwhile, mix together the parsley, dill, and olive oil.
4. Chop the cherry tomato and add the green mixture.
5. Stir the mixture.
6. When the eggs are cooked – chill them and peel.
7. Cut the eggs into the halves.
8. Then place the bacon over the egg halves and add the green mixture.
9. Serve the appetizer immediately!

Nutrition: Calories 192 Fat 14.8 Fiber 0 Carbs 0.7 Protein 13.3

600. Stuffed Figs with Almonds

Preparation Time: 10 minutes
Cooking Time: 5 minutes
Servings: 2

Ingredients:
- 2 figs, dried
- 1 oz. almonds
- ¾ teaspoon ground cinnamon
- 1 teaspoon fresh lemon juice

Directions:
1. Mix up together the ground cinnamon and lemon juice. Stir the mixture.
2. Make the cuts in the figs and fill with the ground cinnamon.
3. Add almonds and place in the air fryer basket.
4. Cook the figs for 5 minutes at 360 F.
5. Then chill the figs and serve!

Nutrition: Calories 132 Fat 7.3 Fiber 4.1 Carbs 15.9 Protein 3.7

601. Pear Chips

Preparation Time: 10 minutes
Cooking Time: 25 minutes
Servings: 6

Ingredients:
- 3 pears
- ¾ teaspoon nutmeg

Directions:
1. Wash the pears and cut into the halves.
2. Remove the seeds and slice.
3. Place the sliced pears on the air fryer rack and sprinkle with the nutmeg.
4. Cook the pears for 25 minutes at 350 F.
5. Flip the sliced pears during cooking if desired.
6. Serve the cooked pear chips and enjoy!

Nutrition: Calories 62 Fat 0.3 Fiber 3.3 Carbs 16.1 Protein 0.4

602. Peach Chips

Preparation Time: 8 minutes
Cooking Time: 6 minutes
Servings: 6

Ingredients:
- 6 peaches
- ¼ teaspoon ground cinnamon
- 1 teaspoon water

Directions:
1. Remove the stones from the peaches.
2. Sprinkle peaches with the ground cinnamon and water.
3. Then place the peaches on the air fryer rack.
4. Cook the peaches for 15 minutes at 380 F.
5. When the time is over – remove the cooked chips from the air fryer and chill well.
6. Serve.

Nutrition: Calories 59 Fat 0.4 Fiber 2.4 Carbs 14.1 Protein 1.4

603. Garlic Tomato Circles

Preparation Time: 10 minutes
Cooking Time: 20 minutes
Servings: 4

Ingredients:
- 2 tomatoes
- ¼ teaspoon salt
- 1 garlic clove, chopped
- 1 teaspoon olive oil
- ¾ teaspoon chili flakes

Directions:
1. Slice the tomatoes into the circles.
2. Then mix up together the chili flakes, olive oil, salt, and chopped garlic.
3. Stir the mixture.
4. Rub the tomato circles with the oil mixture well.
5. Put the tomatoes on the air fryer rack and cook them for 20 minutes at 345 F.

6. Stir the tomatoes every 4 minutes.
7. When the time is over and the tomatoes are cooked – chill them well and serve!

Nutrition: Calories 22 Fat 1.3 Fiber 0.8 Carbs 2.7 Protein 0.6

604. Beef Muffins

Preparation Time: 15 minutes
Cooking Time: 25 minutes
Servings: 6

Ingredients:
- 1 egg
- 10 oz. ground beef
- 1 tablespoon chives
- 1 teaspoon paprika
- ½ teaspoon chili flakes
- 1 tablespoon almond flour
- ¼ teaspoon salt

Directions:
1. Put the ground beef in the bowl and beat the egg in it.
2. Add paprika, chili flakes, and almond flour.
3. After this, add salt and stir it carefully.
4. Place the ground beef mixture in the muffin molds and put them in the air fryer.
5. Cook the beef muffins for 25 minutes at 360 F.
6. Then chill the beef muffins little and discard from the molds.
7. Serve!

Nutrition: Calories 126 Fat 6.1 Fiber 0.6 Carbs 1.3 Protein 16.3

605. Trout Balls

Preparation Time: 10 minutes
Cooking Time: 8 minutes
Servings: 8

Ingredients:
- 10 oz. trout fillet
- ¼ teaspoon minced garlic
- ¼ teaspoon salt
- 1 teaspoon ground coriander
- 1 egg
- 2 tablespoons almond flour
- 1 teaspoon olive oil
- 1 teaspoon dried dill

Directions:
1. Chop the trout into the tiny pieces and combine it together with the minced garlic, salt, and ground coriander.
2. Beat the egg in the mixture and add almond flour and dried dill.
3. Stir it carefully until homogenous.
4. Make the small balls from the fish mixture with the help of 2 spoons.
5. Place the fish balls in the air fryer basket and sprinkle with the olive oil.
6. Cook the trout balls for 8 minutes at 380 F.
7. Chill the fish balls little and serve!

Nutrition: Calories 121 Fat 7.7 Fiber 0.8 Carbs 1.6 Protein 11.7

606. Papaya Sticks

Preparation Time: 10 minutes
Cooking Time: 8 minutes
Servings: 2

Ingredients:
- 12 oz. papaya
- 1 tablespoon almond flour
- 1 teaspoon vanilla extract

Directions:
1. Peel the papaya and cut into the sticks.
2. Sprinkle the papaya sticks with the almond flour and vanilla extract.
3. Put the papaya sticks on the air fryer rack and cook them for 8 minutes at 380 F. Flip the papaya sticks on another side after 4 minutes of cooking.
4. Chill the cooked snack and serve!

Nutrition: Calories 161 Fat 7.5 Fiber 4.5 Carbs 22.4 Protein 3.9

607. Beet Chips

Preparation Time: 5 minutes
Cooking Time: 10 minutes
Servings: 4

Ingredients:
- 14 oz. beet
- 1 teaspoon olive oil
- ½ teaspoon dried oregano

Directions:
1. Peel the beet and slice into the chips.
2. Put the sliced beet on the air fryer rack and sprinkle with the olive oil and dried oregano.
3. Cook the beet chips for 10 minutes at 360 F.
4. Chill the cooked beet chips well and serve!

Nutrition: Calories 54 Fat 1.4 Fiber 2.1 Carbs 10 Protein 1.7

608. Broccoli Steaks

Preparation Time: 9 minutes
Cooking Time: 6 minutes
Servings: 4

Ingredients:
- 10 oz. broccoli head
- 1 tablespoon olive oil
- ¼ teaspoon turmeric
- ½ teaspoon salt
- 1 tablespoon almond flour

Directions:
1. Slice the broccoli into the steaks.
2. Sprinkle the broccoli steaks with the olive oil, turmeric, salt, and almond flour.
3. Stir them gently.
4. After this, put the broccoli in the air fryer basket and cook for 6 minutes at 400 F. Stir the broccoli steaks after 3 minutes.
5. Serve the cooked broccoli steak immediately!

Nutrition: Calories 95 Fat 7.2 Fiber 2.6 Carbs 6.3 Protein 3.5

609. Devil Eggs with Pesto

Preparation Time: 10 minutes
Cooking Time: 15 minutes
Servings: 2

Ingredients:
- 2 eggs
- 1 cup fresh basil
- ¼ cup walnuts
- 2 tablespoons olive oil
- ¼ teaspoon salt
- ¼ teaspoon chili flakes

Directions:
1. Place the eggs on the air fryer rack and cook them at 250 F for 15 minutes.
2. Meanwhile, place the walnuts, olive oil, salt, and chili flakes in the blender.
3. Add the fresh basil and blend the mixture until smooth.
4. When the eggs are cooked – chill them and peel.
5. Cut the eggs into the halves and remove the egg whites.
6. Put the egg whites in the blender and blend the mixture for 30 seconds more.

7. Then fill the egg whites with the egg yolk pesto mixture.
8. Serve and enjoy!

Nutrition: Calories 282 Fat 27.7 Fiber 1.3 Carbs 2.2 Protein 9.7

610. Crab Balls

Preparation Time: 5 minutes
Cooking Time: 20 minutes
Servings: 8

Ingredients:
- ½ cup coconut cream
- 2 tablespoons chives, mined
- 1 egg, whisked
- 1 teaspoon mustard
- 1 teaspoon lemon juice
- 16 ounces lump crabmeat, chopped
- 2/3 cup almond meal
- A pinch of salt and black pepper
- Cooking spray

Directions:
1. In a bowl, mix all the ingredients except the cooking spray and stir well.
2. Shape medium balls out of this mix, place them in the fryer and cook at 390 degrees F for 20 minutes.
3. Serve as an appetizer.

Nutrition: Calories 141 Fat 7 Fiber 2 Carbs 4 Protein 9

DESSERTS RECIPES

611. Tasty Banana Cake
Preparation Time: 40 minutes
Cooking Time: 30 minutes
Servings: 4
Ingredients:
- 1 tbsp. butter, soft
- 1 egg
- 1/3 cup brown sugar
- 2 tbsp. honey
- 1 banana
- 1 cup white flour
- 1 tbsp. baking powder
- ½ tbsp. cinnamon powder
- Cooking spray

Directions:
1. Spurt cake pan with cooking spray.
2. Mix in butter with honey, sugar, banana, cinnamon, egg, flour and baking powder in a bowl then beat.
3. Empty mix in cake pan with cooking spray, put into air fryer and cook at 350°F for 30 minutes.
4. Allow for cooling, slice.
5. Serve.

Nutrition: Calories: 259 kcal Protein: 7.17 g Fat: 7.12 g Carbohydrates: 41.77 g

612. Simple Cheesecake
Preparation Time: 25 minutes
Cooking Time: 20 minutes
Servings: 15
Ingredients:
- 1 lb. cream cheese
- ½ tbsp. vanilla extract
- 2 eggs
- 4 tbsp. sugar
- 1 cup graham crackers
- 2 tbsp. butter

Directions:
1. Mix in butter with crackers in a bowl.
2. Compress crackers blend to the bottom cake pan, put into air fryer and cook at 350° F for 4 minutes.
3. Mix cream cheese with sugar, vanilla, egg in a bowl and beat properly.
4. Sprinkle filling on crackers crust and cook cheesecake in air fryer at 310° F for 15 minutes.
5. Keep cake in fridge for 3 hours, slice.
6. Serve.

Nutrition: Calories: 136 kcal Protein: 3.8 g Fat: 11.93 g Carbohydrates: 3.51 g

613. Bread Pudding
Preparation Time: 20 minutes
Cooking Time: 10 minutes
Servings: 4
Ingredients:
- 6 glazed doughnuts
- 1 cup cherries
- 4 egg yolks
- 1 and ½ cups whipping cream
- ½ cup raisins
- ¼ cup sugar
- ½ cup chocolate chips

Directions:
1. Mix in cherries with whipping cream and egg in a bowl then turn properly.
2. Mix in raisins with chocolate chips, sugar and doughnuts in a bowl then stir.
3. Mix the 2 mixtures, pour into oiled pan then into air fryer and cook at 310° F for 1 hour.
4. Cool pudding before cutting.
5. Serve.

Nutrition: Calories: 452 kcal Protein: 8.43 g Fat: 25.71 g Carbohydrates: 47.34 g

614. Bread Dough And Amaretto Dessert
Preparation Time: 20 minutes
Cooking Time: 10 minutes
Servings: 12
Ingredients:
- 1 lb. bread dough
- 1 cup sugar
- ½ cup butter
- 1 cup heavy cream
- 12 oz. chocolate chips
- 2 tbsp. amaretto liqueur

Directions:
1. Turn dough, cut into 20 slices and cut each piece in halves.
2. Sweep dough pieces with spray sugar, butter, put into air fryer's basket and cook them at 350°F for 5 minutes. Turn them, cook for 3 minutes still. Move to a platter.
3. Melt the heavy cream in pan over medium heat, put chocolate chips and turn until they melt.
4. Put in liqueur, turn and move to a bowl.
5. Serve bread dippers with the sauce.

Nutrition: Calories: 331 kcal Protein: 4.76 g Fat: 13.46 g Carbohydrates: 47.09 g

615. Wrapped Pears
Preparation Time: 15 minutes
Cooking Time: 10 minutes
Servings: 4
Ingredients:
- 4 puff pastry sheets
- 14 oz. vanilla custard
- 2 pears
- 1 egg
- ½ tbsp. cinnamon powder
- 2 tbsp. sugar

Directions:
1. Put wisp pastry slices on flat surface, add spoonful of vanilla custard at the center of each, add pear halves and wrap.
2. Sweep pears with egg, cinnamon and spray sugar, put into air fryer's basket and cook at 320°F for 15 minutes.
3. Split parcels on plates.
4. Serve.

Nutrition: Calories: 171 kcal Protein: 5.57 g Fat: 4.53 g Carbohydrates: 30.04 g

616. Air Fried Bananas
Preparation Time: 15 minutes
Cooking Time: 10 minutes
Servings: 4
Ingredients:

- 3 tbsp. butter
- 2 eggs
- 8 bananas
- ½ cup corn flour
- 3 tbsp. cinnamon sugar
- 1 cup panko

Directions:
1. Warm up pan with the butter over medium heat, put panko, turn and cook for 4 minutes then move to a bowl.
2. Spin each in flour, panko, egg blend, assemble them in air fryer's basket, grime with cinnamon sugar and cook at 280° F for 10 minutes.
3. Serve immediately.

Nutrition: Calories: 238 kcal Protein: 7.19 g Fat: 15.54 g Carbohydrates: 17.74 g

617. Cocoa Cake

Preparation Time: 15 minutes
Cooking Time: 10 minutes
Servings: 6

Ingredients:
- 3.5 oz. butter
- 3 eggs
- 3 oz. sugar
- 1 tbsp. cocoa powder
- 3 oz. flour
- ½ tbsp. lemon juice

Directions:
1. Mix in 1 tablespoon butter with cocoa powder in a bowl and beat.
2. Mix in the rest of the butter with eggs, flour, sugar and lemon juice in another bowl, blend properly and move half into a cake pan
3. Put half of the cocoa blend, spread, add the rest of the butter layer and crest with remaining cocoa.
4. Put into air fryer and cook at 360° F for 17 minutes.
5. Allow to cool before slicing.
6. Serve.

Nutrition: Calories: 306 kcal Protein: 7.32 g Fat: 19.5 g Carbohydrates: 26.1 g

618. Apple Bread

Preparation Time: 15 minutes
Cooking Time: 10 minutes
Servings: 6

Ingredients:
- 3 cups apples
- 1 cup sugar
- 1 tbsp. vanilla
- 2 eggs
- 1 tbsp. apple pie spice
- 2 cups white flour
- 1 tbsp. baking powder
- 1 stick butter
- 1 cup water

Directions:
1. Mix in egg with 1 butter stick, sugar, apple pie spice and turn using mixer.
2. Put apples and turn properly.
3. Mix baking powder with flour in another bowl and turn.
4. Blend the 2 mixtures, turn and move it to spring form pan.
5. Get spring form pan into air fryer and cook at 320°F for 40 minutes
6. Slice. Serve.

Nutrition: Calories: 443 kcal Protein: 8.66 g Fat: 20 g Carbohydrates: 56.57 g

619. Mini Lava Cakes

Preparation Time: 15 minutes
Cooking Time: 10 minutes
Servings: 3

Ingredients:
- 1 egg
- 4 tbsp. sugar
- 2 tbsp. olive oil
- 4 tbsp. milk
- 4 tbsp. flour
- 1 tbsp. cocoa powder
- ½ tbsp. baking powder
- ½ tbsp. orange zest

Directions:
1. Mix in egg with sugar, flour, salt, oil, milk, orange zest, baking powder and cocoa powder, turn properly. Move it to oiled ramekins.
2. Put ramekins in air fryer and cook at 320°F for 20 minutes.
3. Serve warm.

Nutrition: Calories: 249 kcal Protein: 7.17 g Fat: 15.24 g Carbohydrates: 22.39 g

620. Crispy Apples

Preparation Time: 20 minutes
Cooking Time: 10 minutes
Servings: 4

Ingredients:
- 2 tbsp. cinnamon powder
- 5 apples
- ½ tbsp. nutmeg powder
- 1 tbsp. maple syrup
- ½ cup water
- 4 tbsp. butter
- ¼ cup flour
- ¾ cup oats
- ¼ cup brown sugar

Directions:
1. Get the apples in a pan, put in nutmeg, maple syrup, cinnamon and water.
2. Mix in butter with flour, sugar, salt and oat, turn, put spoonful of blend over apples, get into air fryer and cook at 350°F for 10 minutes.
3. Serve while warm.

Nutrition: Calories: 392 kcal Protein: 6.4 g Fat: 15.1 g Carbohydrates: 69.48 g

621. Ginger Cheesecake

Preparation Time: 2 hours and 30 minutes
Cooking Time: 20 minutes
Servings: 6

Ingredients:
- 2 tbsp. butter
- ½ cup ginger cookies
- 16 oz. cream cheese
- 2 eggs
- ½ cup sugar
- 1 tbsp. rum
- ½ tbsp. vanilla extract
- ½ tbsp. nutmeg

Directions:
1. Spread pan with the butter and sprinkle cookie crumbs on the bottom.

2. Whisk cream cheese with rum, vanilla, nutmeg and eggs, beat properly and sprinkle the cookie crumbs.
3. Put in air fryer and cook at 340° F for 20 minutes.
4. Allow cheese cake to cool in fridge for 2 hours before slicing.
5. Serve.

Nutrition: Calories: 364 kcal Protein: 9.64 g Fat: 29.96 g Carbohydrates: 13.15 g

622. Cocoa Cookies

Preparation Time: 15 minutes
Cooking Time: 10 minutes
Servings: 12
Ingredients:
- 6 oz. coconut oil
- 6 eggs
- 3 oz. cocoa powder
- 2 tbsp. vanilla
- ½ tbsp. baking powder
- 4 oz. cream cheese
- 5 tbsp. sugar

Directions:
1. Mix in eggs with coconut oil, baking powder, cocoa powder, cream cheese, vanilla in a blender and sway and turn using a mixer.
2. Get it into a lined baking dish and into the fryer at 320°F and bake for 14 minutes.
3. Split cookie sheet into rectangles.
4. Serve.

Nutrition: Calories: 136 kcal Protein: 6.89 g Fat: 8.27 g Carbohydrates: 7.03 g

623. Special Brownies

Preparation Time: 10 minutes
Cooking Time: 20 minutes
Servings: 4
Ingredients:
- 1 egg
- 1/3 cup cocoa powder
- 1/3 cup sugar
- 7 tbsp. butter
- ½ tbsp. vanilla extract
- ¼ cup white flour
- ¼ cup walnuts
- ½ tbsp. baking powder
- 1 tbsp. peanut butter

Directions:
1. Warm pan with 6 tablespoons butter and the sugar over medium heat, turn, cook for 5 minutes, move to a bowl, put salt, egg, cocoa powder, vanilla extract, walnuts, baking powder and flour, turn mix properly and into a pan.
2. Mix peanut butter with one tablespoon butter in a bowl, heat in microwave for some seconds, turn properly and sprinkle brownies blend over.
3. Put in air fryer and bake at 320° F and bake for 17 minutes.
4. Allow brownies to cool, cut.
5. Serve.

Nutrition: Calories: 358 kcal Protein: 7.19 g Fat: 29.08 g Carbohydrates: 21.37g

624. Blueberry Scones

Preparation Time: 20 minutes
Cooking Time: 10 minutes
Servings:10
Ingredients:
- 1 cup white flour
- 1 cup blueberries
- 2 eggs
- ½ cup heavy cream
- ½ cup butter
- 5 tbsp. sugar
- 2 tbsp. vanilla extract
- 2 tbsp. baking powder

Directions:
1. Mix in flour, baking powder, salt and blueberries in a bowl and turn.
2. Mix heavy cream with vanilla extract, sugar, butter and eggs and turn properly.
3. Blend the 2 mixtures, squeeze till dough is ready, obtain 10 triangles from mix, put on baking sheet into air fryer and cook them at 320°F for 10 minutes.
4. Serve cold.

Nutrition: Calories: 227 kcal Protein: 4.11 g Fat: 14.17 g Carbohydrates: 19.88 g

625. Half Dipped Chocolate Biscuits

Preparation Time: 20 minutes
Cooking Time: 15 minutes
Servings: 6
Ingredients:
- 4 oz. butter
- 4 oz. white sugar
- 8 oz. self-raising flour
- 1 tsp vanilla essence
- 1 small egg beaten
- 2 oz. milk chocolate

Directions:
1. Get a clean mixing bowl, and in it, combine the butter, sugar, and flour. Rub the butter into the flour until you have the mixture appearing like breadcrumbs.
2. Now pour in the vanilla essence and the egg, gradually, until the mixture turns into a dough.
3. Shape the dough into walnut-sized balls. Transfer the balls into the air fryer.
4. Allow cooking at 360 F for 15 minutes.
5. With the biscuits cooling, melt the milk chocolate in the air fryer - at 360 F for 4 minutes. While melting, stir constantly, the mixture is clearly in the liquid form.
6. Dip one side of the cool biscuits in the chocolate. Transfer them into the fridge and allow them to refrigerate for an hour.
7. Serve the set biscuits.

Nutrition: Calories: 377 kcal Protein: 6.09 g Fat: 17.68 g Carbohydrates: 48.3 g

626. Chocolate Cake

Preparation Time: 30 minutes
Cooking Time: 15 minutes
Servings: 4
Ingredients:
- Cooking spray
- 3 ½ tbsp. butter, softened
- ¼ cup white sugar
- 1 tbsp. apricot jam leg
- 6 tbsp. all-purpose flour
- Salt to taste
- 1 tbsp. unsweetened cocoa powder

Directions:
1. Ensure that your air fryer is preheated to 320 F.

DESSERTS RECIPES

2. Get a small fluted pan and spray with some cooking spray.
3. Combine butter and sugar into a clean bowl. Beat the mixture with an electric mixer until you have a creamy and light mixture. Now toss in the jam and egg, and mix thoroughly. Sift in the flour, salt, cocoa powder and mix well again.
4. Transfer the batter into the sprayed pan, and return it into the air fryer basket.
5. Cook in the air fryer until a toothpick inserted into the center of the cake comes out unstained - this takes about 15 minutes.

Nutrition: Calories: 195 kcal Protein: 3.56 g Fat: 14.31 g Carbohydrates: 14.54 g

627. Chocolate Cupcakes With Cream Cheese Frosting

Preparation Time: 25 minutes
Cooking Time: 25 minutes
Servings: 8
Ingredients:
- ¼ of the mixture chocolate cake batter
- 3 oz. butter
- 9 oz. brown sugar
- 14 oz. soft cheese
- 1 tbsp. vanilla essence
- 3 tbsp. organic cocoa powder

Directions:
1. The first step is to make the cake batter - simply mix it like you were making a chocolate cake. Set aside when ready.
2. Get eight small cupcake cases. Flour the base of each, as well as the sides. This prevents them from getting sticky.
3. Pour in the cake batter into each of the cases until they are ¾-filled.
4. Transfer them into the air fryer and allow cooking at 400 F for 7 minutes.
5. To make the cream frosting, combine the butter, brown sugar, soft cheese, and vanilla in a clean mixing bowl. Use a hand mixer to mix until the mixture is creamy and smooth.
6. Transfer the frosting into the freezer and leave for an hour. This makes it firm up a bit.
7. With the aid of the cake decorating kit, add ¼ of the set frosting cake into the cake decorator.
8. Using a fork, mix in the cocoa powder in the bowl until the mixture appears nice and chocolate in color.
9. Add the rest of the mixture into the cake decorating kit, and swirl the cupcake layer right on the top of the buns.
10. Keep the buns in the fridge for 20 minutes before serving.

Nutrition: Calories: 351 kcal Protein: 10.45 g Fat: 20.11 g Carbohydrates: 33.22

628. Almost Guilt-Free Cinnamon Doughnut

Preparation Time: 10 minutes
Cooking Time: 5 minutes
Servings: 2 to 3
Ingredients:
- 14 oz. plan flour/all-purpose flour
- 1 cup milk
- 1½ tsp instant yeast
- 1½ oz. butter
- 4 oz. brown sugar
- ½ tsp ground cinnamon

Directions:
1. Combine all your ingredients in the bread maker pan in the order provided by your manufacturer.
2. With the bread maker set to DOUGH setting, allow it to run till it stops.
3. Roll dough out until you have a thickness of ¼ - inch. Cut the doughnuts using your doughnuts cutter.
4. Ensure that your air fryer is preheated to 305 F. Bake 3-4 doughnuts at once, for 5 minutes or until they are golden brown.

Nutrition: Calories: 814 kcal Protein: 19.22 g Fat: 17.5 g Carbohydrates: 143.53 g

629. Donuts Recipe

Preparation Time: 20 minutes
Cooking Time: 5 minutes
Servings: 8
Ingredients:
- 1/3 cup granulated sugar
- ½ to 1 tsp cinnamon (adjust to your taste)
- 4 tbsp. dark brown sugar (try to remove or break up any clumps)
- Pinch of allspice
- 1 can Pillsbury Grands Flaky Layers biscuits (8 biscuits)
- 3 tbsp. butter, melted

Directions:
1. Combine the sugar, cinnamon, brown sugar and allspice in a cereal- or soup-sized bowl. Mix and keep.
2. Without flattening the biscuits, remove them from the can. Cut holes out of the center of each of the biscuits using a 1- inch circle biscuit cutter.
3. Move the donuts into the air fryer basket, and air fry for 5 minutes at 350 F. For the holes, fry for 3 minutes at the same temperature. You may divide the donuts and holes into batches, depending on the size of your air fryer.
4. Withdraw each hole or donut and immediately paint butter over their entire surface using a pastry brush.
5. Drop the painted holes and donuts into the sugar mixture, submerging them to ensure an even and generous coating. Shake off the excess gently.
6. Serve the holes and donuts while warm.

Nutrition: Calories: 77 kcal Protein: 1.11 g Fat: 5.56 g Carbohydrates: 6.05 g

630. Peach Hand Pies

Preparation Time: 55 minutes
Cooking Time: 12 to 14 minutes
Servings: 8
Ingredients:
- 2 (5-oz) fresh peaches, peeled and chopped
- ¼ tsp table salt
- 1 tsp vanilla extract
- 3 tbsp. granulated sugar
- 1 tbsp. fresh lemon juice (from 1 lemon)
- 1 tsp cornstarch
- 1 pkg (14-oz) refrigerated piecrusts
- Cooking spray

Directions:
1. Get a clean medium bowl, and in it, combine peaches, salt, vanilla, sugar, and lemon juice. Stir well. Leave for 15 minutes but stir occasionally. Drain the peaches, keeping one tablespoon liquid. Now stir cornstarch into the reserved liquid, and add the mixture into the drained peaches.
2. Make eight 4-inch circles out of the piecrusts. Add the filling in the center of each circle - about one tablespoon

per cir-cle. Brush the edges with water before folding the dough over the filling. This forms half-moons. Seal by crimping the edges with a fork. On the top of the pies, cut three small slits. Now spray the pies generously with cooking spray.
3. Transfer the pies into the air fryer basket - 3 at once in a single layer. Allow cooking for 12-14 minutes at 350 F, until the pies are golden brown.
4. Do the same for the other pies.

Nutrition: Calories: 55 kcal Protein: 0.99 g Fat: 0.8 g Carbohydrates: 11.66 g

631. Honey Glazed Pineapple Fries
Preparation Time: 15 minutes
Cooking Time: 10 minutes
Servings: 2
Ingredients:
- 4 oz. fresh pineapple
- 2 tsp cinnamon
- 2 tbsp. honey

Directions:
1. Chip the peeled pineapple into chunky chip sizes.
2. Arrange the fries in the grill pan placed in your air fryer. Maintain a long neat row, without gaps.
3. Allow cooking in the air fryer for 390 F for 3 minutes.
4. Turn the fries over using thongs and allow cooking for another 3 minutes at 390 F.
5. Withdraw the grill pan and sprinkle the pineapple fries with cinnamon, before glazing them with honey using a pastry brush.
6. Serve immediately while warm.

Nutrition: Calories: 145 kcal Protein: 3.61 g Fat: 3.11 g Carbohydrates: 28.3 g

632. Baked Apple
Preparation Time: 40 minutes
Cooking Time: 20 minutes
Servings: 2
Ingredients:
- 1 medium apple or pear
- ¼ tsp cinnamon
- 2 tbsp. raisins
- 2 tbsp. chopped walnuts
- ¼ tsp nutmeg
- 1½ tsp light margarine, melted
- ¼ cup water

Directions:
1. Ensure that your air fryer is preheated to 350 F.
2. Cut the pear or apple in half, around the middle, to gain access to scrape out some of the flesh.
3. Place the pear or apple at the base of the air fryer, or in the frying pan of the air fryer (if available).
4. Get a clean small bowl, and in it, combine the cinnamon, raisins, walnuts, nutmeg, and margarine.
5. Add the mixture to the center of the pear or apple halves.
6. Add some water into the pan, and bake the halves for 20 minutes.

Nutrition: Calories: 156 kcal Protein: 5.44 g Fat: 9.25 g Carbohydrates: 15.33 g

633. Mini Apple Pie
Preparation Time: 30 minutes
Cooking Time: 18 minutes
Servings: 8
Ingredients:
- 1 oz. butter
- 3 oz. plain flour
- ½ oz. caster sugar
- Water
- 2 medium red apples
- Pinch cinnamon
- Pinch caster sugar

Directions:
1. The first step is to make your pastry. Do this by combining the butter and plain flour in a mixing bowl, while rubbing the fat into the flour. Add the sugar and stir thoroughly. Add water to moisten the in-gredients, so that they can form into a nice dough.
2. Once the dough is formed, knead it well until you have a nice smooth texture.
3. Cover your pastry tins with butter, to pre-vent sticking.
4. Roll out the pastry, and fill the tins with the pastry.
5. Place your peeled and diced apples into the tins too.
6. Add sprinkles of cinnamon and sugar.
7. Add an extra pastry layer to the top. In-clude a few fork markings to leave some breathing spaces.
8. Allow cooking for 18 minutes in the air fryer.

Nutrition: Calories: 105 kcal Protein: 2.05 g Fat: 3.82 g Carbohydrates: 16.17 g

634. Flourless Chocolate Cake
Preparation Time: 2 hours
Cooking Time: 35 minutes
Servings: 1
Ingredients:
- 10 bananas
- 4 tbsp. honey
- 10 tsp organic cocoa powder
- 8 large eggs
- 1 large avocado

Directions:
1. Ensure that your air fryer is preheated to 360 F.
2. Combine all ingredients into the blender (except the avocado) and blend until a smooth chocolate cake mixture is formed.
3. Divide the mixture into two - set aside one half, and divide the other half into two cake baking tins. Transfer the tins into the air fryer and leave for 3 5 minutes at 360 F.
4. After 35 minutes, withdraw the cake tins and let them rest on the wire rack and cool.
5. To the other half of the cake mixture, add the avocado until the paste is of your pre-ferred thickness.
6. Sandwich a small layer in between two cakes. You may use the rest as a lovely chocolate icing around the cake.
7. Keep the cake in the fridge for about an hour to set the icing.
8. Serve.

Nutrition: Calories: 1136 kcal Protein: 35.48 g Fat: 73.97 g Carbohydrates: 101.68 g

635. Butter Cake
Preparation Time: 35 minutes
Cooking Time: 15 minutes
Servings: 4
Ingredients:
- Cooking spray
- 7 tbsp. butter, at room temperature
- ¼ cup and 2 tbsp. white sugar leg
- 1 pinch salt, or to taste
- 1 and 2/3 cups all-purpose flour
- 6 tbsp. milk

Directions:

DESSERTS RECIPES

1. Ensure that your air fryer is preheated to 350 F.
2. Get a small fluted tube pan and spray with some cooking spray.
3. In a clean bowl, use your electric mixer to mix butter and ¼ cup white sugar plus two tablespoons of white sugar until you have a light and creamy mixture. Add the egg and mix lightly until the batter is soft and smooth. Stir in salt and flour. Add the milk and mix batter thoroughly.
4. Move the batter into the sprayed pan, and level the surface with the back of a spoon.
5. Transfer the pan into the air fryer basket and allow baking for 15 minutes, or until an inserted toothpick comes out clean of the cake.
6. Remove the cake from the pan and set aside to cool for about 5 minutes.

Nutrition: Calories: 339 kcal Protein: 7.29 g Fat: 23.37 g Carbohydrates: 24.94 g

636. Lime Mousse
Preparation Time: 15 minutes
Cooking Time: 12 minutes
Servings: 2
Ingredients:
- 4 ounces cream cheese, softened
- ½ cup heavy cream
- 2 tablespoon fresh lime juice
- 5-6 drops liquid stevia
- Pinch of salt

Directions:
1. In a bowl, add all the ingredients and mix until well combined.
2. Transfer the mixture into 2 ramekins.
3. Arrange a sheet pan in the center of Instant Omni Plus Toaster Oven.
4. Place the ramekins over the sheet pan.
5. Select "Air Fry" and then adjust the temperature to 350 degrees F.
6. Set the timer for 12 minutes and press "Start".
7. When the display shows "Turn Food" do nothing.
8. When cooking time is complete, remove the muffin molds from Toaster Oven
9. Place the ramekins onto a wire rack to cool.
10. Refrigerate for at least 3 hours before serving.

Nutrition: Calories 302 Total Fat 30.2 g Saturated Fat 19.4 g Cholesterol 103 mg Sodium 257 mg Total Carbs 2.4 g Fiber 0 g Sugar 0.1 g Protein 4.9 g

637. Mini Cheesecakes
Preparation Time: 15 minutes
Cooking Time: 10 minutes
Servings: 4
Ingredients:
- ¾ cup sugar
- 2 eggs
- 1 teaspoon vanilla extract
- ½ teaspoon fresh lime juice
- 16 ounces cream cheese, softened
- 2 tablespoon heavy cream

Directions:
1. In a blender, add the sugar, eggs, vanilla extract and lime juice and pulse until smooth.
2. Add the cream cheese and sour cream and pulse until smooth.
3. Place the mixture into 2 (4-inch) springform pans evenly.
4. Arrange a sheet pan in the center of Instant Omni Plus Toaster Oven.
5. Place the ramekins over the sheet pan.
6. Select "Air Fry" and then adjust the temperature to 350 degrees F.
7. Set the timer for 10 minutes and press "Start".
8. When the display shows "Turn Food" do nothing.
9. When cooking time is complete, remove the muffin molds from Toaster Oven
10. Place the ramekins onto a wire rack to cool.
11. Refrigerate overnight before serving.

Nutrition: Calories 496 Total Fat 31.5 g Saturated Fat 19.2 g Cholesterol 178 mg Sodium 486 mg Total Carbs 41.4 g Fiber 0 g Sugar 41.4 g Protein 14.2 g

638. Cherry Crumble
Preparation Time: 15 minutes
Cooking Time: 25 minutes
Servings: 4
Ingredients:
- 1 (14-ounce) can cherry pie filling
- ¼ cup butter, softened
- 9 tablespoons self-rising flour
- 7 tablespoons powdered sugar
- Pinch of salt

Directions:
1. Lightly, grease a baking dish.
2. Place the cherry pie filling into the prepared baking dish evenly.
3. In a bowl, add the remaining ingredients and mix until a crumbly mixture forms.
4. Spread the mixture over pie filling evenly.
5. Arrange a wire rack in the center of Instant Omni Plus Toaster Oven.
6. Place the baking dish onto the wire rack.
7. Select "Air Fry" and then adjust the temperature to 320 degrees F.
8. Set the timer for 25 minutes and press "Start".
9. When the display shows "Turn Food" do nothing.
10. When cooking time is complete, remove the muffin molds from Toaster Oven
11. Place the ramekins onto a wire rack to cool.
12. Refrigerate overnight before serving.
13. Place the baking dish onto a wire rack to cool for about 10 minutes.
14. Serve warm.

Nutrition: Calories 334 Total Fat 11.8 g Saturated Fat 7.3 g Cholesterol 31 mg Sodium 139 mg Total Carbs 55.2 g Fiber 1.1 g Sugar 13.8 g Protein 2.3 g

639. Blackberries Cobbler
Preparation Time: 15 minutes
Cooking Time: 20 minutes
Servings: 6
Ingredients:
For Filling:
- 2½ cups fresh blackberries
- 1 teaspoon vanilla extract
- 1 teaspoon fresh lime juice
- 1 cup sugar
- 1 teaspoon all-purpose flour
- 1 tablespoon butter, melted

For Topping:
- 1¾ cups all-purpose flour
- 6 tablespoons sugar
- 4 teaspoons baking powder
- 1 cup milk
- 5 tablespoons butter

Directions:

1. For filling: in a bowl, add all the ingredients and mix until well combined.
2. In another large bowl, mix together the flour, baking powder, and sugar.
3. Add the milk and butter and mix until a crumbly mixture form.
4. In the bottom of a greased baking dish place the blueberries mixture and top with the flour mixture evenly.
5. Arrange the baking dish in the center of Instant Omni Plus Toaster Oven.
6. Select "Air Fry" and then adjust the temperature to 320 degrees F.
7. Set the timer for 20 minutes and press the "Start".
8. When the display shows "Add Food" place the baking pan over the drip pan.
9. When the display shows "Turn Food" do nothing.
10. When cooking time is complete, remove the pan from Toaster Oven and place onto a wire rack to cool for about 10 minutes before serving.

Nutrition: Calories 453 Total Fat 13 g Saturated Fat 7.9 g Cholesterol 34 mg Sodium 105 mg Total Carbs 81.7 g Fiber 4.2 g Sugar 49.4 g Protein 6.1 g

640. Glazed Bananas

Preparation Time: 10 minutes
Cooking Time: 10 minutes
Servings: 2

Ingredients:
- 1 ripe banana, peeled and sliced lengthwise
- ½ teaspoon fresh lime juice
- 2 teaspoons maple syrup
- 1/8 teaspoon ground cinnamon

Directions:
1. Coat each banana half with lime juice.
2. Arrange the banana halves onto the greased sheet pan, cut sides up.
3. Drizzle the banana halves with maple syrup and sprinkle with cinnamon.
4. Arrange the baking dish in the center of Instant Omni Plus Toaster Oven.
5. Select "Air Fry" and then adjust the temperature to 350 degrees F.
6. Set the timer for 10 minutes and press the "Start".
7. When the display shows "Add Food" place the baking pan over the drip pan.
8. When the display shows "Turn Food" do nothing.
9. When cooking time is complete, remove the pan from Toaster Oven. Serve immediately.

Nutrition: Calories 70 Total Fat 0.2 g Saturated Fat 0.1 g Cholesterol 0 mg Sodium 1 mg Total Carbs 18.1 g Fiber 1.6 g Sugar 11.2 g Protein 0.7 g

641. Banana Muffins

Preparation Time: 15 minutes
Cooking Time: 25 minutes
Servings: 12

Ingredients:
- 1 2/3 cups all-purpose flour
- 1 teaspoon baking soda
- 1 teaspoon baking powder
- ½ teaspoon ground cinnamon
- ¼ teaspoon ground nutmeg
- ¼ teaspoon ground ginger
- ½ teaspoon salt
- 4 ripe bananas, peeled and mashed
- 2 eggs
- ½ cup brown sugar
- 1 teaspoon vanilla extract
- 3 tablespoon milk
- 1 tablespoon Nutella
- ¼ cup almonds, chopped

Directions:
1. In a large bowl, sift together the flour, baking soda, baking powder, spices and salt.
2. In another bowl, mix together the remaining ingredients except walnuts.
3. Add the banana mixture into flour mixture and mix until just combined.
4. Fold in the almonds.
5. Place the mixture into 12 greased muffin molds evenly.
6. Arrange a sheet pan in the center of Instant Omni Plus Toaster Oven.
7. Place the muffin molds over the sheet pan.
8. Select "Air Fry" and then adjust the temperature to 248 degrees F.
9. Set the timer for 25 minutes and press "Start".
10. When the display shows "Turn Food" do nothing.
11. When cooking time is complete, remove the muffin molds from Toaster Oven and place the pan onto a wire rack for about 10 minutes.
12. Carefully, invert the muffins onto the wire rack to completely cool before serving.

Nutrition: Calories 223 Total Fat 6.1 g Saturated Fat 1.5 g Cholesterol 45 mg Sodium 267 mg Total Carbs 38.3 g Fiber 2.4 g Sugar 15.8 g Protein 5 g

642. Chocolate Muffins

Preparation Time: 15 minutes
Cooking Time: 10 minutes
Servings: 9

Ingredients:
- 1½ cups all-purpose flour
- ¼ cup sugar
- 2 teaspoons baking powder
- ½ teaspoon salt
- 1 cup plain Greek yogurt
- 1/3 cup olive oil
- 1 egg
- 1½ teaspoons vanilla extract
- ¼ cup semi-sweet mini chocolate chips
- ¼ cup walnuts, chopped

Directions:
1. In a bowl, mix well flour, sugar, baking powder, and salt.
2. In another bowl, add the yogurt, oil, egg, and vanilla extract and whisk until well combined.
3. Add the flour mixture and mix until just combined.
4. Fold in the chocolate chips and walnuts.
5. Place the mixture into 9 greased muffin molds evenly.
6. Arrange a sheet pan in the center of Instant Omni Plus Toaster Oven.
7. Place the muffin molds over the sheet pan.
8. Select "Air Fry" and then adjust the temperature to 355 degrees F.
9. Set the timer for 10 minutes and press "Start".
10. When the display shows "Turn Food" do nothing.
11. When cooking time is complete, remove the muffin molds from Toaster Oven and place the pan onto a wire rack for about 10 minutes.
12. Carefully, invert the muffins onto the wire rack to completely cool before serving.

DESSERTS RECIPES

Nutrition: Calories 247 Total Fat 12.3 g Saturated Fat 2.8 g Cholesterol 20 mg Sodium 155 mg Total Carbs 28.8 g Fiber 0.8 g Sugar 11.3 g Protein 5.6 g

643. Banana-Choco Brownies

Preparation Time: 15 minutes
Cooking Time: 30 minutes
Servings: 12
Ingredients:
- 2 cups almond flour
- 2 teaspoons baking powder
- ½ teaspoon baking powder
- ½ teaspoon baking soda
- ½ teaspoon salt
- 1 over-ripe banana
- 3 large eggs
- ½ teaspoon stevia powder
- ¼ cup coconut oil
- 1 tablespoon vinegar
- 1/3 cup almond flour
- 1/3 cup cocoa powder

Directions:
1. Preheat the air fryer for 5 minutes.
2. Combine all ingredients in a food processor and pulse until well-combined.
3. Pour into a baking dish that will fit in the air fryer.
4. Place in the air fryer basket and cook for 30 minutes at 3500F or if a toothpick inserted in the middle comes out clean.

Nutrition: Calories: 75 Carbohydrates: 2.1g Protein: 1.7g Fat: 6.6g

644. Blueberry & Lemon Cake

Preparation Time: 10 minutes
Cooking Time: 12 minutes
Servings: 4
Ingredients:
- 2 eggs
- 1 cup blueberries
- zest from 1 lemon
- juice from 1 lemon
- 1 tsp. vanilla
- brown sugar for topping (a little sprinkling on top of each muffin-less than a teaspoon)
- 2 1/2 cups self-rising flour
- 1/2 cup Monk Fruit (or use your preferred sugar)
- 1/2 cup cream
- 1/4 cup avocado oil (any light cooking oil)

Directions:
1. In mixing bowl, beat well wet Ingredients. Stir in dry ingredients and mix thoroughly.
2. Lightly grease baking pan of air fryer with cooking spray. Pour in batter.
3. For 12 minutes, cook on 330oF.
4. Let it stand in air fryer for 5 minutes.
5. Serve and enjoy.

Nutrition: Calories 589 Carbs: 76.7g Protein: 13.5g Fat: 25.3g

645. Bread Pudding with Cranberry

Preparation Time: 15 minutes
Cooking Time: 35 minutes
Servings: 4
Ingredients:
- 1-1/2 cups milk
- 2-1/2 eggs
- 1/2 cup cranberries1 teaspoon butter
- 1/4 cup and 2 tablespoons white sugar
- 1/4 cup golden raisins
- 1/8 teaspoon ground cinnamon
- 3/4 cup heavy whipping cream
- 3/4 teaspoon lemon zest
- 3/4 teaspoon kosher salt
- 3/4 French baguettes, cut into 2-inch slices
- 3/8 vanilla bean, split and seeds scraped away

Directions:
1. Lightly grease baking pan of air fryer with cooking spray. Spread baguette slices, cranberries, and raisins.
2. In blender, blend well vanilla bean, cinnamon, salt, lemon zest, eggs, sugar, and cream. Pour over baguette slices. Let it soak for an hour.
3. Cover pan with foil.
4. For 35 minutes, cook on 330oF.
5. Let it rest for 10 minutes.
6. Serve and enjoy.

Nutrition: Calories: 581 Carbs: 76.1g Protein: 15.8g Fat: 23.7g

646. Cherries 'n Almond Flour Bars

Preparation Time: 15 minutes
Cooking Time: 35 minutes
Servings: 12
Ingredients:
- ¼ cup water
- ½ cup butter, softened
- ½ teaspoon salt
- ½ teaspoon vanilla
- 1 ½ cups almond flour
- 1 cup erythritol
- 1 cup fresh cherries, pitted
- 1 tablespoon xanthan gum
- 2 eggs

Directions:
1. In a mixing bowl, combine the first 6 ingredients until you form a dough.
2. Press the dough in a baking dish that will fit in the air fryer.
3. Place in the air fryer and bake for 10 minutes at 3750F.
4. Meanwhile, mix the cherries, water, and xanthan gum in a bowl.
5. Take the dough out and pour over the cherry mixture.
6. Return to the air fryer and cook for 25 minutes more at 3750F.

Nutrition: Calories: 99 Carbohydrates: 2.1g Protein: 1.8g Fat: 9.3g

647. Cherry-Choco Bars

Preparation Time: 10 minutes
Cooking Time: 15 minutes
Servings: 8
Ingredients:
- ¼ teaspoon salt
- ½ cup almonds, sliced
- ½ cup chia seeds
- ½ cup dark chocolate, chopped
- ½ cup dried cherries, chopped
- ½ cup prunes, pureed
- ½ cup quinoa, cooked
- ¾ cup almond butter
- 1/3 cup honey
- 2 cups old-fashioned oats
- 2 tablespoon coconut oil

Directions:
1. Preheat the air fryer to 375oF.
2. In a mixing bowl, combine the oats, quinoa, chia seeds, almond, cherries, and chocolate.
3. In a saucepan, heat the almond butter, honey, and coconut oil.
4. Pour the butter mixture over the dry mixture. Add salt and prunes.
5. Mix until well combined.
6. Pour over a baking dish that can fit inside the air fryer.
7. Cook for 15 minutes.
8. Let it cool for an hour before slicing into bars.

Nutrition: Calories: 321 Carbohydrates: 35g Protein: 7g Fat: 17g

648. Coffee 'n Blueberry Cake

Preparation Time: 10 minutes
Cooking Time: 35 minutes
Servings: 6
Ingredients:
- 1 cup white sugar
- 1 egg
- 1/2 cup butter, softened
- 1/2 cup fresh or frozen blueberries
- 1/2 cup sour cream
- 1/2 teaspoon baking powder
- 1/2 teaspoon ground cinnamon
- 1/2 teaspoon vanilla extract
- 1/4 cup brown sugar
- 1/4 cup chopped pecans
- 1/8 teaspoon salt
- 1-1/2 teaspoons confectioners' sugar for dusting
- 3/4 cup and 1 tablespoon all-purpose flour

Directions:
1. In a small bowl, whisk well pecans, cinnamon, and brown sugar.
2. In a blender, blend well all wet Ingredients. Add dry Ingredients except for confectioner's sugar and blueberries. Blend well until smooth and creamy.
3. Lightly grease baking pan of air fryer with cooking spray.
4. Pour half of batter in pan. Sprinkle half of pecan mixture on top. Pour the remaining batter. And then topped with remaining pecan mixture.
5. Cover pan with foil.
6. For 35 minutes, cook on 330oF.
7. Serve and enjoy with a dusting of confectioner's sugar.

Nutrition: Calories: 471 Carbs: 59.5g Protein: 4.1g Fat: 24.0g

649. Crisped 'n Chewy Chonut Holes

Preparation Time: 10 minutes
Cooking Time: 10 minutes
Servings: 6
Ingredients:
- ¼ cup almond milk
- ¼ cup coconut sugar
- ¼ teaspoon cinnamon
- ½ teaspoon salt
- 1 cup white all-purpose flour
- 1 tablespoon coconut oil, melted
- 1 teaspoon baking powder
- 2 tablespoon aquafaba or liquid from canned chickpeas

Directions:
1. In a mixing bowl, mix the flour, sugar, and baking powder. Add the salt and cinnamon and mix well.
2. In another bowl, mix together the coconut oil, aquafaba, and almond milk.
3. Gently pour the dry ingredients to the wet ingredients. Mix together until well combined or until you form a sticky dough.
4. Place the dough in the refrigerator to rest for at least an hour.
5. Preheat the air fryer to 370oF.
6. Create small balls of the dough and place inside the air fryer and cook for 10 minutes. Do not shake the air fryer.
7. Once cooked, sprinkle with sugar and cinnamon.
8. Serve with your breakfast coffee.

Nutrition: Calories: 120 Carbohydrates: 21.62g Protein: 2.31g Fat: 2.76g

650. Leche Flan Filipino Style

Preparation Time: 10 minutes
Cooking Time: 30 minutes
Servings: 4
Ingredients:
- 1 cup heavy cream
- 1 teaspoon vanilla extract
- 1/2 (14 ounce) can sweetened condensed milk
- 1/2 cup milk
- 2-1/2 eggs
- 1/3 cup white sugar

Directions:
1. In blender, blend well vanilla, eggs, milk, cream, and condensed milk.
2. Lightly grease baking pan of air fryer with cooking spray. Add sugar and heat for 10 minutes at 370oF until melted and caramelized. Lower heat to 300oF and continue melting and swirling.
3. Pour milk mixture into caramelized sugar. Cover pan with foil.
4. Cook for 20 minutes at 330oF.
5. Let it cool completely in the fridge.
6. Place a plate on top of pan and invert pan to easily remove flan.
7. Serve and enjoy.

Nutrition: Calories: 498 Carbs: 46.8g Protein: 10.0g Fat: 30.0g

651. Maple Cinnamon Buns

Preparation Time: 20 minutes
Cooking Time: 30 minutes
Servings: 9
Ingredients:
- ¼ cup icing sugar
- ½ cup pecan nuts, toasted
- ¾ cup tablespoon unsweetened almond milk
- 1 ½ cup plain white flour, sifted
- 1 ½ tablespoon active yeast
- 1 cup wholegrain flour, sifted
- 1 tablespoon coconut oil, melted
- 1 tablespoon ground flaxseed
- 2 ripe bananas, sliced
- 2 teaspoons cinnamon powder
- 4 Medjool dates, pitted
- 4 tablespoons maple syrup

Directions:
1. Heat the ¾ cup almond milk to lukewarm and add the maple syrup and yeast. Allow the yeast to activate for 5 to 10 minutes.
2. Meanwhile, mix together flaxseed and 3 tablespoons of water to make the egg replacement. Allow flaxseed to soak for 2 minutes. Add the coconut oil.

DESSERTS RECIPES

3. Pour the flaxseed mixture to the yeast mixture.
4. In another bowl, combine the two types of flour and the 1 tablespoon cinnamon powder. Pour the yeast-flaxseed mixture and combine until dough forms.
5. Knead the dough on a floured surface for at least 10 minutes.
6. Place the kneaded dough in a greased bowl and cover with a kitchen towel. Leave in a warm and dark area for the bread to rise for 1 hour.
7. While the dough is rising, make the filling by mixing together the pecans, banana slices, and dates. Add 1 tablespoon of cinnamon powder.
8. Preheat the air fryer to 3900F.
9. Roll the risen dough on a floured surface until it is thin. Spread the pecan mixture on to the dough.
10. Roll the dough and cut into nine slices.
11. Place inside a dish that will fit in the air fryer and cook for 30 minutes.
12. Once cooked, sprinkle with icing sugar.

Nutrition: Calories: 293 Carbohydrates: 44.9g Protein: 5.6g Fat:10.1 g

652. Poppy Seed Pound Cake
Preparation Time: 10 minutes
Cooking Time: 20 minutes
Servings: 8
Ingredients:
- ¼ cup erythritol powder
- ¼ teaspoon vanilla extract
- ½ cup coconut milk
- 1 ½ cups almond flour
- 1 ½ teaspoon baking powder
- 1/3 cup butter, unsalted
- 2 large eggs, beaten
- 2 tablespoon psyllium husk powder
- 2 tablespoons poppy seeds

Directions:
1. Preheat the air fryer for 5 minutes.
2. In a mixing bowl, combine all ingredients.
3. Use a hand mixer to mix everything.
4. Pour into a small loaf pan that will fit in the air fryer.
5. Bake for 20 minutes at 3750F or until a toothpick inserted in the middle comes out clean.

Nutrition: Calories:145 Carbohydrates: 3.6 Protein: 2.1g Fat: 13.6g

653. Banana Smores
Preparation Time: 10 minutes
Cooking Time: 6 minutes
Servings: 4
Ingredients:
- 4 Bananas
- 3 tbsp. Mini-peanut butter chips
- 3 tbsp. Graham cracker cereal
- 3 tbsp. Mini-chocolate chips - semi-sweet

Directions:
1. Heat the Air Fryer in advance at 400° Fahrenheit.
2. Slice the un-peeled bananas lengthwise along the inside of the curve. Don't slice through the bottom of the peel. Open slightly - forming a pocket.
3. Fill each pocket with chocolate chips, peanut butter chips, and marshmallows. Poke the cereal into the filling.
4. Arrange the stuffed bananas in the fryer basket, keeping them upright with the filling facing up.
5. Air-fry until the peel has blackened, and the chocolate and marshmallows have toasted (6 minutes).
6. Chill for 1-2 minutes. Spoon out the filling to serve.

Nutrition: Calories: 28 kcal Protein: 1.79 g Fat: 1.6 g Carbohydrates: 1.57 g

654. Fluffy Peanut Butter Marshmallow Turnovers
Preparation Time: 10 minutes
Cooking Time: 5 minutes
Servings: 4
Ingredients:
- 4 Defrosted Sheets Filo pastry
- 4 tbsp. Chunky peanut butter
- 2 oz. Melted butter
- 4 tsp. Marshmallow fluff
- pinch Sea salt

Directions:
1. Set the temperature of the Air Fryer at 360° Fahrenheit.
2. Use the melted butter to brush one sheet of the filo. Put the second sheet on top and brush it also with butter. Continue the process until you have completed all four sheets.
3. Cut the layers into four—12-inch x 3-inch strips.
4. Place one teaspoon of the marshmallow fluff on the underside and one tablespoon of the peanut butter.
5. Fold the tip over the filo strip to form a triangle, making sure the filling is completely wrapped.
6. Seal the ends with a small amount of butter. Place the completed turnovers into the Air Fryer for three to five minutes.
7. When done, they will be fluffy and golden brown.
8. Add a touch of sea salt for the sweet/salty combo.

Nutrition: Calories: 221 kcal Protein: 3.2 g Fat: 17.35 g Carbohydrates: 14.48 g

655. Yogurt Pineapple Sticks
Preparation Time: 5 minutes
Cooking Time: 10 minutes
Servings: 4
Ingredients:
- Half of 1 Pineapple
- .25 cup Desiccated coconut
- The Dip:
- small sprig Fresh mint
- 1 cup Vanilla yogurt

Directions:
1. Warm the Air Fryer to reach 392° Fahrenheit.
2. Slice the pineapple into stick segments. Dip the chunks of pineapple into the coconut. Arrange the sticks of pineapple into the cooker basket and air-fry for ten minutes.
3. Dice the mint into fine pieces and mix in with the yogurt.
4. Empty the dip into a serving dish. Arrange the baked sticks around the dip to serve.

Nutrition: Calories: 106 kcal Protein: 4.01 g Fat: 4.79 g Carbohydrates: 11.76 g

656. Low Carb Snickerdoodle Cookies
Preparation Time: 10 minutes
Cooking Time: 15 minutes
Servings: 16
Ingredients:
Cookies:
- 2 cups superfine almond flour
- ½ tsp. baking soda
- ¾ cup erythritol sweetener
- ½ cup salted butter softened

- Salt

Coating:
- 1 tsp. ground cinnamon
- 2 tbsp. erythritol

Directions:
1. Switch on oven to 350 degrees.
2. Combine all the ingredients until you form a stiff dough.
3. Then roll the cookie dough into 16 equal-sized balls, about 1 ½ inches wide.
4. Mix the sweetener and cinnamon in a small bowl to create the coating.
5. Then roll the balls generously in the cinnamon coating.
6. Place the coated cookie balls on a cookie sheet covered in parchment paper. Then gently smash with a flat round surface.
7. Bake for 15 minutes and then let cool before serving.

Nutrition: Calories: 131 Protein: 3g Net Carbs: 1.5g Fat 13g

657. White Chocolate Raspberry Fat Bombs

Preparation Time: 5 minutes + 1 hour chilling
Cooking Time: 0 minutes
Servings: 10-12

Ingredients:
- ½ cup coconut oil
- 2 oz. cacao butter
- ½ cup freeze-dried raspberries
- ¼ powdered erythritol sweetener

Directions:
1. Put paper liners into a 12 cup muffin pan or use a silicone muffin pan with no liners.
2. In a small saucepan, heat coconut oil and cacao butter over the lowest setting until completely melted. Then remove the saucepan from the heat.
3. Use a food processor, blender, or coffee grinder to blend the freeze-dried raspberries.
4. Add the blended berries and sweetener to the saucepan and then stir until sweetener is dissolved.
5. Evenly divide the mixture into the muffin cups. Keep stirring mixture while pouring into the cups. The raspberry mixture will sink to the bottom.
6. Chill in the refrigerator for 1 hour or until firm.

Nutrition: Calories: 70 Protein: 2g Net Carbs: 2g Fat 7g

658. Sponge Ricotta Cake

Preparation Time: 5 minutes
Cooking Time: 30 minutes
Servings: 8

Ingredients:
- 3 eggs, whisked
- 1 cup almond flour
- 1 cup ricotta, soft
- 1/3 swerve
- 7 tbsp. ghee; melted
- 1 tsp. baking powder
- Cooking spray

Directions:
1. In a bowl, combine all the ingredients except the cooking spray and stir them very well.
2. Grease a cake pan that fits the air fryer with the cooking spray and pour the cake mix inside.
3. Put the pan in the fryer and cook at 350°F for 30 minutes.
4. Cool the cake down, slice and serve.

Nutrition: Calories: 210 Fat: 12g Fiber: 3g Carbs: 6g Protein: 9g

659. Plum Cake

Preparation Time: 10 minutes
Cooking Time: 30 minutes
Servings: 8

Ingredients:
- 4 plums, pitted and chopped.
- 1 ½ cups almond flour
- ½ cup coconut flour
- ¾ cup almond milk
- ½ cup butter, soft
- 3 eggs
- ½ cup swerve
- 1 tbsp. vanilla extract
- 2 tsp. baking powder
- ¼ tsp. almond extract

Directions:
1. Take a bowl and mix all the ingredients and whisk well.
2. Pour this into a cake pan that fits the air fryer after you've lined it with parchment paper, put the pan in the machine and cook at 370°F for 30 minutes.
3. Cool the cake down, slice and serve

Nutrition: Calories: 183 Fat: 4g Fiber: 3g Carbs: 4g Protein: 7g

660. Baked Plums

Preparation Time: 5 minutes
Cooking Time: 20 minutes
Servings: 6

Ingredients:
- 6 plums; cut into wedges
- 10 drops stevia
- Zest of 1 lemon, grated
- 2 tbsp. water
- 1 tsp. ginger, ground
- ½ tsp. cinnamon powder

Directions:
1. In a pan that fits the air fryer, combine the plums with the rest of the ingredients, toss gently.
2. Put the pan in the air fryer and cook at 360°F for 20 minutes. Serve cold

Nutrition: Calories: 170 Fat: 5g Fiber: 1g Carbs: 3g Protein: 5g

661. Walnut and Vanilla Bars

Preparation Time: 5 minutes
Cooking Time: 16 minutes
Servings: 4

Ingredients:
- 1 egg
- ¼ cup almond flour
- ¼ cup walnuts; chopped.
- 1/3 cup cocoa powder
- 7 tbsp. ghee; melted
- 3 tbsp. swerve
- ½ tsp. baking soda
- 1 tsp. vanilla extract

Directions:
1. Take a bowl and mix all the ingredients and stir well.
2. Spread this on a baking sheet that fits your air fryer lined with parchment paper.
3. Put it in the fryer and cook at 330°F and bake for 16 minutes
4. Leave the bars to cool down, cut and serve

Nutrition: Calories: 182 Fat: 12g Fiber: 1g Carbs: 3g Protein: 6g

662. Plum Cream

Preparation Time: 5 minutes
Cooking Time: 20 minutes
Servings: 4

DESSERTS RECIPES

Ingredients:
- 1 lb. plums, pitted and chopped.
- 1 ½ cups heavy cream
- ¼ cup swerve
- 1 tbsp. lemon juice

Directions:
1. Take a bowl and mix all the ingredients and whisk really well.
2. Divide this into 4 ramekins, put them in the air fryer and cook at 340°F for 20 minutes. Serve cold

Nutrition: Calories: 171 Fat: 4g Fiber: 2g Carbs: 4g Protein: 4g

663. Currant Pudding
Preparation Time: 5 minutes
Cooking Time: 20 minutes
Servings: 6

Ingredients:
- 1 cup red currants, blended
- 1 cup coconut cream
- 1 cup black currants, blended
- 3 tbsp. stevia

Directions:
1. In a bowl, combine all the ingredients and stir well.
2. Divide into ramekins, put them in the fryer and cook at 340°F for 20 minutes
3. Serve the pudding cold.

Nutrition: Calories: 200 Fat: 4g Fiber: 2g Carbs: 4g Protein: 6g

664. Currant Cookies
Preparation Time: 5 minutes
Cooking Time: 30 minutes
Servings: 6

Ingredients:
- ½ cup currants
- ½ cup swerve
- 2 cups almond flour
- ½ cup ghee; melted
- 1 tsp. vanilla extract
- 2 tsp. baking soda

Directions:
1. Take a bowl and mix all the ingredients and whisk well.
2. Spread this on a baking sheet lined with parchment paper, put the pan in the air fryer and cook at 350°F for 30 minutes
3. Cool down; cut into rectangles and serve.

Nutrition: Calories: 172 Fat: 5g Fiber: 2g Carbs: 3g Protein: 5g

665. Fruity Oreo Muffins
Preparation Time: 15 minutes
Cooking Time: 10 minutes
Servings: 6

Ingredients:
- 1 cup milk
- 1 pack Oreo biscuits, crushed
- ¾ teaspoon baking powder
- 1 banana, peeled and chopped
- 1 apple, peeled, cored and chopped
- 1 teaspoon cocoa powder
- 1 teaspoon honey
- 1 teaspoon fresh lemon juice
- A pinch of ground cinnamon

Directions:
1. Preheat the Air fryer to 320 degree F and grease 6 muffin cups lightly.
2. Mix milk, biscuits, cocoa powder, baking soda, and baking powder in a bowl until well combined.
3. Transfer the mixture into the muffin cups and cook for about 10 minutes.
4. Remove from the Air fryer and invert the muffin cups onto a wire rack to cool.
5. Meanwhile, mix the banana, apple, honey, lemon juice, and cinnamon in another bowl.
6. Scoop some portion of muffins from the center and fill with fruit mixture to serve.

Nutrition: Calories: 182 Fat: 3.1g Carbohydrates: 31.4g Sugar: 19.5g Protein: 3.1g Sodium: 196mg

666. Doughnuts Pudding
Preparation Time: 15 minutes
Cooking Time: 1 hour
Servings: 4

Ingredients:
- 6 glazed doughnuts, cut into small pieces
- ¾ cup frozen sweet cherries
- ½ cup raisins
- ½ cup semi-sweet chocolate baking chips
- 4 egg yolks
- ¼ cup sugar
- 1 teaspoon ground cinnamon
- 1½ cups whipping cream

Directions:
1. Preheat the Air fryer to 310 degree F and grease a baking dish lightly.
2. Mix doughnut pieces, cherries, raisins, chocolate chips, sugar, and cinnamon in a large bowl.
3. Whisk the egg yolks with whipping cream in another bowl until well combined.
4. Combine the egg yolk mixture into the doughnut mixture and mix well.
5. Arrange the doughnuts mixture evenly into the baking dish and transfer into the Air fryer basket.
6. Cook for about 60 minutes and dish out to serve warm.

Nutrition: Calories: 786 Fat: 43.2g Carbohydrates: 9.3g Sugar: 60.7g Protein: 11g Sodium: 419mg

667. Marshmallow Pastries
Preparation Time: 20 minutes
Cooking Time: 5 minutes
Servings: 8

Ingredients:
- 4-ounce butter, melted
- 8 phyllo pastry sheets, thawed
- ½ cup chunky peanut butter
- 8 teaspoons marshmallow fluff
- Pinch of salt

Directions:
1. Preheat the Air fryer to 360 degree F and grease an Air fryer basket.
2. Brush butter over 1 filo pastry sheet and top with a second filo sheet.
3. Brush butter over second filo pastry sheet and repeat with all the remaining sheets.
4. Cut the phyllo layers in 8 strips and put 1 tablespoon of peanut butter and 1 teaspoon of marshmallow fluff on the underside of a filo strip.
5. Fold the tip of the sheet over the filling to form a triangle and fold repeatedly in a zigzag manner.
6. Arrange the pastries into the Air fryer basket and cook for about 5 minutes.
7. Season with a pinch of salt and serve warm.

Nutrition: Calories: 283 Fat: 20.6g Carbohydrates: 20.2g Sugar: 3.4g Protein: 6g Sodium: 320mg

668. Cinnamon Doughnuts

Preparation Time: 10 minutes
Cooking Time: 12 minutes
Servings: 6
Ingredients:
- 1 cup white almond flour
- 1 teaspoon baking powder
- 2 tablespoons water
- ¼ cup almond milk
- ¼ cup swerve
- ½ teaspoon salt
- 1 tablespoon coconut oil, melted
- 2 teaspoons cinnamon

Directions:
1. Preheat the Air fryer to 360 degree F and grease an Air fryer basket.
2. Mix flour, swerve, salt, cinnamon and baking powder in a bowl.
3. Stir in the coconut oil, water, and soy milk until a smooth dough is formed.
4. Cover this dough and refrigerate for about 1 hour.
5. Mix ground cinnamon with 2 tablespoons swerve in another bowl and keep aside.
6. Divide the dough into 12 equal balls and roll each ball in the cinnamon swerve mixture.
7. Transfer 6 balls in the Air fryer basket and cook for about 6 minutes.
8. Repeat with the remaining balls and dish out to serve.

Nutrition: Calories: 166 Fat: 4.9g Carbohydrates: 9.3g Sugar: 2.7g Protein: 2.4g Sodium: 3mg

669. Tea Cookies

Preparation Time: 15 minutes
Cooking Time: 25 minutes
Servings: 15
Ingredients:
- ½ cup salted butter, softened
- 2 cups almond meal
- 1 organic egg
- 1 teaspoon ground cinnamon
- 2 teaspoons sugar
- 1 teaspoon organic vanilla extract

Directions:
1. Preheat the Air fryer to 370 degree F and grease an Air fryer basket.
2. Mix all the ingredients in a bowl until well combined.
3. Make equal sized balls from the mixture and transfer in the Air fryer basket.
4. Cook for about 5 minutes and press down each ball with fork.
5. Cook for about 20 minutes and allow the cookies cool to serve with tea.

Nutrition: Calories: 291 Fat: 14g Carbohydrates: 30.3g Sugar: 2.3g Protein: 11.9g Sodium: 266mg

670. Zucchini Brownies

Preparation Time: 5 minutes
Cooking Time: 35 minutes
Servings: 12
Ingredients:
- 1 cup butter
- 1 cup dark chocolate chips
- 1½ cups zucchini, shredded
- ¼ teaspoon baking soda
- 1 egg
- 1 teaspoon vanilla extract
- 1/3 cup applesauce, unsweetened
- 1 teaspoon ground cinnamon
- ½ teaspoon ground nutmeg

Directions:
1. Preheat the Air fryer to 345°F and grease 3 large ramekins.
2. Mix all the ingredients in a large bowl until well combined.
3. Pour evenly into the prepared ramekins and smooth the top surface with the back of spatula.
4. Transfer the ramekin in the Air fryer basket and cook for about 35 minutes.
5. Dish out and cut into slices to serve.

Nutrition: Calories: 195 Fat: 18.4g Carbohydrates: 8.2g Sugar: 6.4g Protein: 1.5g Sodium: 143mg

671. Lemon Mousse

Preparation Time: 15 minutes
Cooking Time: 10 minutes
Servings: 6
Ingredients:
- 12-ounces cream cheese, softened
- ¼ teaspoon salt
- 1 teaspoon lemon liquid stevia
- 1/3 cup fresh lemon juice
- 1½ cups heavy cream

Directions:
1. Preheat the Air fryer to 345 degrees F and grease a large ramekin lightly.
2. Mix all the ingredients in a large bowl until well combined.
3. Pour into the ramekin and transfer into the Air fryer.
4. Cook for about 10 minutes and pour into the serving glasses.
5. Refrigerate to cool for about 3 hours and serve chilled.

Nutrition: Calories: 305 Fat: 31g Carbohydrates: 2.6g Sugar: 0.4g Protein: 5g Sodium: 279mg

672. Pear Delight

Preparation Time: 5 minutes
Cooking Time: 20 minutes
Servings: 4
Ingredients:
- 4 pears; peeled and roughly cut into cubes
- 1/4 cup brown sugar
- 4 tbsp. butter; melted
- 1 tbsp. maple syrup
- 2 tsp. cinnamon powder

Directions:
1. In a pan that fits your air fryer, place all the ingredients and toss.
2. Place the pan in the air fryer and cook at 300°F for 20 minutes. Divide into cups, refrigerate and serve cold

Nutrition: Calories: 191 kcal Protein: 1.79 g Fat: 13.05 g Carbohydrates: 17.9 g

673. Pumpkin Muffins

Preparation Time: 10 minutes
Cooking Time: 15 minutes
Servings: 12
Ingredients:
- 2 cups gluten free oats
- 1 cup pumpkin puree
- ½ cup honey
- 1 tsp coconut butter

DESSERTS RECIPES

- 2 medium eggs beaten
- 1 tbsp. cocoa nibs
- 1 tsp nutmeg
- 1 tbsp. vanilla essence

Directions:
1. Combine all ingredients into the blender and blend until the mixture is smooth.
2. Add the mixture into little muffin cases, filling up 12 different cases.
3. Transfer the filled cases into the air fryer.
4. Allow cooking for 15 minutes at 360 F.
5. Serve when cool.

Nutrition: Calories: 163 kcal Protein: 7.24 g Fat: 7.57 g Carbohydrates: 24 g

674. Cranberry Muffins

Preparation Time: 10 minutes
Cooking Time: 15 minutes
Servings: 12

Ingredients:
- 3 oz. flour
- tsp cinnamon
- 1½ tsp baking powder
- Pinch of salt
- tbsp. sugar
- 1 small egg, beaten
- oz. melted butter
- oz. milk
- 3 oz. dried cranberries
- 8 paper muffin cups

Directions:
1. Ensure that the air fryer is preheated to 390 F.
2. Double up the muffin cups so that you have a total of four cups.
3. Get a clean bowl, and in it, sift in the flour and add cinnamon, baking powder, a pinch of salt, and sugar. Mix thoroughly.
4. Get another bowl, and in it, beat the egg lightly, adding the melted butter, and the milk. Mix well.
5. Stir the egg mixture into the flour, and add the cranberries. Mix well.
6. Place the batter into the doubled muffin cups, and move them into the air fryer basket carefully.
7. Return the basket into the air fryer, and allow baking for 15 minutes, or until you have golden brown, cooked muffins. Leave the muffins to cool in the cups.

Nutrition: Calories: 497 kcal Protein: 8.59 g Fat: 24.82 g Carbohydrates: 60.45 g

675. Apple Cinnamon Dessert Empanadas

Preparation Time: 10 minutes
Cooking Time: 50 minutes
Servings: 12

Ingredients:
- 2 tbsp. raw honey
- 1/8 tsp nutmeg
- tsp cinnamon
- 1 tsp vanilla extract
- apples, diced
- 1 tsp water
- tsp cornstarch
- 12 empanada wrappers
- 1 tsp olive oil spray

Directions:
1. In a saucepan on medium-high heat, combine honey, nutmeg, cinnamon, vanilla, and apples. Cook for 2-3 minutes while stirring until you have soft apples.
2. In a different bowl, combine water and the cornstarch. Transfer the mixture into the pan and cook for an extra 30 seconds while stirring.
3. On a clean flat surface, lay out the empanada wrappers, adding the apple mixture to each wrapper.
4. Close and roll each empanada into a half, pinching the crust along the edges. Now roll each side inward and continue twisting until you have a closed crust.
5. Brush empanadas with olive oil.
6. Transfer the wrapped empanadas into the air fryer basket. Feel free to stack them.
7. Allow cooking for 8 minutes at 400 F.
8. Turn and flip the empanadas after 8 minutes, then allow cooking for an extra 10 minutes.
9. Allow to cool and serve.

Nutrition: Calories: 133 kcal Protein: 3.77 g Fat: 1.42 g Carbohydrates: 26.24 g

676. Apple Dumplings

Preparation Time: 15 minutes
Cooking Time: 25 minutes
Servings: 8

Ingredients:
- 2 tbsp. sultana raisins
- tbsp. brown sugar
- sheets puff pastry
- small apples, peeled and cored
- 2 tbsp. butter, melted

Directions:
1. Ensure that your air fryer is preheated to 320 F.
2. Apply some aluminum foil as lining for the air fryer basket.
3. Get a clean bowl, and in it, combine the sultanas and brown sugar.
4. On a clean work surface, place a soft pastry sheet and with the apple placed on the sheet, fill the core with the sultana mixture. Fold the pastry around the apple such that it is entirely covered. Do the same for the remaining filling, apple, and pastry.
5. Transfer the dumplings into the already-prepared air fryer basket.
6. Brush the dumplings with melted butter before cooking for 25 minutes or until you have soft, golden brown apples.

Nutrition: Calories: 68 kcal Protein: 1.06 g Fat: 4.23 g Carbohydrates: 7.13 g

677. Pineapple with Honey and Coconut

Preparation Time: 15 minutes
Cooking Time: 12 minutes
Servings: 4

Ingredients:
- ½ small fresh pineapple
- ½ tbsp. lime juice
- tbsp. honey
- ¼ liter ice cream or mango sorbet
- Parchment paper

Directions:
1. Ensure that your air fryer is preheated to 390 F.
2. Leaving ½ inch of the edge unlined, line the base of the basket with baking parchment.

3. Cut the pineapple into eight sections by cutting lengthways. Remove the skin, alongside the deep crowns, as well as the tough core.
4. Combine, in a bowl, the lime juice, and the honey. Now brush the pineapple sec-tions with the mixture before transferring them into the air fryer basket. Add sprin-kles of coconut on top.
5. With the basket in the air fryer, set the cooking time to 12 minutes or until the pineapple and the coconut appear golden brown.
6. Place the pineapple sections on plates, alongside a sufficient amount of ice cream.

Nutrition: Calories: 49 kcal Protein: 1.8 g Fat: 1.56 g Carbohydrates: 7.06 g

678. Tasty Cheese Bites

Preparation Time: 10 minutes
Cooking Time: 2 minutes
Servings: 16
Ingredients:
- 8 oz. cream cheese, softened
- 2 tbsp. erythritol
- 1/2 cup almond flour
- 1/2 tsp vanilla
- 4 tbsp. heavy cream
- 1/2 cup erythritol

Directions:
1. Add cream cheese, vanilla, 1/2 cup erythritol, and 2 tbsp. heavy cream in a stand mixer and mix until smooth.
2. Scoop cream cheese mixture onto the parchment lined plate and place in the refrigerator for 1 hour.
3. In a small bowl, mix together almond flour and 2 tbsp. erythritol.
4. Dip cheesecake bites in remaining heavy cream and coat with almond flour mixture.
5. Place prepared cheesecake bites in air fryer basket and air fry for 2 minutes at 350 F.
6. Make sure cheesecake bites are frozen before air fry otherwise they will melt.
7. Drizzle with chocolate syrup and serve.

Nutrition: Calories 80 Fat 7 g Carbohydrates 2 g Sugar 1 g Protein 2 g Cholesterol 16 mg

679. Coconut Pie

Preparation Time: 10 minutes
Cooking Time: 12 minutes
Servings: 6
Ingredients:
- 2 eggs
- 1/2 cup coconut flour
- 1/2 cup erythritol
- 1 cup shredded coconut
- 1 1/2 tsp vanilla
- 1/4 cup butter
- 1 1/2 cups coconut milk

Directions:
1. Add all ingredients into the large bowl and mix until well combined.
2. Spray a 6-inch baking dish with cooking spray.
3. Pour batter into the prepared dish and place in the air fryer basket.
4. Cook at 350 F for 10-12 minutes.
5. Slice and serve.

Nutrition: Calories 282 Fat 28.9 g Carbohydrates 6.3 g Sugar 3.2 g Protein 4 g Cholesterol 75 mg

680. Pecan Muffins

Preparation Time: 10 minutes
Cooking Time: 15 minutes
Servings: 12
Ingredients:
- 4 eggs
- 1 tsp vanilla
- 1/4 cup almond milk
- 2 tbsp. butter, melted
- 1/2 cup swerve
- 1 tsp psyllium husk
- 1 tbsp. baking powder
- 1/2 cup pecans, chopped
- 1/2 tsp ground cinnamon
- 2 tsp allspice
- 1 1/2 cups almond flour

Directions:
1. Preheat the air fryer to 370 F.
2. Beat eggs, almond milk, vanilla, sweetener, and butter in a bowl using a hand mixer until smooth.
3. Add remaining ingredients and mix until well combined.
4. Pour batter into the silicone muffin molds and place into the air fryer basket in batches.
5. Cook muffins for 15 minutes.
6. Serve and enjoy.

Nutrition: Calories 204 Fat 18 g Carbohydrates 6 g Sugar 1.2 g Protein 5 g Cholesterol 60 mg

681. Cappuccino Muffins

Preparation Time: 10 minutes
Cooking Time: 20 minutes
Servings: 12
Ingredients:
- 4 eggs
- 2 cups almond flour
- 1/2 tsp vanilla
- 1 tsp espresso powder
- 1/2 cup sour cream
- 1 tsp cinnamon
- 2 tsp baking powder
- 1/4 cup coconut flour
- 1/2 cup Swerve
- 1/4 tsp salt

Directions:
1. Preheat the air fryer to 325 F.
2. Add sour cream, vanilla, espresso powder, and eggs in a blender and blend until smooth.
3. Add almond flour, cinnamon, baking powder, coconut flour, sweetener, and salt. Blend again until smooth.
4. Pour batter into the silicone muffin molds and place into the air fryer basket. (Cook in batches)
5. Cook muffins for 20 minutes.
6. Serve and enjoy.

Nutrition: Calories 150 Fat 13 g Carbohydrates 5.3 g Sugar 0.8 g Protein 6 g Cholesterol 59 mg

682. Almond Bars

Preparation Time: 10 minutes
Cooking Time: 35 minutes
Servings: 12
Ingredients:
- 2 eggs, lightly beaten
- 1 cup erythritol
- ½ tsp vanilla
- ¼ cup water
- ½ cup butter, softened

- ¾ cup cherries, pitted
- 1 ½ cup almond flour
- 1 tbsp. xanthan gum
- ½ tsp salt

Directions:
1. In a bowl, mix together almond flour, erythritol, eggs, vanilla, butter, and salt until dough is formed.
2. Press dough in air fryer baking dish.
3. Place in the air fryer and cook at 375 F for 10 minutes.
4. Meanwhile, mix together cherries, xanthan gum, and water.
5. Pour cherry mixture over cooked dough and cook for 25 minutes more.
6. Slice and serve.

Nutrition: Calories 168 Fat 15 g Carbohydrates 5 g Sugar 1.8 g Protein 4 g Cholesterol 48 mg

683. Coffee Cookies

Preparation Time: 10 minutes
Cooking Time: 15 minutes
Servings: 12

Ingredients:
- 1 cup almond flour
- 2 eggs, lightly beaten
- 2 tsp baking powder
- ½ tbsp. cinnamon
- ¼ cup erythritol
- ¼ cup brewed espresso
- ½ cup ghee, melted

Directions:
1. Add all ingredients into the bowl and mix until well combined.
2. Place cookie sheet into the air fryer basket.
3. Make small cookies from mixture and place into the air fryer basket on cookie sheet.
4. Cook at 350 F for 15 minutes.
5. Serve and enjoy.

Nutrition: Calories 141 Fat 14 g Carbohydrates 2.8 g Sugar 0.4 g Protein 3 g Cholesterol 49 mg

684. Berry Cobbler

Preparation Time: 10 minutes
Cooking Time: 10 minutes
Servings: 6

Ingredients:
- 1 egg, lightly beaten
- 1 tbsp. butter, melted
- 2 tsp swerve
- ½ tsp vanilla
- 1 cup almond flour
- ½ cup raspberries, sliced
- ½ cup strawberries, sliced

Directions:
1. Preheat the air fryer to 360 F.
2. Add sliced strawberries and raspberries into the air fryer baking dish.
3. Sprinkle sweetener over berries.
4. Mix together almond flour, vanilla, and butter in the bowl.
5. Add egg in almond flour mixture and stir well to combine.
6. Spread almond flour mixture over sliced berries. Cover dish with foil and place into the air fryer and cook for 10 minutes.
7. Serve and enjoy.

Nutrition: Calories 66 Fat 5 g Carbohydrates 3 g Sugar 1 g Protein 2 g Cholesterol 32 mg

685. Cashew Pie

Preparation Time: 10 minutes
Cooking Time: 18 minutes
Servings: 8

Ingredients:
- 1 egg
- 2 oz cashews, crushed
- ½ tsp baking soda
- 1/3 cup heavy cream
- 1 oz. dark chocolate, melted
- 1 tbsp. butter
- 1 tsp vinegar
- 1 cup coconut flour

Directions:
1. Add egg in a bowl and beat using a hand mixer. Add coconut flour and stir well.
2. Add butter, vinegar, baking soda, heavy cream, and melted chocolate and stir well.
3. Add cashews and mix well.
4. Preheat the air fryer to 350 F.
5. Add prepared dough in air fryer baking dish and flatten it into a pie shape.
6. Cook for 18 minutes.
7. Slice and serve.

Nutrition: Calories 105 Fat 8 g Carbohydrates 5 g Sugar 2.4 g Protein 2.4 g Cholesterol 32 mg

686. Almond Pumpkin Cookies

Preparation Time: 10 minutes
Cooking Time: 8 minutes
Servings: 8

Ingredients:
- ¼ cup almond flour
- ½ cup pumpkin puree
- 3 tbsp. swerve
- ½ tsp baking soda
- 1 tbsp. coconut flakes
- ½ tsp cinnamon
- Pinch of salt

Directions:
1. Preheat the air fryer to 360 F.
2. Add all ingredients into the bowl and mix until well combined.
3. Spray air fryer basket with cooking spray.
4. Make cookies from bowl mixture and place into the air fryer and cook for 8 minutes.
5. Serve and enjoy.

Nutrition: Calories 30 Fat 2 g Carbohydrates 3 g Sugar 0.7 g Protein 1 g Cholesterol 0 mg

687. Vanilla Butter Pie

Preparation Time: 10 minutes
Cooking Time: 20 minutes
Servings: 8

Ingredients:
- 1 egg
- 2 tbsp. erythritol
- ½ cup butter, melted
- 1 tsp vanilla
- 1 cup almond flour
- 1 tsp baking soda
- 1 tbsp. vinegar

Directions:

1. Mix together almond flour and baking soda in a bowl.
2. In a separate bowl, whisk the egg with sweetener and vanilla.
3. Pour whisk egg, vinegar, and butter in almond flour and mix until dough is formed.
4. Preheat the air fryer to 340 F.
5. Roll dough using the rolling pin in air fryer baking dish size.
6. Place rolled dough in air fryer baking dish. Place in the air fryer and cook for 20 minutes.
7. Slice and serve.

Nutrition: Calories 132 Fat 13.8 g Carbohydrates 0.9 g Sugar 0.3 g Protein 1.6 g Cholesterol 51 mg

688. Poppy seed Muffins

Preparation Time: 10 minutes
Cooking Time: 14 minutes
Servings: 12
Ingredients:
- 3 eggs
- 4 true lemon packets
- 2 tbsp poppy seeds
- 1/4 cup coconut oil
- 1/4 cup ricotta cheese
- 1 tsp baking powder
- 1 cup almond flour
- 1 tsp lemon extract
- 1/4 cup heavy whipping cream
- 1/3 cup swerve

Directions:
1. Add all ingredients into the large bowl and beat using a hand mixer until fluffy.
2. Pour batter into the silicone muffin molds and place in the air fryer. In batches.
3. Cook at 320 F for 14 minutes.
4. Serve and enjoy.

Nutrition: Calories 90 Fat 8 g Carbohydrates 3 g Sugar 2 g Protein 3 g Cholesterol 35 mg

689. Chia Chocolate Cookies

Preparation Time: 5 minutes
Cooking Time: 8 minutes
Servings: 20
Ingredients:
- 2 1/2 tbsps. ground chia
- 2 tbsp. chocolate protein powder
- 1 cup sunflower seed butter
- 1 cup almond flour

Directions:
1. Preheat the air fryer to 325 F.
2. In a large bowl, add all ingredients and mix until combined.
3. Make cookies from bowl mixture and place into the air fryer and cook for 8 minutes.
4. Serve and enjoy.

Nutrition: Calories 110 Fat 9 g Carbohydrates 5 g Sugar 0.5 g Protein 4 g Cholesterol 35 mg

690. Cinnamon Ginger Cookies

Preparation Time: 10 minutes
Cooking Time: 12 minutes
Servings: 8
Ingredients:
- 1 egg
- 1/2 tsp vanilla
- 1/8 tsp ground cloves
- 1 tsp baking powder
- 3/4 cup erythritol
- 2/4 cup butter, melted
- 1 1/2 cups almond flour
- 1/4 tsp ground nutmeg
- 1/4 tsp ground cinnamon
- 1/2 tsp ground ginger
- Pinch of salt

Directions:
1. In a large bowl, mix together all dry ingredients.
2. In a separate bowl, mix together all wet ingredients.
3. Add dry ingredients to the wet ingredients and mix until dough is formed. Cover and place in the fridge for 30 minutes.
4. Preheat the air fryer to 325 F.
5. Make cookies from dough and place into the air fryer and cook for 12 minutes.
6. Serve and enjoy.

Nutrition: Calories 230 Fat 22 g Carbohydrates 4 g Sugar 1 g Protein 5 g Cholesterol 24 mg

691. Crustless Pie

Preparation Time: 10 minutes
Cooking Time: 24 minutes
Servings: 4
Ingredients:
- 3 eggs
- 1/2 cup pumpkin puree
- 1/2 tsp cinnamon
- 1 tsp vanilla
- 1/4 cup erythritol
- 1/2 cup cream
- 1/2 cup unsweetened almond milk

Directions:
1. Preheat the air fryer to 325 F.
2. Spray air fryer baking dish with cooking spray and set aside.
3. In a large bowl, add all ingredients and beat until smooth.
4. Pour pie mixture into the prepared dish and place into the air fryer and cook for 24 minutes.
5. Let it cool completely and place into the refrigerator for 1-2 hours.
6. Slice and serve.

Nutrition: Calories 85 Fat 5 g Carbohydrates 4 g Sugar 1 g Protein 5 g Cholesterol 35 mg

692. Tasty Peanut Butter Bars

Preparation Time: 10 minutes
Cooking Time: 24 minutes
Servings: 9
Ingredients:
- 2 eggs
- 1 tbsp. coconut flour
- 1/2 cup butter, softened
- 1/2 cup peanut butter
- 1/4 cup almond flour
- 1/2 cup swerve

Directions:
1. Spray air fryer baking pan with cooking spray and set aside.
2. In a bowl, beat together butter, eggs, and peanut butter until well combined.
3. Add dry ingredients and mix until a smooth batter is formed.

DESSERTS RECIPES

4. Spread batter evenly in prepared pan and place into the air fryer and cook at 325 F for 24 minutes.
5. Slice and serve.

Nutrition: Calories 215 Fat 20 g Carbohydrates 4 g Sugar 2 g Protein 6 g Cholesterol 26 mg

693. Apple Fritters

Preparation Time: 10 minutes
Cooking Time: 10 minutes
Servings: 24
Ingredients:
- egg
- t. baking powder
- 1 ¾ c flour
- Vegetable oil
- Powder Sugar, for garnish
- 1 cup Milk
- 1 cup Apple, chopped

Directions:
1. In mixing bowl size medium mix flour and baking powder
2. In small mixing bowl mix milk, and eggs until combined
3. In the medium mixing bowl, add apples to flour mixture and then milk mixture. Stir until flour is moist.
4. Line the bottom of air fryer basket with parchment paper
5. Depending on the size of your air fryer you may be able to cook 2 -3 at a time, but be sure not to overcrowd.
6. Place a dollop of batter onto the parchment-lined basket, then lightly dab the top of the fritters with oil
7. Pre-heat air fryer to 400
8. Cooking until deep golden brown about 6 minutes.
9. Sprinkle with powder sugar and serve.

Nutrition: Calories: 49 Net Carbs: 9.6 g Fat: 0.5 g Protein: 1.5 g

694. Churros

Preparation Time: 20 minutes
Cooking Time: 10 minutes
Servings: 8
Ingredients:
- tbsp. cinnamon
- 8 oz. crescent rolls
- tbsp. Sugar
- tbsp. Butter, melted

Directions:
1. Begin by whisking together sugar and cinnamon
2. Next unroll the crescent dough on a well-floured cutting board. And separate into 4 rectangles
3. Press the perforations to seal the dough together
4. Next brush each rectangle with the melted butter
5. Then sprinkle on 2 teaspoons of cinnamon sugar coating one side of two of the rectangle dough
6. Next take the dough without the cinnamon and sugar and place on top of the other rectangles butter side up.
7. Using a pizza cutter or sharp knife cut each dough into 4 strips.
8. Twist the strips and place on parchment-lined baking sheet
9. Next, working batches place each strip into the air fryer and fry at 330 for 5 minutes or until crisp and golden brown.
10. Remove from fryer and place back on parchment, brush again with butter and sprinkle remaining cinnamon-sugar mixture across churros

Nutrition: Calories: 127 Net Carbs: 18.4 g Fat: 4.7 g Protein: 3.1 g

695. Beignets

Preparation Time: 20 minutes
Cooking Time: 6 minutes
Servings: 24
Ingredients:
- c. coconut milk
- ½ t. yeast
- tbsp. powdered sugar
- tbsp. melted coconut oil
- tbsp. aquafaba, from chickpeas
- t. vanilla
- c. flour

Directions:
1. Begin by mixing coconut milk, powdered sugar, and yeast in a small bowl.
2. Next start heating the coconut milk until it is warm to the touch but not hot. Then add to your mixture from the small bowl and let sit 10 minutes to allow the yeast to foam.
3. Next using the paddle attachment on a stand mixer add the vanilla, aquafaba, coconut oil, and mix. Then add flour one cup at a time.
4. As flour is missing the dough should begin to come away from the sides, if you have a dough hook switch from paddle to the dough hook.
5. Allow dough to knead in the mixer for about 3 minutes dough will be wet, but you should be able to scrape it out and form into balls with your hands.
6. Place the dough in mixing bowl and cover with a clean towel and allow to rise for 1 hour.
7. On a large clean cutting board sprinkle some flour and pat out the dough into a rectangle shape about 1/3-inch thick. Then Cut into 24 squares and allow to proof for 30 minutes.
8. Cooking in batches add 3 to 6 beignets at a time cook at 390 for 3 minutes then turn and allow to fry 3 more minutes or until golden brown.
9. Sprinkle with powdered sugar and enjoy.

Nutrition: Calories: 102 Net Carbs: 15 g Fat: 3 g Protein: 3 g

696. Cinnamon Rolls

Preparation Time: 20 minutes
Cooking Time: 10 minutes
Servings: 6
Ingredients:
- ½ t. cinnamon ground
- 1/3 c. brown sugar, packed
- 8 oz. Crescent rolls
- 2 tbsp. butter, melted
- ½ c. powdered sugar
- 2 oz. cream cheese, softened
- tbsp. milk

Directions:
1. Begin by lining the bottom of the air fryer basket with parchment paper and then brushing with butter.
2. In a mixing bowl medium-size mix together cinnamon, brown sugar, butter, and a pinch of salt and mix until smooth and fluffy
3. Next lightly flour your work surface, and roll out crescent rolls into one rectangular piece approximately 9"X7".
4. Spread butter mixture over dough leaving ¼ inch border on the long edge.
5. Roll dough towards the long edge that has not butter mixture and press to seal.
6. Cut dough into 6 equal rolls.
7. Arrange rolls in prepared air fryer cut side up and spaced evenly.
8. Fry for 10 minutes until golden at temperature 350.

9. While frying make your glaze by whisking together milk, powdered sugar, and cream cheese. If the glaze is to thick use teaspoons of milk until desired consistency.
10. Spread glaze over warm rolls and serve.

Nutrition: Calories: 255 Net Carbs: 38.1 g Protein: 5 g Fat: 9.7 g

697. S'more

Preparation Time: 10 minutes
Cooking Time: 6 minutes
Servings: 8

Ingredients:
- 4 marshmallows
- Heresy bar
- 8 graham cracker squares

Directions:
1. Begin by placing a marshmallow on a graham cracker
2. Place in the air fryer and roast marshmallow at 400 for 6 minutes
3. Remove from air fryer and top with chocolate and graham cracker square and enjoy

Nutrition: Calories: 225 Net Carbs: 38 g Fat: 7 g Protein: 2 g

698. Fried Oreos

Preparation Time: 10 minutes
Cooking Time: 5 minutes
Servings: 9

Ingredients:
- 9 Oreo cookies
- Crescent roll sheet

Directions:
1. Begin by opening crescent roll and spreading it on a work surface then cut 9 even squares.
2. Place one Oreo into each square and wrap dough around the cookie.
3. Lightly spray the outside of the wrapped cookies with cooking spray and place in the fryer and fry at 360 for 2 minutes, then flip and fry an additional 2 minutes.
4. Sprinkle tops of Oreos with powdered sugar and enjoy.

Nutrition: Calories: 58 Net Carbs: 8.4 g Fat: 2.6 g Protein: 0.6 g

699. Fig Egg Rolls

Preparation Time: 15 minutes
Cooking Time: 5 minutes
Servings: 15

Ingredients:
- ¼ c. sugar
- 2 tbsp. butter, melted
- 15 egg roll wrappers
- 8.5 oz. jar fig jam
- 16 oz. cream cheese
- ½ c. sugar
- tsp. Cinnamon
- tsp. Lemon Juice
- 1 tsp. Vanilla extract

Directions:
1. Begin by adding lemon juice, sugar, cream cheese, and vanilla extract into a mixer and whipping about 2 minutes to combine.
2. Remove the mixture and place into a pastry bag
3. Next stir the jam in the jar so it is loosened and easy to be scooped with a spoon.
4. Next layout the egg roll wrappers in a diamond shape with the point facing you.
5. In the center of the egg roll pipe approximately 2 tablespoons of cream cheese mixture then top with a tablespoon of jam.
6. Using a pastry brush to coat the edges of the egg roll wrapper with water.
7. Fold the bottom over the filling and secure tightly, then fold each side in and roll the egg roll up the rest of the way.
8. Next spray both sides with cooking spray.
9. Then allow the egg rolls to rest at room temperature
10. Next place 4-5 egg rolls in air fryer basket and fry at 370 for 5 minutes or until egg rolls are golden brown.
11. Remove egg rolls and allow to cool
12. After all egg rolls are cooked brush the tops with melted butter and sprinkle with cinnamon and sugar.
13. Serve at room temperature.

Nutrition: Calories: 297 Net Carbs: 41.5 g Fat: 12.6 g Protein: 5.5 g

700. Grilled Pineapple

Preparation Time: 10 minutes
Cooking Time: 10 minutes
Servings: 4

Ingredients:
- 3 tbsp. melted butter
- 2 t. cinnamon, ground
- ½ c. brown sugar
- pineapple, peeled – cored and cut into spears

Directions:
1. Begin by using a small bowl to mix together cinnamon and brown sugar.
2. Next brush pineapple with melted butter to coat all sides then toss in cinnamon sugar until spears are well coated.
3. Spray air fryer with cooking spray and add pineapple fry at 400 for 5 minutes.
4. Brush with additional butter and fry another 5 minutes or until sugar is bubbling.

Nutrition: Calories: 295 Net Carbs: 57 g Fat: 8 g Protein: 1 g

701. Chocolate Covered Strawberry S'more

Preparation Time: 10 minutes
Cooking Time: 6 minutes
Servings: 8

Ingredients:
- 4 marshmallows
- 4 t. Nutella
- 8 strawberries sliced
- 8 chocolate graham cracker squares

Directions:
1. Begin by placing a marshmallow on the chocolate graham cracker
2. Place in the basket of air fryer and roast marshmallow for 6 minutes with a temperature of 400
3. Remove from air fryer, and top with 2 slices of strawberry and Nutella then add top graham cracker square and enjoy.

Nutrition: Calories: 225 Net Carbs: 38 g Protein: 2 g Fat: 7 g

CONCLUSION

Throughout this book, we have learned a lot about owning and using an air fryer. We can confidently say that the air fryer is one of the best inventions of kitchen appliances.

Healthy food should not be a fad or an impossibility to choose; it should be part of everyone's life. To get it, certain appliances can help you and a lot: like an air fryer. It will give you more excitement to cook more delicious and healthy dishes.

An air fryer will cook different foods in a similar way as a traditional one would. But thanks to its special operation, you can do it without using a single drop of oil. In this way, you can prepare exquisite dishes without added fats and with considerably lower caloric intake.

Now you know some of the many functions and recipes of an air fryer. We hope that this eBook has helped you discover some exciting features.

Having an air fryer is a great option. You can enjoy a healthier meal and save a good part of the oil expense without giving up enjoyable, fried foods.

www.ingramcontent.com/pod-product-compliance
Ingram Content Group UK Ltd.
Pitfield, Milton Keynes, MK11 3LW, UK
UKHW051332300825
7654UKWH00025B/350